T0290234

NETTER'S PHOTOGRAPHIC ANATOMY COMPANION

NOTE TO INSTRUCTORS:
Contact your Elsevier Sales Representative for an image bank for *Netter's Photographic Anatomy Companion*, 1e, or request these supporting materials at: http://evolve.elsevier.com/Netter/photographic/

NETTER'S PHOTOGRAPHIC ANATOMY COMPANION

Marios Loukas, MD, PhD
Professor
Department of Anatomical Sciences
Dean, School of Medicine
St. George's University
Grenada, West Indies

R. Shane Tubbs, MS, PA-C, PhD
Professor of Neurosurgery, Neurology, Surgery, and Structural and Cellular Biology
Director of Surgical Anatomy, Tulane University School of Medicine, New Orleans, Louisiana
Program Director of Anatomical Research, Clinical Neuroscience Research Center, Center for Clinical Neurosciences
Department of Neurosurgery, Tulane University School of Medicine, New Orleans, Louisiana
Department of Neurology, Tulane University School of Medicine, New Orleans, Louisiana
Department of Structural and Cellular Biology, Tulane University School of Medicine, New Orleans, Louisiana
Professor, Department of Neurosurgery, and Ochsner Neuroscience Institute, Ochsner Health System, New Orleans, Louisiana
Professor of Anatomy, Department of Anatomical Sciences, St. George's University, Grenada, West Indies
Honorary Professor, University of Queensland, Brisbane, QLD, Australia
Faculty, National Skull Base Center of California, Thousand Oaks, California

Illustrations by
Frank H. Netter, MD

Contributing Illustrator
Carlos A.G. Machado, MD

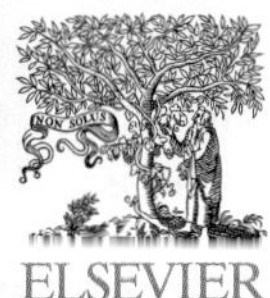
ELSEVIER

Elsevier
1600 John F. Kennedy Blvd.
Ste 1800
Philadelphia, PA 19103-2899

NETTER'S PHOTOGRAPHIC ANATOMY COMPANION ISBN: 978-0-323-82540-5

Publisher: Elyse W. O'Grady
Senior Content Strategist: Marybeth Thiel
Publishing Services Manager: Deepthi Unni
Project Manager: Gayathri S
Design Direction: Patrick C. Ferguson

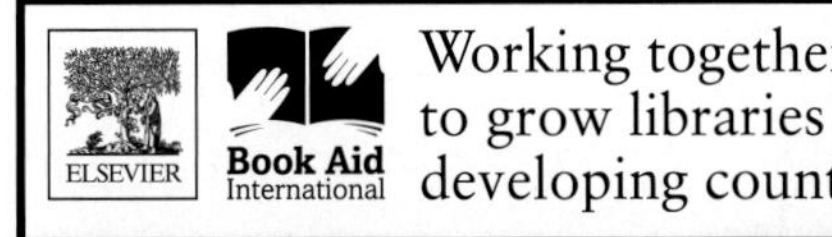
ELSEVIER
Book Aid International
Working together to grow libraries in developing countries
www.elsevier.com • www.bookaid.org

Printed in India

Last digit is the print number: 9 8 7 6 5 4 3 2 1

DEDICATION

To my wife Joanna, for her support and unconditional love for the past 25 years.

Marios Loukas, MD, PhD

I dedicate *Netter's Photographic Anatomy Companion* to the memory of Sherry Stone, Eddie Dodd, and Frankie Miles.

R. Shane Tubbs, MS, PA-C, PhD

ABOUT THE AUTHORS

Marios Loukas, MD, PhD

Marios Loukas, MD, PhD, received his medical degree from Warsaw University School of Medicine, and a PhD from the Institute of Rheumatology at the Department of Pathology in Warsaw, Poland. He held a postdoctoral position at Ulm University Clinic in Germany and studied arteriogenesis.

Dr. Loukas began his academic career at Harvard Medical School, where he served as a lecturer and a laboratory instructor for the Human Body Course. In 2005 he joined St. George's University in Grenada and shortly after became Professor and Chair of the Department of Anatomical Sciences. Under his leadership, the department developed a unique division of Ultrasound in Medical Education that instructs faculty members in how to teach the use and interpret ultrasound to medical students and residents and how to provide effective continuing medical education (CME) courses.

In 2012 Dr. Loukas was appointed as the Dean of Research for the School of Medicine at St. George's University. One of his main responsibilities is to develop a transdisciplinary research infrastructure to support translational research and to bridge basic science and clinical departments with the aim of enhancing student research.

Dr. Loukas' research has been continuously funded from St. George's University. He has been the recipient of numerous teaching and research awards, such as the 2007 Herbert M. Stauffer Award from the Association of University Radiologists and the Harvard Excellence in Tutoring Award from Harvard Medical School.

Dr. Loukas has published more than 900 papers in peer-reviewed journals and authored 12 books, including *Gray's Anatomy Review*, *Gray's Clinical Photographic Dissector of the Human Body*, *McMinn and Abrahams' Clinical Atlas of Human Anatomy*, *History of Anatomy*, and *Bergman's Comprehensive Textbook of Human Variation*, and 18 chapters in various medical and surgical textbooks, including *Gray's Anatomy*. He has also served as an editor and co-editor for 12 journals and as a reviewer for more than 50 journals. He is the co-editor of the journal *Clinical Anatomy*. With this background, Dr. Loukas has been able to provide his medical knowledge in the anatomical sciences to a larger audience as the past President of the American Association of Clinical Anatomists. His scientific interests include surgical anatomy and techniques and cardiovascular pathology. Recently, his focus has been directed toward issues of integrated curriculum and faculty development in medical education with an emphasis on simulation and technology and effective teaching and testing. In 2021 Dr. Loukas was appointed as the Dean at St. George's University School of Medicine.

R. Shane Tubbs, MS, PA-C, PhD

R. Shane Tubbs, MS, PA-C, PhD, is a native of Birmingham, Alabama and a clinical anatomist. His research interests are centered around clinical/surgical problems identified and solved with anatomical studies. This investigative paradigm in anatomy has resulted in over 2000 peer-reviewed publications. Dr. Tubbs' laboratory has made novel discoveries in human anatomy including a new nerve to the skin of the lower eyelid, a new space of the face, a new venous sinus of the skull base, new connections between the parts of the sciatic nerve, new ligaments of the neck, a previously undescribed cutaneous branch of the inferior gluteal nerve, and an etiology for postoperative C5 nerve palsies. Moreover, many anatomical feasibility studies from Dr. Tubbs' laboratory have gone on to be used by surgeons from around the world and have thus resulted in new surgical/clinical procedures such as treating hydrocephalus by shunting cerebrospinal fluid into various bones, restoration of upper limb function in paralyzed patients with neurotization procedures using the contralateral spinal accessory nerve, and harvesting of clavicle for anterior cervical discectomy and fusion procedures in patients with cervical instability or degenerative spine disease. He was recently listed in the top 2% of international researchers.

Dr. Tubbs sits on the editorial board of over 25 journals and has reviewed for over 200 scientific journals. He has been a visiting professor to major institutions in the United States and worldwide. Dr. Tubbs has authored over 60 books and over 100 book chapters. His published books by Elsevier include *Gray's Anatomy Review*, *Gray's Clinical Photographic Dissector of the Human Body*, *Netter's Introduction to Clinical Procedures*, and *Nerves and Nerve Injuries* volumes I and II. He is an editor for the 41st and 42nd editions of the over 150-year-old *Gray's Anatomy* and the 5th through 8th editions of *Netter's Atlas of Anatomy*, and is the editor-in-chief of the journal *Clinical Anatomy*. He is the Chair of the Federative International Programme on Anatomical Terminologies (FIPAT). Dr. Tubbs is now co-editor-in-chief of the 43rd edition of *Gray's Anatomy* and president of the American Association of Clinical Anatomists.

ABOUT THE ARTISTS

Frank H. Netter, MD

Frank H. Netter, MD, was born in 1906 in New York City. He studied art at the Art Student's League and the National Academy of Design before entering medical school at New York University, where he received his MD degree in 1931. During his student years, Dr. Netter's notebook sketches attracted the attention of the medical faculty and other physicians, allowing him to augment his income by illustrating articles and textbooks. He continued illustrating as a sideline after establishing a surgical practice in 1933, but he ultimately opted to give up his practice in favor of a full-time commitment to art. After service in the US Army during World War II, Dr. Netter began his long collaboration with the CIBA Pharmaceutical Company (now Novartis Pharmaceuticals). This 45-year partnership resulted in the production of the extraordinary collection of medical art so familiar to physicians and other medical professionals worldwide.

In 2005 Elsevier, Inc. purchased the Netter Collection and all publications from Icon Learning Systems. There are now over 50 publications featuring the art of Dr. Netter available through Elsevier, Inc.

Dr. Netter's works are among the finest examples of the use of illustration in the teaching of medical concepts. The 13-book *Netter Collection of Medical Illustrations*, which includes the greater part of the more than 4000 paintings created by Dr. Netter, became and remains one of the most famous medical works ever published. *Netter's Atlas of Human Anatomy*, first published in 1989, presents the anatomical paintings from the Netter Collection. Now translated into 16 languages, it is the anatomy atlas of choice among medical and health professions students worldwide.

The Netter illustrations are appreciated not only for their aesthetic qualities but also, more importantly, for their intellectual content. As Dr. Netter wrote in 1949, "... clarification of a subject is the aim and goal of illustration. No matter how beautifully painted, how delicately and subtly rendered a subject may be, it is of little value as a medical illustration if it does not serve to make clear some medical point." Dr. Netter's planning, conception, point of view, and approach are what inform his paintings and what makes them so intellectually valuable.

Frank H. Netter, MD, physician and artist, died in 1991.

Learn more about the physician-artist whose work has inspired the Netter Reference collection: https://netterimages.com/artist-frank-h-netter.html

Carlos A.G. Machado, MD

Carlos Machado was chosen by Novartis to be Dr. Netter's successor. He continues to be the main artist who contributes to the *Netter Collection of Medical Illustrations*.

Self-taught in medical illustration, cardiologist Carlos Machado has contributed meticulous updates to some of Dr. Netter's original plates and has created many paintings of his own in the style of Netter as an extension of the Netter collection. Dr. Machado's photorealistic expertise and his keen insight into the physician/patient relationship inform his vivid and unforgettable visual style. His dedication to researching each topic and subject he paints places him among the premier medical illustrators at work today.

Learn more about his background and see more of his art at: https://netterimages.com/artist-carlos-a-g-machado.html

PREFACE

Some students often find that their cadaveric dissections look different from the drawings in their anatomical atlases. Therefore creating an atlas of anatomy that contrasts anatomical drawings with cadaveric dissections would be a valuable resource for students of any anatomy course, as it would help bridge the gap between theoretical knowledge and practical application in the dissection lab. Such an atlas would enhance the student's understanding of the human body by providing two different modalities of visualizing human anatomy.

Within this atlas, the reader will find a unique juxtaposition – a visual dialogue between the reality of cadaveric imagery and the artistry of world-renowned drawings from the *Atlas of Human Anatomy* by Frank N. Netter. *Netter's Photographic Anatomy Companion* aims to provide a unique and comprehensive perspective that intertwines the art of illustration with signature Netter artwork with the authenticity of cadaveric dissection, including anatomical variations.

Netter's Photographic Anatomy Companion uses high-yield plates from the *Atlas of Human Anatomy*, and the cadaveric images have the same label placement as the adjacent drawings. These labels identify all relevant anatomical structures, including muscles, bones, nerves, blood vessels, and organs. Used together, these annotations serve as a guide for students to understand the structures and their relationships.

Ideally, *Netter's Photographic Anatomy Companion* will be integrated with dissection or prosection lab curricula. Additionally, instructors can use *Netter's Photographic Anatomy Companion* to prepare students before lab sessions and use it as a reference during dissections. Lastly, courses that do not have access to cadaveric specimens will be exposed to this material via the included cadaveric dissections. Additional benefits of *Netter's Photographic Anatomy Companion* include the following:

- **Enhanced Learning:** Students can visualize and understand anatomical structures more effectively by comparing drawings to real-life dissections. Allow students to correlate these drawings with cadaveric structures more easily.
- **Improved Preparation:** It prepares students for dissection labs by familiarizing them with annotated drawings and dissections.
- **Efficient Study:** The atlas provides a comprehensive and structured resource for studying anatomy, which can save students time and help them retain information more effectively.

In summary, an atlas of anatomy that contrasts drawings with cadaveric dissections can be a powerful educational tool that can significantly benefit students in their study of anatomy and their preparation for dissection labs, ultimately helping them become more proficient and confident in their understanding of the intricacies of the human body.

Each section is thoughtfully organized to facilitate an in-depth exploration of the anatomy of the human body. This approach enhances understanding and reinforces retention, making it an invaluable resource for students, educators, and professionals in medicine and biology.

Marios Loukas, MD, PhD
R. Shane Tubbs, MS, PA-C, PhD

ACKNOWLEDGMENTS

This prosection book is the collaborative effort incorporating the expertise and valuable input from various scientific and clinical peers. The authors express gratitude to the colleagues and friends who generously shared their knowledge, provided significant feedback, and offered assistance. The completion of the prosection book owes much to the contributions of the individuals mentioned below, without whom it would not have achievable.

The two main contributors, **Nelson Davis** and **Damion Richards**, provided superb dissections and technical expertise for this project.

We would also like to thank the following colleagues for their technical expertise in dissections and their enormous help with this project:

- *Dr. Kevlian Andrew, Department of Anatomical Sciences, St. George's University, Grenada, West Indies*
- *Dr. Anna Carrera, Department of Medical Sciences; Clinical Anatomy, Embryology and Neurosciences Research Group (NEOMA), University of Girona, Girona, Spain*
- *Dr. Rachael George, Department of Anatomical Sciences, St. George's University, Grenada, West Indies*
- *Dr. Vasavi Gorantla, Department of Anatomical Sciences, St. George's University, Grenada, West Indies*
- *Dr. Robert Hage, Department of Anatomical Sciences, St. George's University, Grenada, West Indies*
- *Dr. Joe Iwanaga, Tulane University School of Medicine, New Orleans, Louisiana, USA*
- *Dr. Ewarld Marshall, Department of Pathology, St. George's University, Grenada, West Indies*
- *Dr. Michael Montalbano, Department of Anatomical Sciences, St. George's University, Grenada, West Indies*
- *Dr. Francisco Reina, Department of Medical Sciences; Clinical Anatomy, Embryology and Neurosciences Research Group (NEOMA), University of Girona, Girona, Spain*
- *Dr. Ramesh Rao, Department of Anatomical Sciences, St. George's University, Grenada, West Indies*
- *Dr. Deepak Sharma, Department of Anatomical Sciences, St. George's University, Grenada, West Indies*

We are also grateful to the following members of St. George's University for their photographic, technical, academic and administrative expertise:

- *Dr. Kazzara Raeburn (chair Department of Anatomical Sciences)*
- *Dr. Ewarld Marshal, (chair, Department of Pathology)*
- *Dr. Maira DuPlessis (research director, Department of Anatomical Sciences)*
- *Dr. Sasha Lake (vice chair, Department of Pathology)*
- *Yvonne James (administrative assistant)*
- *Joanna Loukas (photography)*
- *Ryan Jacobs (senior technician)*
- *Tyan Mitchell (laboratory technician)*
- *Sarah Logie (laboratory technician)*

A special thanks to David Nahabedian MSc, CMI, an instructor at the Department of Anatomical Sciences, at St. George's University, School of Medicine in Grenada, for his medical illustration assistance and contribution throughout the book.

The following St. George's University alumni and current research fellows of the Department of Anatomical Sciences have been great friends and colleagues. Their continuous support, comments, criticism, and enthusiasm have contributed enormously to the completion of this project:

- Shanado Williams, MD
- Ali Walji, MD
- Fawwaz Safi, MD
- Sanyukta Dudhat, MD
- Kadesha Fergsuon, MD
- Yuvedha Velan, MD
- Kachina Morgan, MD
- Kelsey Dowers, MD
- Ji Hyun Park, MD
- Alice Nasser, MD
- Eric Hallquist, MD

The authors would also like to thank Marybeth Thiel and Elyse O'Grady, our editors, and all the team at Elsevier for guiding us through the preparation of this book.

The authors state that every effort was made to follow all local and international laws and ethical guidelines that pertain to the use of human cadaveric donors in anatomical education and research. The authors extend their appreciation and gratitude to those who generously donated their bodies to science. This contribution facilitated this anatomical educational project to enhance students' learning and, ultimately, contribute to the improvement of patient care. Therefore these donors and their families deserve our outmost gratitude.

Iwanaga, J., Singh, V., Takeda, S., Ogeng'o, J., Kim, H. J., Moryś, J., Ravi, K. S., Ribatti, D., Trainor, P. A., Sañudo, J. R., Apaydin, N., Sharma, A., Smith, H. F., Walocha, J. A., Hegazy, A. M. S., Duparc, F., Paulsen, F., Del Sol, M., Adds, P., Louryan, S., Fazan, V. P. S., Boddeti, R. K., & Tubbs, R. S. (2022). Standardized statement for the ethical use of human cadaveric tissues in anatomy research papers: Recommendations from Anatomical Journal Editors-in-Chief. *Clinical Anatomy*, 35(4), 526–528.

Iwanaga, J., Singh, V., Ohtsuka, A., Hwang, Y., Kim, H. J., Morys', J., Ravi, K. S., Ribatti, D., Trainor, P.A., Sañudo, J. R., Apaydin, N., S¸engül, G., Albertine, K. H., Walocha, J. A., Loukas, M., Duparc, F.,Paulsen, F., Del Sol, M., Adds, P., Hegazy, A., & Tubbs, R. S. (2021). Acknowledging the use of humancadaveric tissues in research papers: Recommendations from anatomical journal editors. Clinical Anatomy, 34(1), 2–4.

CONTENTS

CHAPTER 1

HEAD AND NECK

Alternate Version Available in Appendix

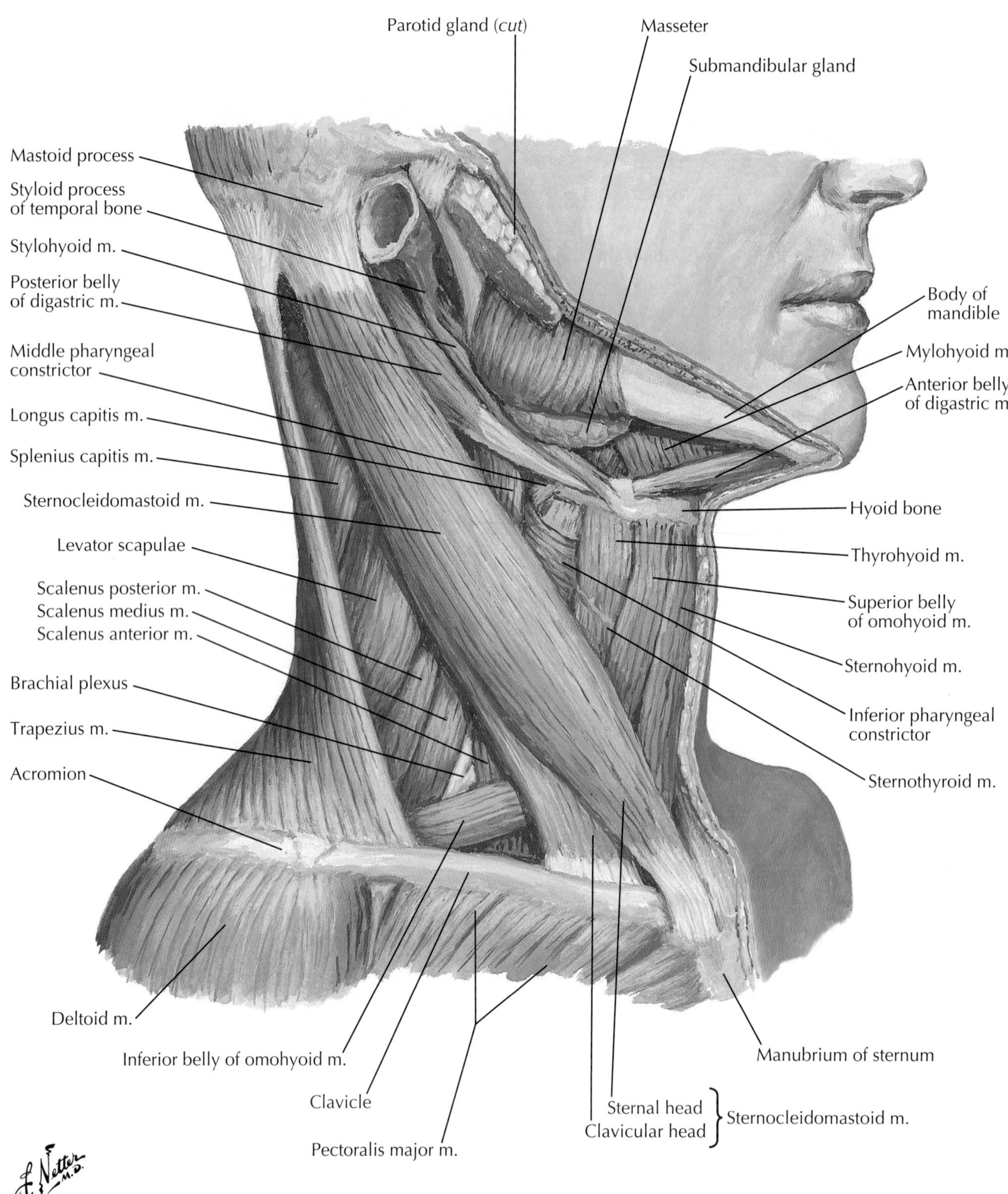

Parotid gland (*cut*)
Masseter
Submandibular gland
Mastoid process
Styloid process of temporal bone
Stylohyoid m.
Posterior belly of digastric m.
Middle pharyngeal constrictor
Longus capitis m.
Splenius capitis m.
Sternocleidomastoid m.
Levator scapulae
Scalenus posterior m.
Scalenus medius m.
Scalenus anterior m.
Brachial plexus
Trapezius m.
Acromion
Body of mandible
Mylohyoid m.
Anterior belly of digastric m.
Hyoid bone
Thyrohyoid m.
Superior belly of omohyoid m.
Sternohyoid m.
Inferior pharyngeal constrictor
Sternothyroid m.
Deltoid m.
Inferior belly of omohyoid m.
Clavicle
Pectoralis major m.
Manubrium of sternum
Sternal head
Clavicular head
Sternocleidomastoid m.
F. Netter M.D.

Fig. 1.1 Muscles of Neck: Lateral View (Illustration)

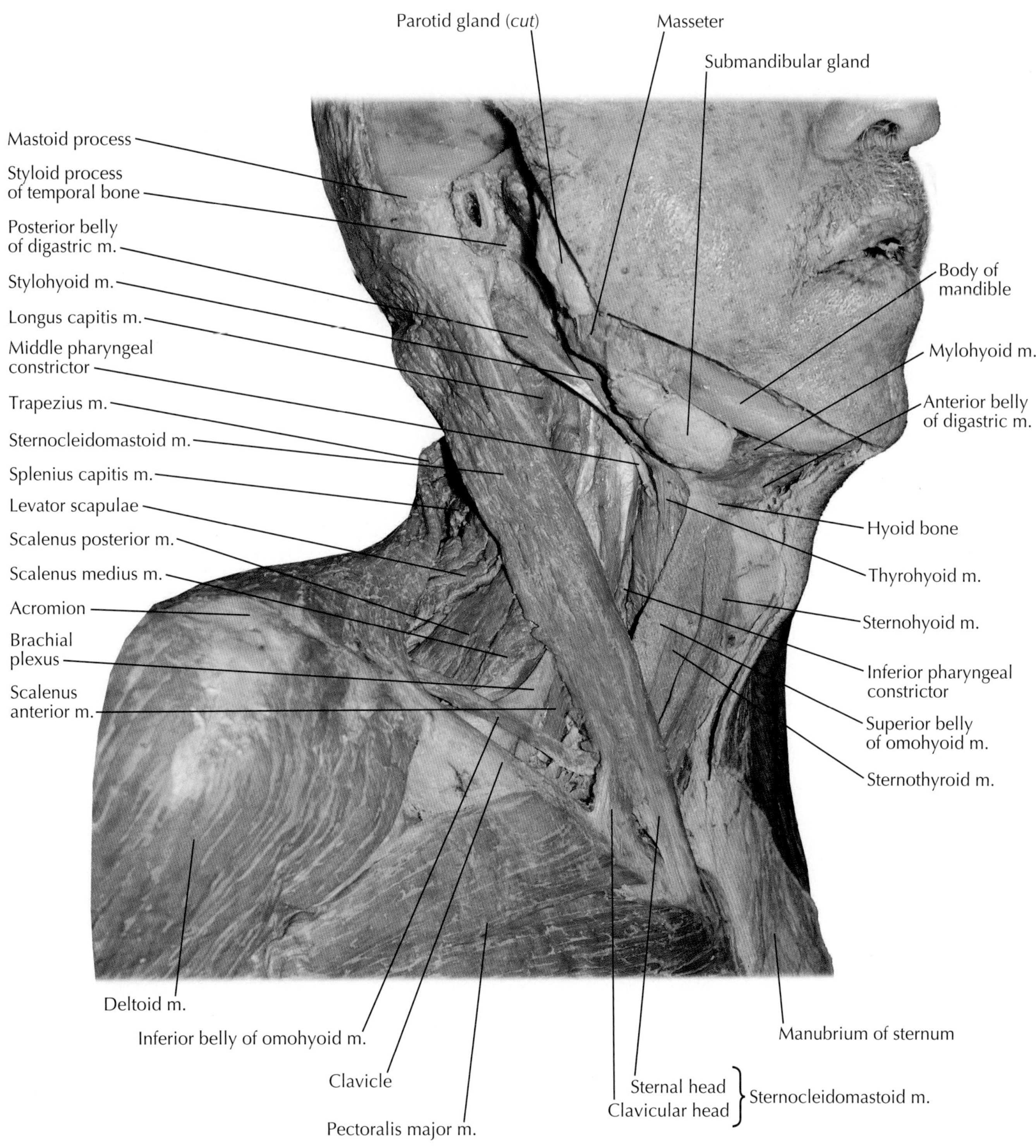
Parotid gland (*cut*)
Masseter
Submandibular gland
Mastoid process
Styloid process of temporal bone
Posterior belly of digastric m.
Stylohyoid m.
Longus capitis m.
Middle pharyngeal constrictor
Trapezius m.
Sternocleidomastoid m.
Splenius capitis m.
Levator scapulae
Scalenus posterior m.
Scalenus medius m.
Acromion
Brachial plexus
Scalenus anterior m.
Body of mandible
Mylohyoid m.
Anterior belly of digastric m.
Hyoid bone
Thyrohyoid m.
Sternohyoid m.
Inferior pharyngeal constrictor
Superior belly of omohyoid m.
Sternothyroid m.
Deltoid m.
Inferior belly of omohyoid m.
Clavicle
Pectoralis major m.
Sternal head
Clavicular head
Sternocleidomastoid m.
Manubrium of sternum

Fig. 1.2 Muscles of Neck: Lateral View (Photograph)

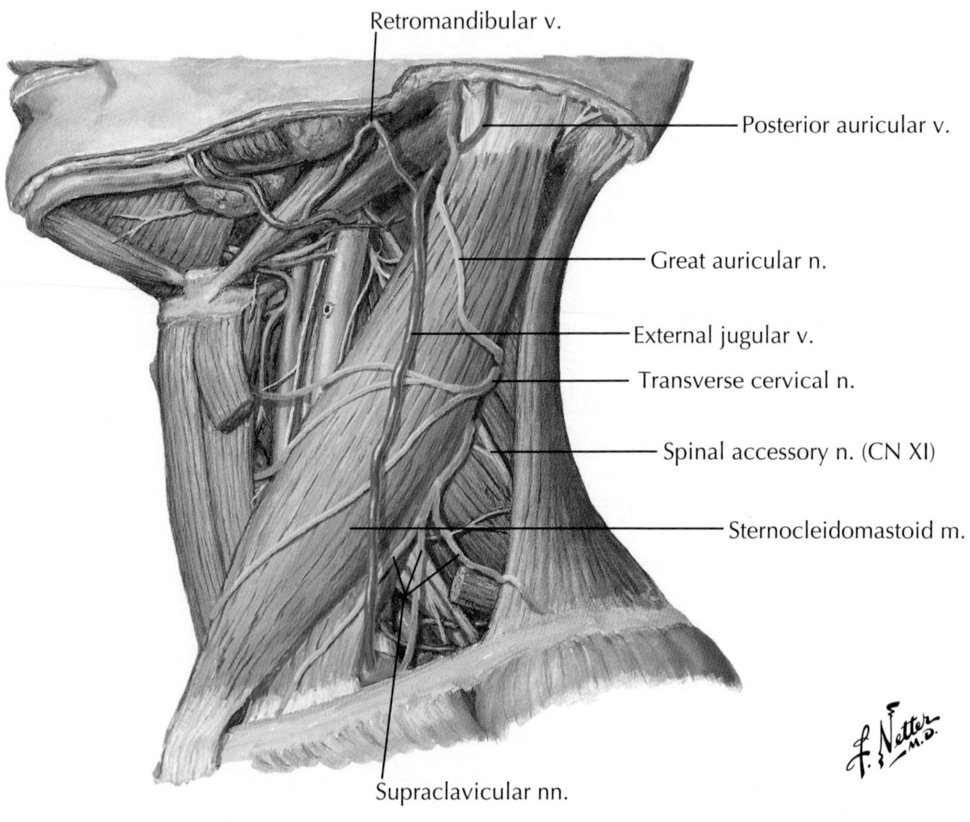
Retromandibular v.
Posterior auricular v.
Great auricular n.
External jugular v.
Transverse cervical n.
Spinal accessory n. (CN XI)
Sternocleidomastoid m.
Supraclavicular nn.
F. Netter M.D.

Fig. 1.3 Nerves of Neck (Illustration)

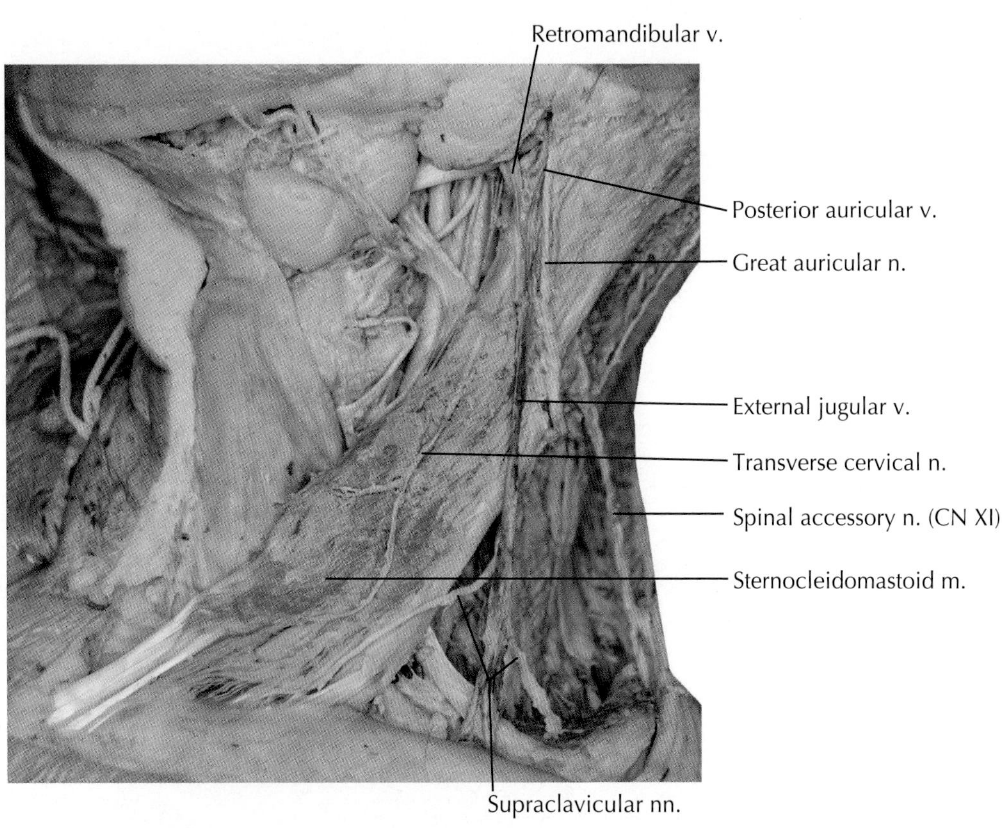
Retromandibular v.
Posterior auricular v.
Great auricular n.
External jugular v.
Transverse cervical n.
Spinal accessory n. (CN XI)
Sternocleidomastoid m.
Supraclavicular nn.

Fig. 1.4 Nerves of Neck (Photograph)

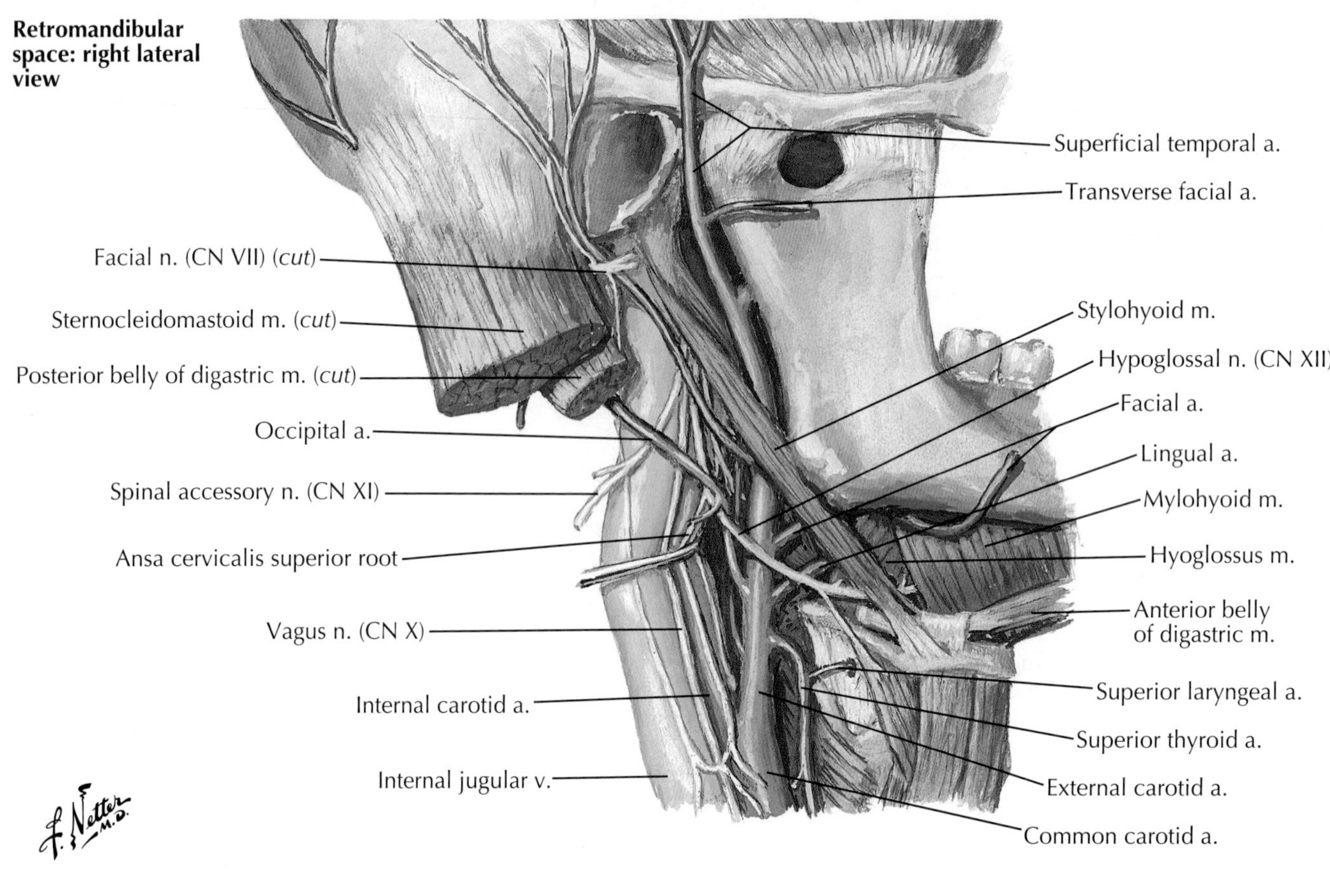
Retromandibular space: right lateral view
Superficial temporal a.
Transverse facial a.
Facial n. (CN VII) (*cut*)
Sternocleidomastoid m. (*cut*)
Posterior belly of digastric m. (*cut*)
Occipital a.
Spinal accessory n. (CN XI)
Ansa cervicalis superior root
Vagus n. (CN X)
Internal carotid a.
Internal jugular v.
Stylohyoid m.
Hypoglossal n. (CN XII)
Facial a.
Lingual a.
Mylohyoid m.
Hyoglossus m.
Anterior belly of digastric m.
Superior laryngeal a.
Superior thyroid a.
External carotid a.
Common carotid a.
F. Netter M.D.

Fig. 1.5 Carotid Arteries (Illustration)

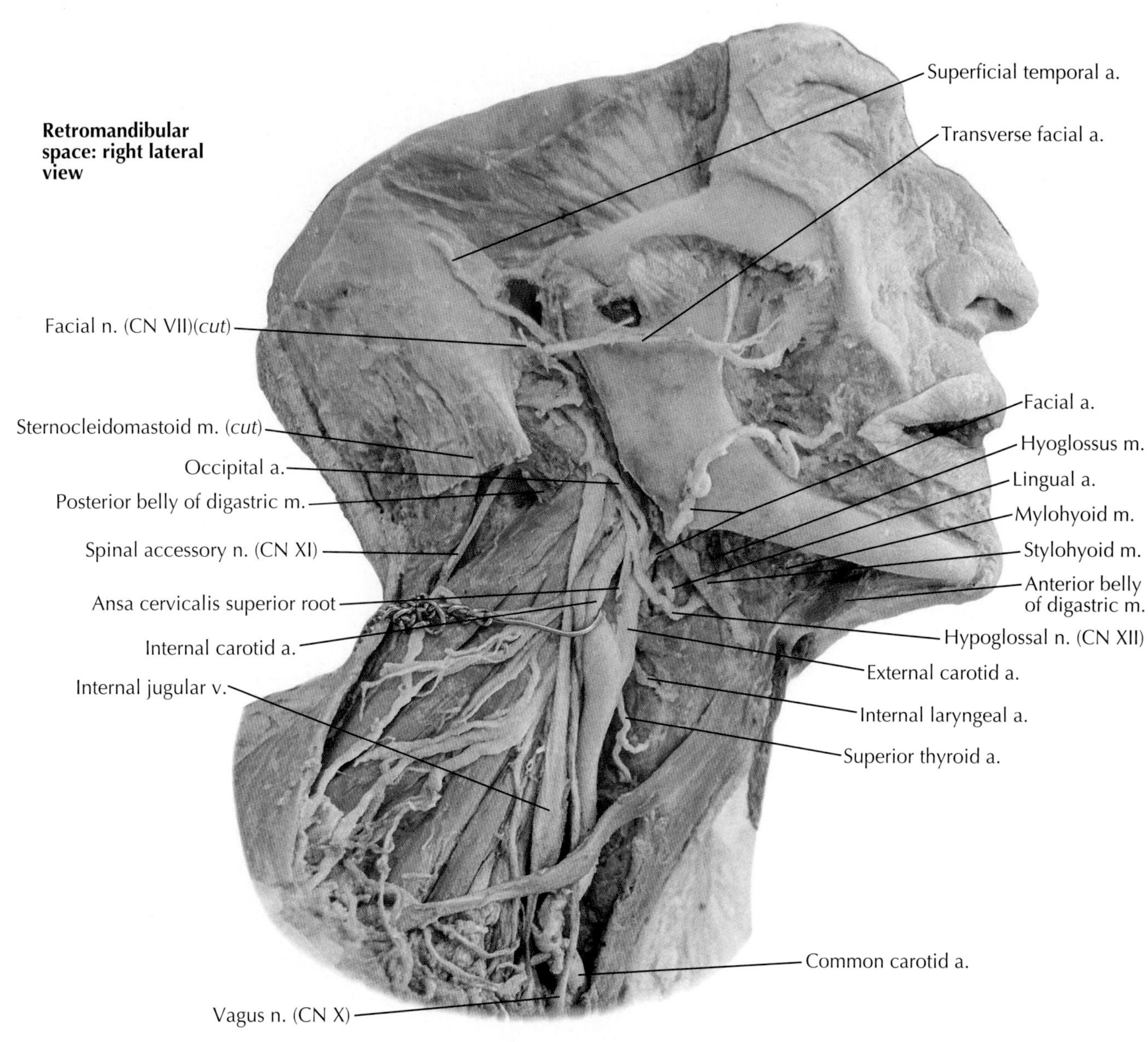
Retromandibular space: right lateral view
Superficial temporal a.
Transverse facial a.
Facial n. (CN VII)(cut)
Facial a.
Sternocleidomastoid m. (cut)
Hyoglossus m.
Occipital a.
Lingual a.
Posterior belly of digastric m.
Mylohyoid m.
Spinal accessory n. (CN XI)
Stylohyoid m.
Ansa cervicalis superior root
Anterior belly of digastric m.
Internal carotid a.
Hypoglossal n. (CN XII)
Internal jugular v.
External carotid a.
Internal laryngeal a.
Superior thyroid a.
Common carotid a.
Vagus n. (CN X)

Fig. 1.6 Carotid Arteries (Photograph)

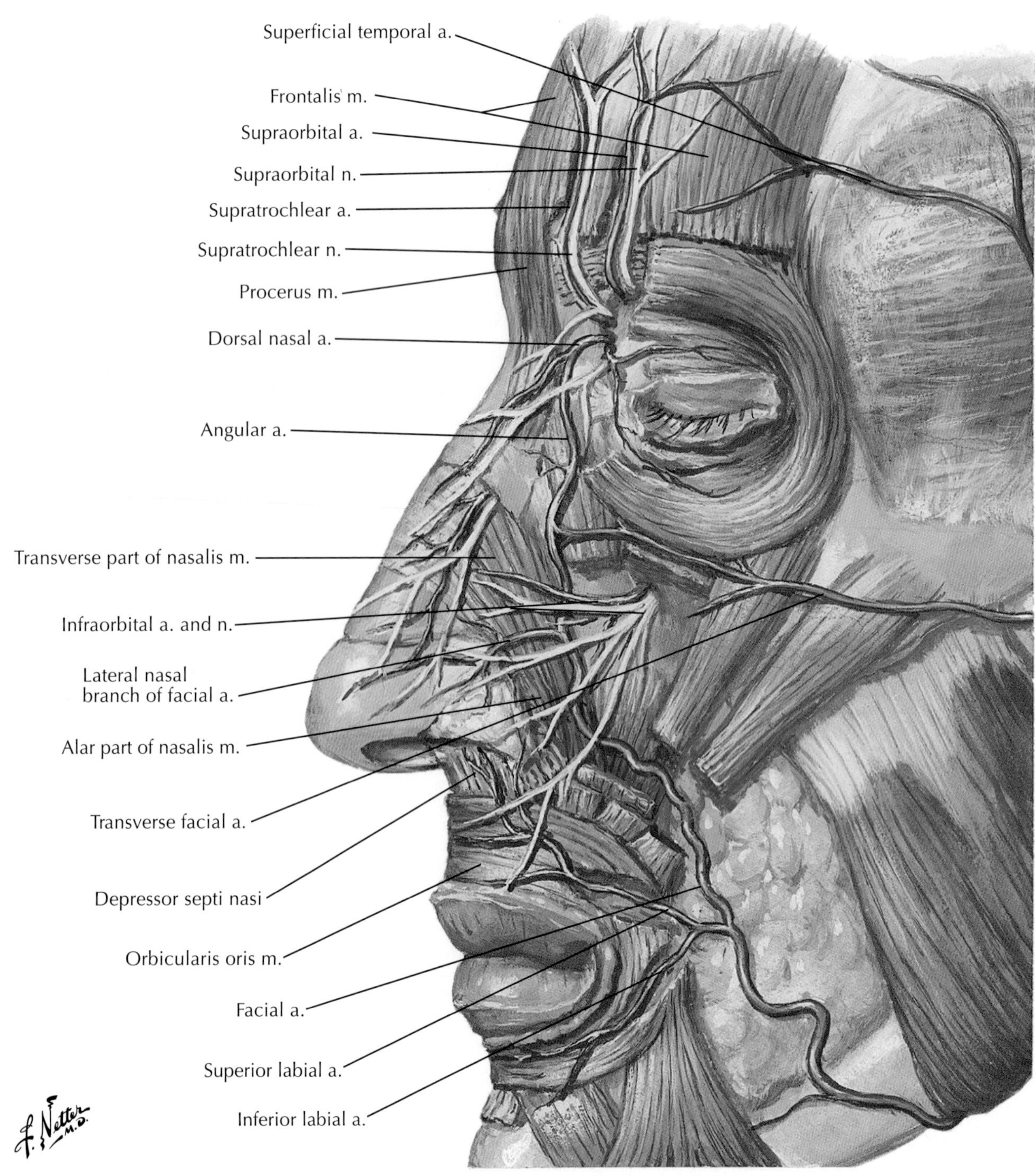
Superficial temporal a.
Frontalis m.
Supraorbital a.
Supraorbital n.
Supratrochlear a.
Supratrochlear n.
Procerus m.
Dorsal nasal a.
Angular a.
Transverse part of nasalis m.
Infraorbital a. and n.
Lateral nasal
branch of facial a.
Alar part of nasalis m.
Transverse facial a.
Depressor septi nasi
Orbicularis oris m.
Facial a.
Superior labial a.
Inferior labial a.
F. Netter M.D.

Fig. 1.7 Muscles, Nerves, and Arteries of Face (Illustration)

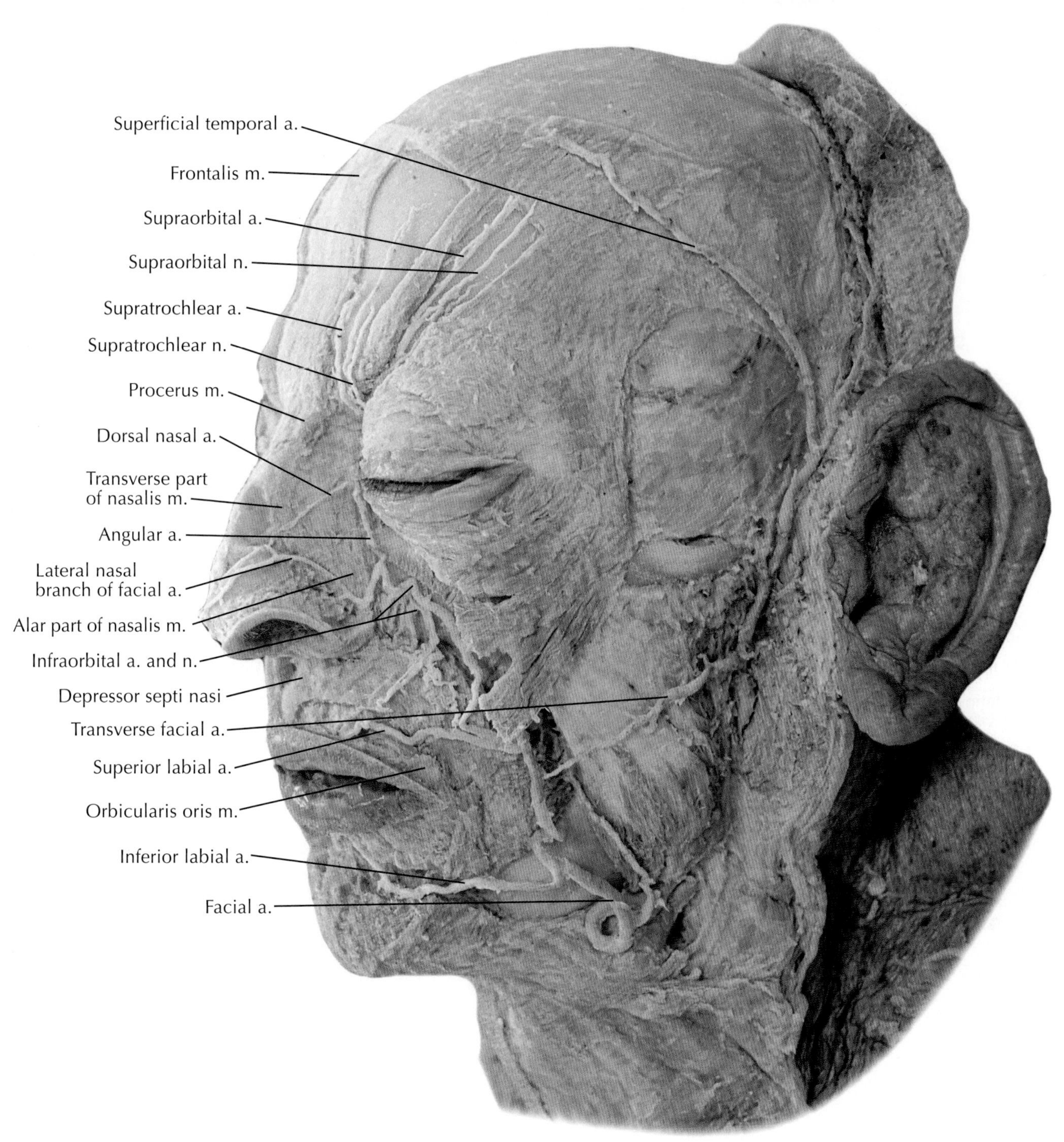
Superficial temporal a.
Frontalis m.
Supraorbital a.
Supraorbital n.
Supratrochlear a.
Supratrochlear n.
Procerus m.
Dorsal nasal a.
Transverse part of nasalis m.
Angular a.
Lateral nasal branch of facial a.
Alar part of nasalis m.
Infraorbital a. and n.
Depressor septi nasi
Transverse facial a.
Superior labial a.
Orbicularis oris m.
Inferior labial a.
Facial a.

Fig. 1.8 Muscles, Nerves, and Arteries of Face (Photograph)

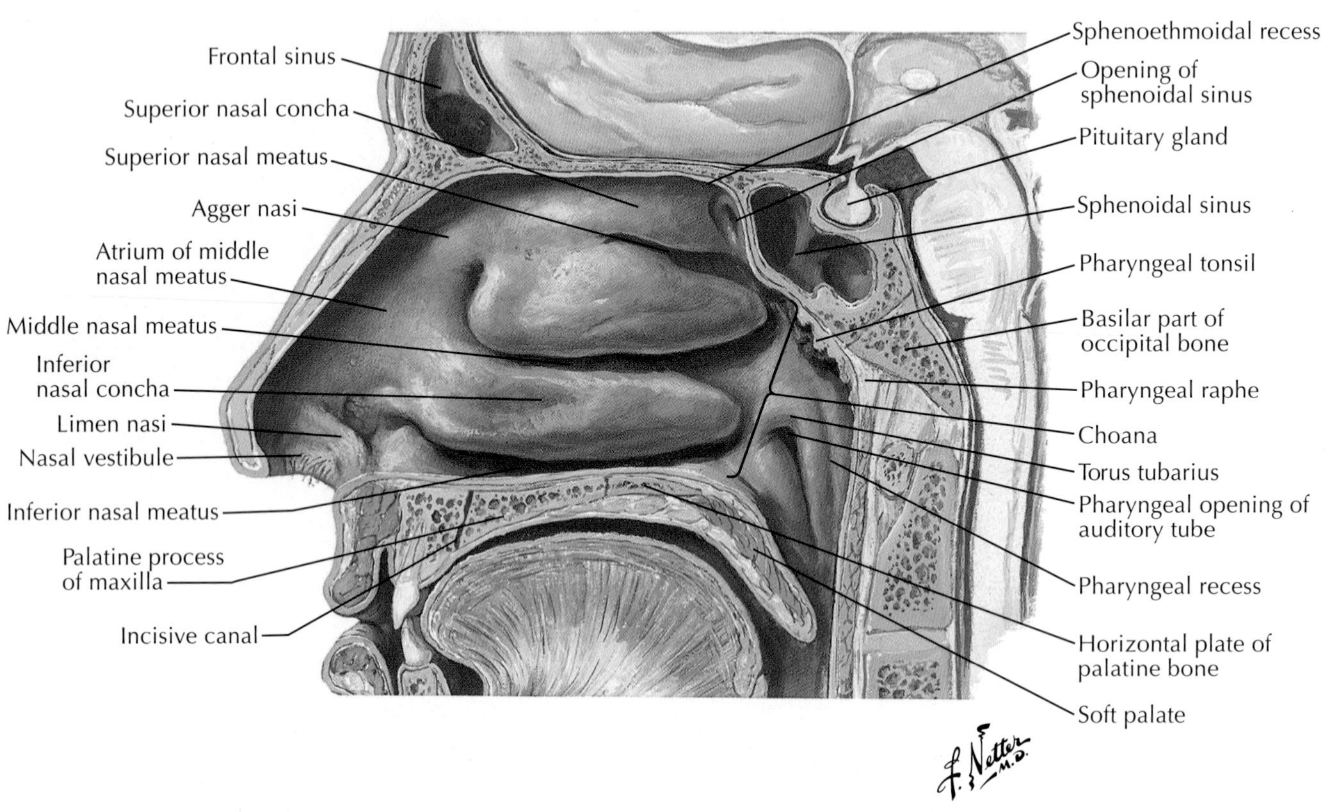
Frontal sinus
Superior nasal concha
Superior nasal meatus
Agger nasi
Atrium of middle nasal meatus
Middle nasal meatus
Inferior nasal concha
Limen nasi
Nasal vestibule
Inferior nasal meatus
Palatine process of maxilla
Incisive canal
Sphenoethmoidal recess
Opening of sphenoidal sinus
Pituitary gland
Sphenoidal sinus
Pharyngeal tonsil
Basilar part of occipital bone
Pharyngeal raphe
Choana
Torus tubarius
Pharyngeal opening of auditory tube
Pharyngeal recess
Horizontal plate of palatine bone
Soft palate
F. Netter M.D.

Fig. 1.9 Lateral Wall of Nasal Cavity (Illustration)

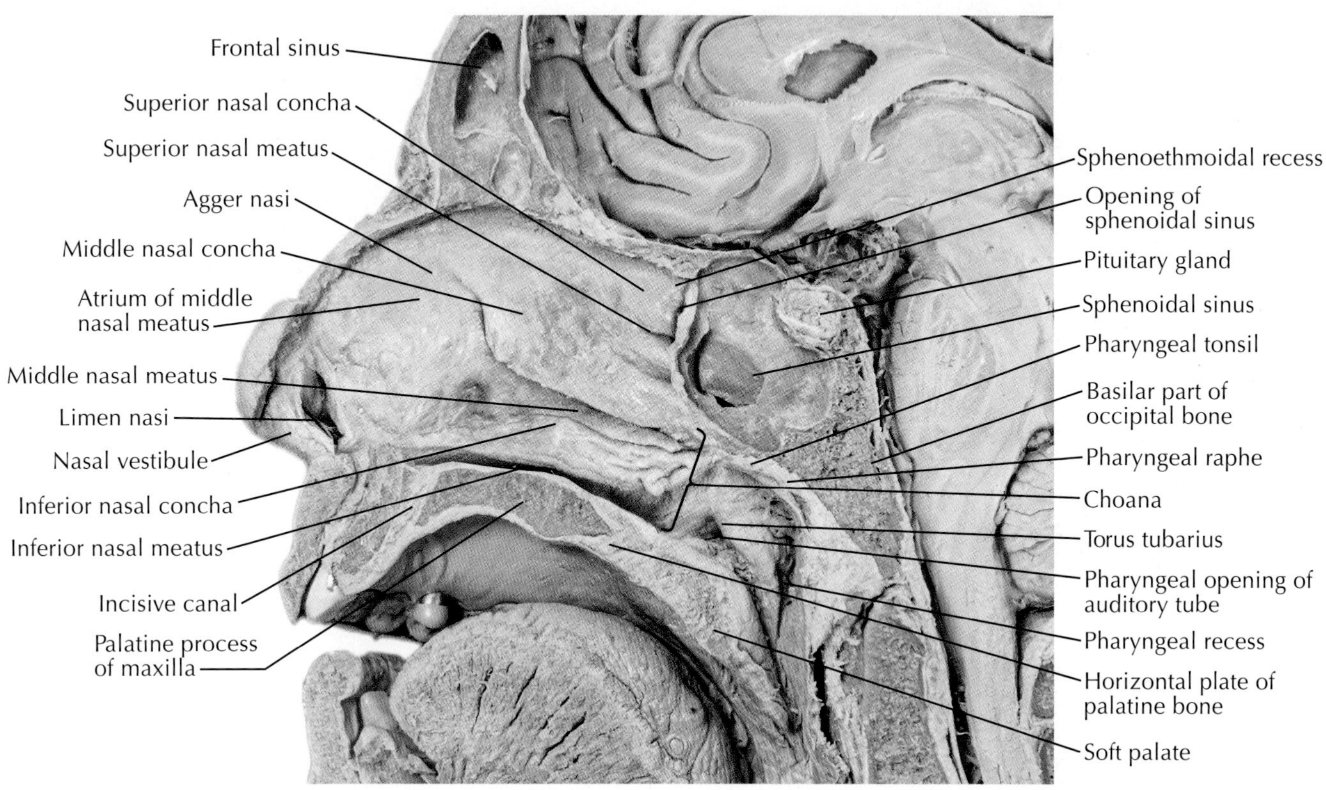
Frontal sinus
Superior nasal concha
Superior nasal meatus
Agger nasi
Middle nasal concha
Atrium of middle nasal meatus
Middle nasal meatus
Limen nasi
Nasal vestibule
Inferior nasal concha
Inferior nasal meatus
Incisive canal
Palatine process of maxilla
Sphenoethmoidal recess
Opening of sphenoidal sinus
Pituitary gland
Sphenoidal sinus
Pharyngeal tonsil
Basilar part of occipital bone
Pharyngeal raphe
Choana
Torus tubarius
Pharyngeal opening of auditory tube
Pharyngeal recess
Horizontal plate of palatine bone
Soft palate

Fig. 1.10 Lateral Wall of Nasal Cavity (Photograph)

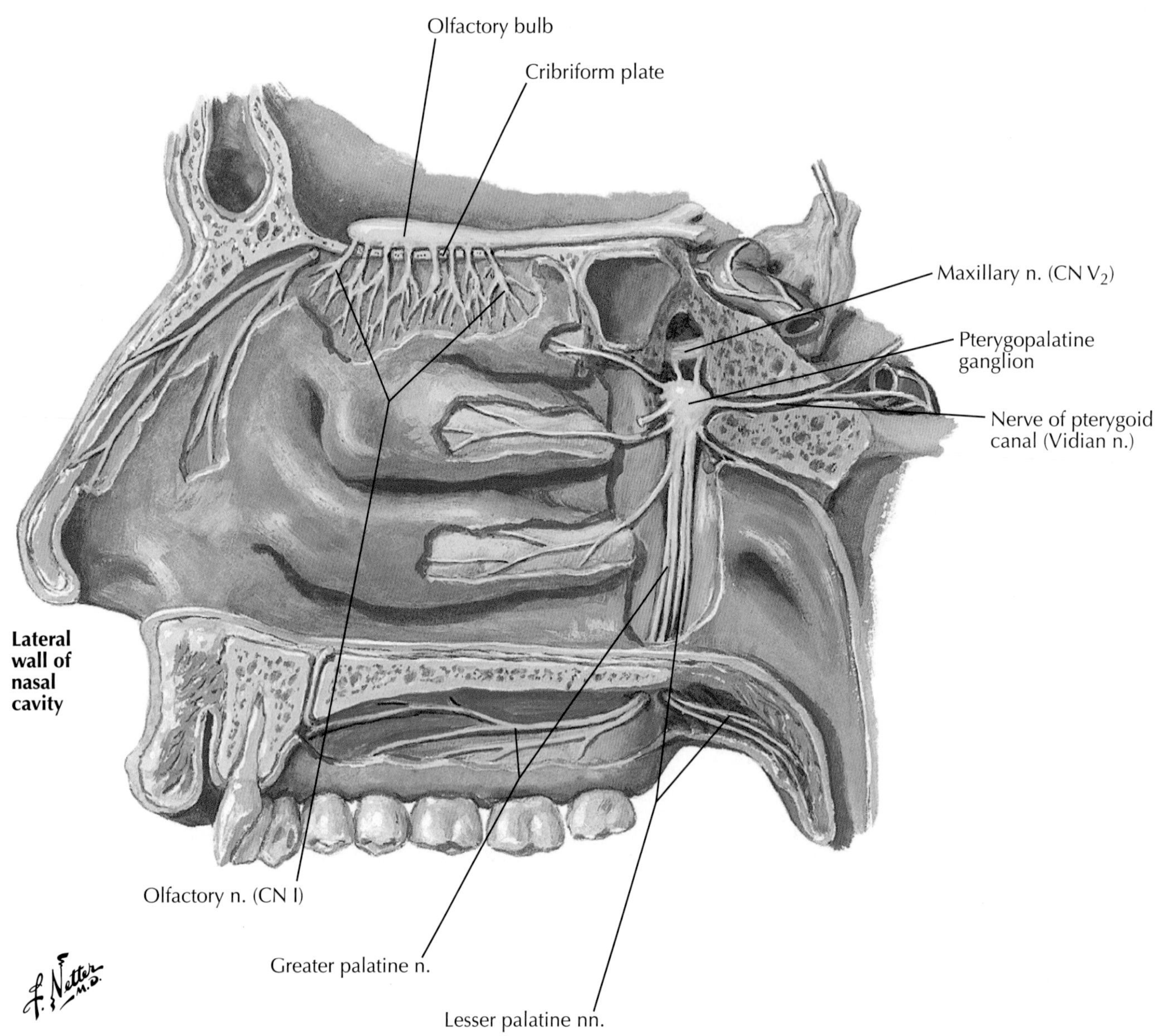
Olfactory bulb
Cribriform plate
Maxillary n. (CN V_2)
Pterygopalatine ganglion
Nerve of pterygoid canal (Vidian n.)
Lateral wall of nasal cavity
Olfactory n. (CN I)
Greater palatine n.
Lesser palatine nn.
F. Netter M.D.

Fig. 1.11 Nerves of Nasal Cavity (Illustration)

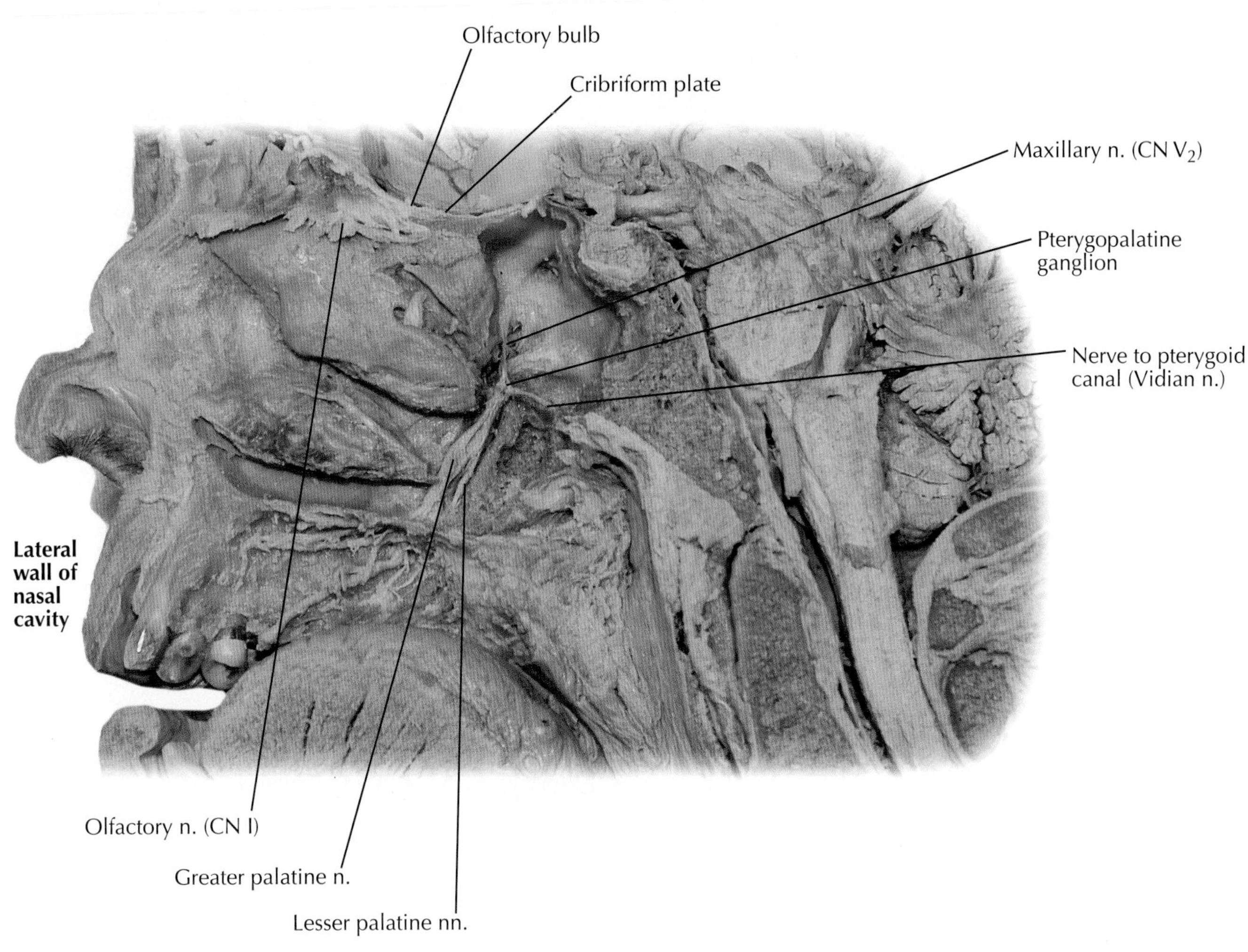
Olfactory bulb
Cribriform plate
Maxillary n. (CN V_2)
Pterygopalatine ganglion
Nerve to pterygoid canal (Vidian n.)
Lateral wall of nasal cavity
Olfactory n. (CN I)
Greater palatine n.
Lesser palatine nn.

Fig. 1.12 Nerves of Nasal Cavity (Photograph)

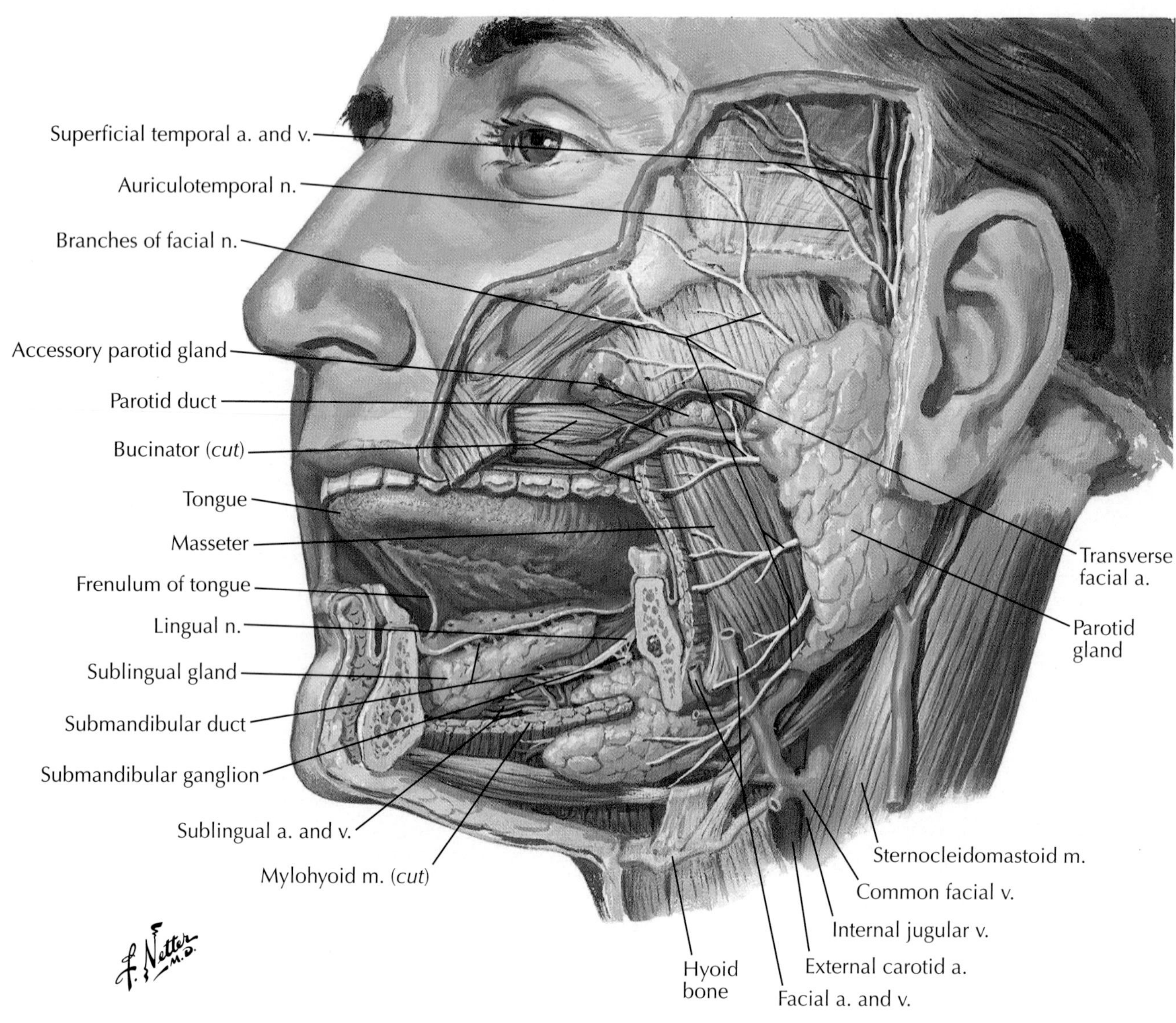
Superficial temporal a. and v.
Auriculotemporal n.
Branches of facial n.
Accessory parotid gland
Parotid duct
Bucinator (cut)
Tongue
Masseter
Frenulum of tongue
Lingual n.
Sublingual gland
Submandibular duct
Submandibular ganglion
Sublingual a. and v.
Mylohyoid m. (cut)
Transverse facial a.
Parotid gland
Sternocleidomastoid m.
Common facial v.
Internal jugular v.
External carotid a.
Hyoid bone
Facial a. and v.
F. Netter M.D.

Fig. 1.13 Salivary Glands (Illustration)

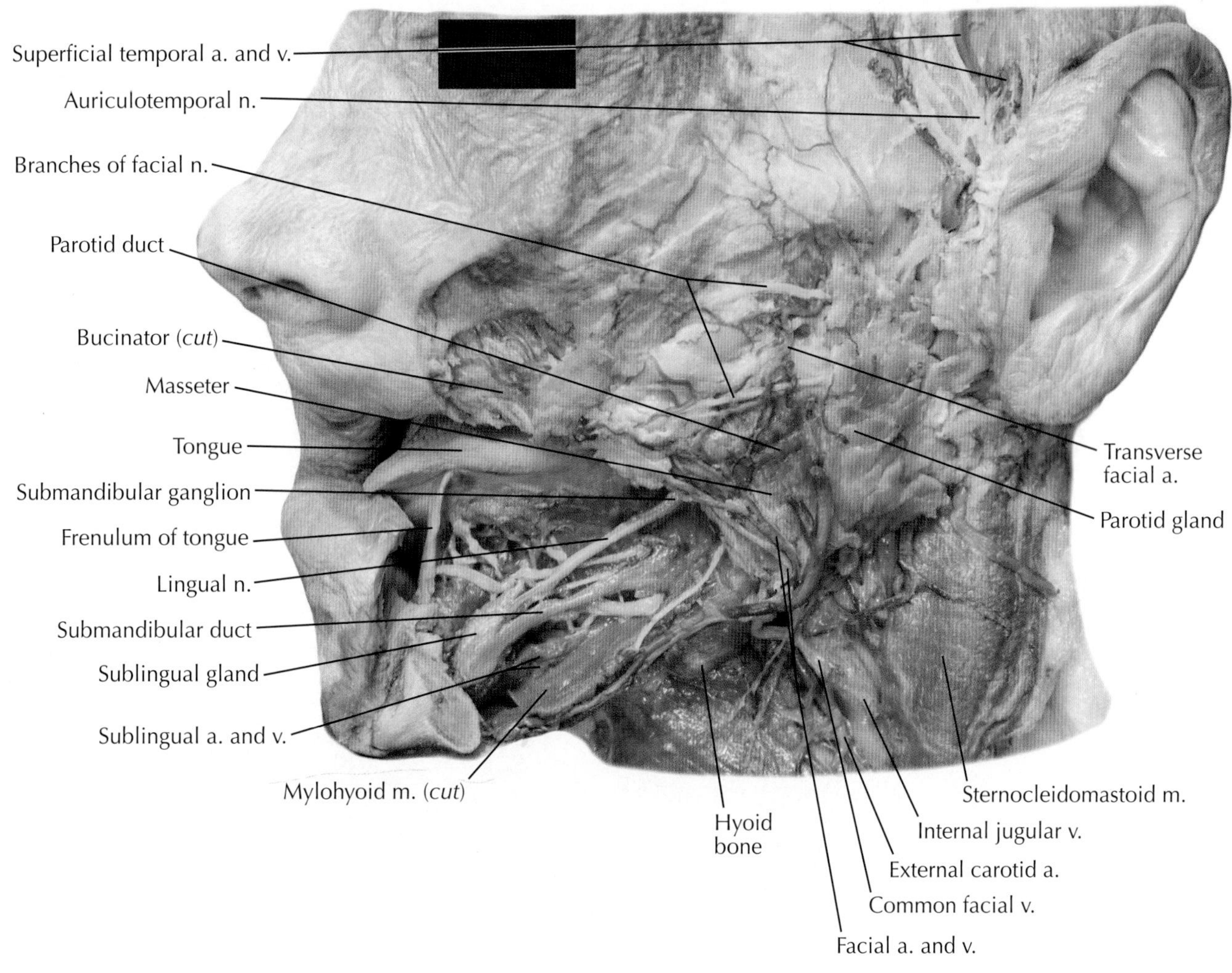
Superficial temporal a. and v.
Auriculotemporal n.
Branches of facial n.
Parotid duct
Bucinator (cut)
Masseter
Tongue
Submandibular ganglion
Frenulum of tongue
Lingual n.
Submandibular duct
Sublingual gland
Sublingual a. and v.
Mylohyoid m. (cut)
Hyoid bone
Transverse facial a.
Parotid gland
Sternocleidomastoid m.
Internal jugular v.
External carotid a.
Common facial v.
Facial a. and v.

Fig. 1.14 Salivary Glands (Photograph)

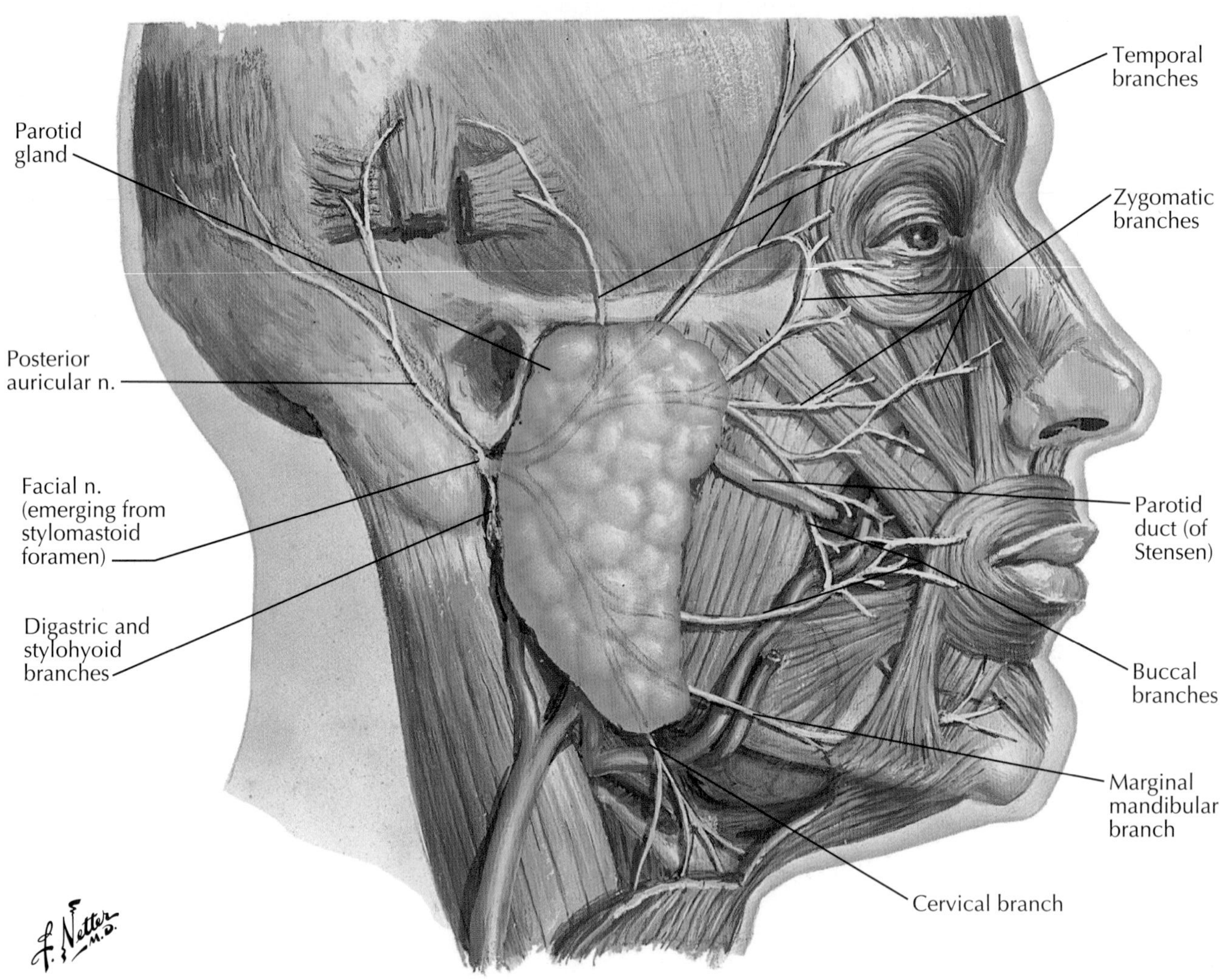
Temporal branches
Parotid gland
Zygomatic branches
Posterior auricular n.
Facial n. (emerging from stylomastoid foramen)
Parotid duct (of Stensen)
Digastric and stylohyoid branches
Buccal branches
Marginal mandibular branch
Cervical branch

Fig. 1.15 Facial Nerve Branches and Parotid Gland (Illustration)

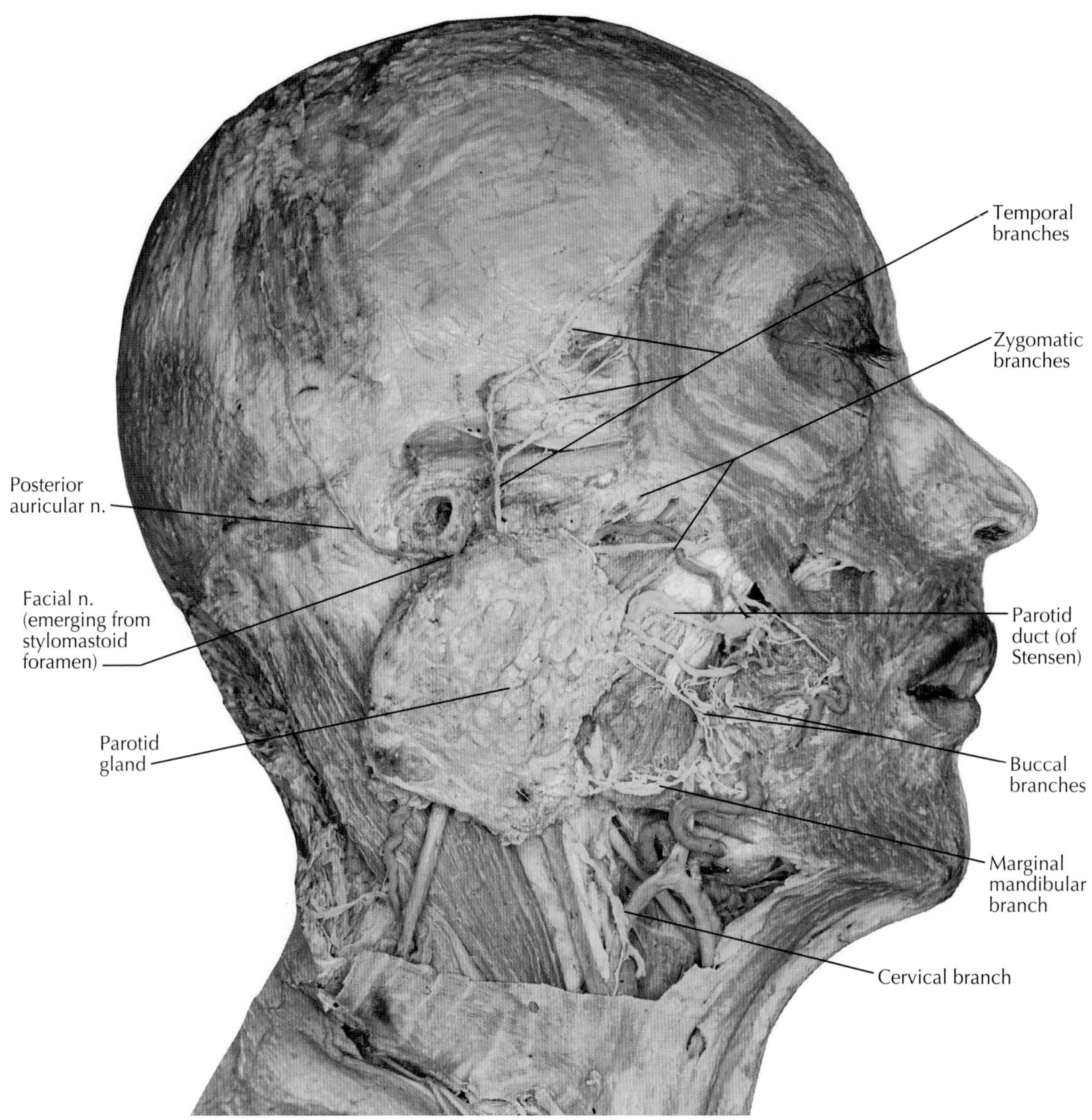
Temporal branches
Zygomatic branches
Posterior auricular n.
Facial n. (emerging from stylomastoid foramen)
Parotid duct (of Stensen)
Parotid gland
Buccal branches
Marginal mandibular branch
Cervical branch

Fig. 1.16 Facial Nerve Branches and Parotid Gland (Photograph) (see Fig. A.1)

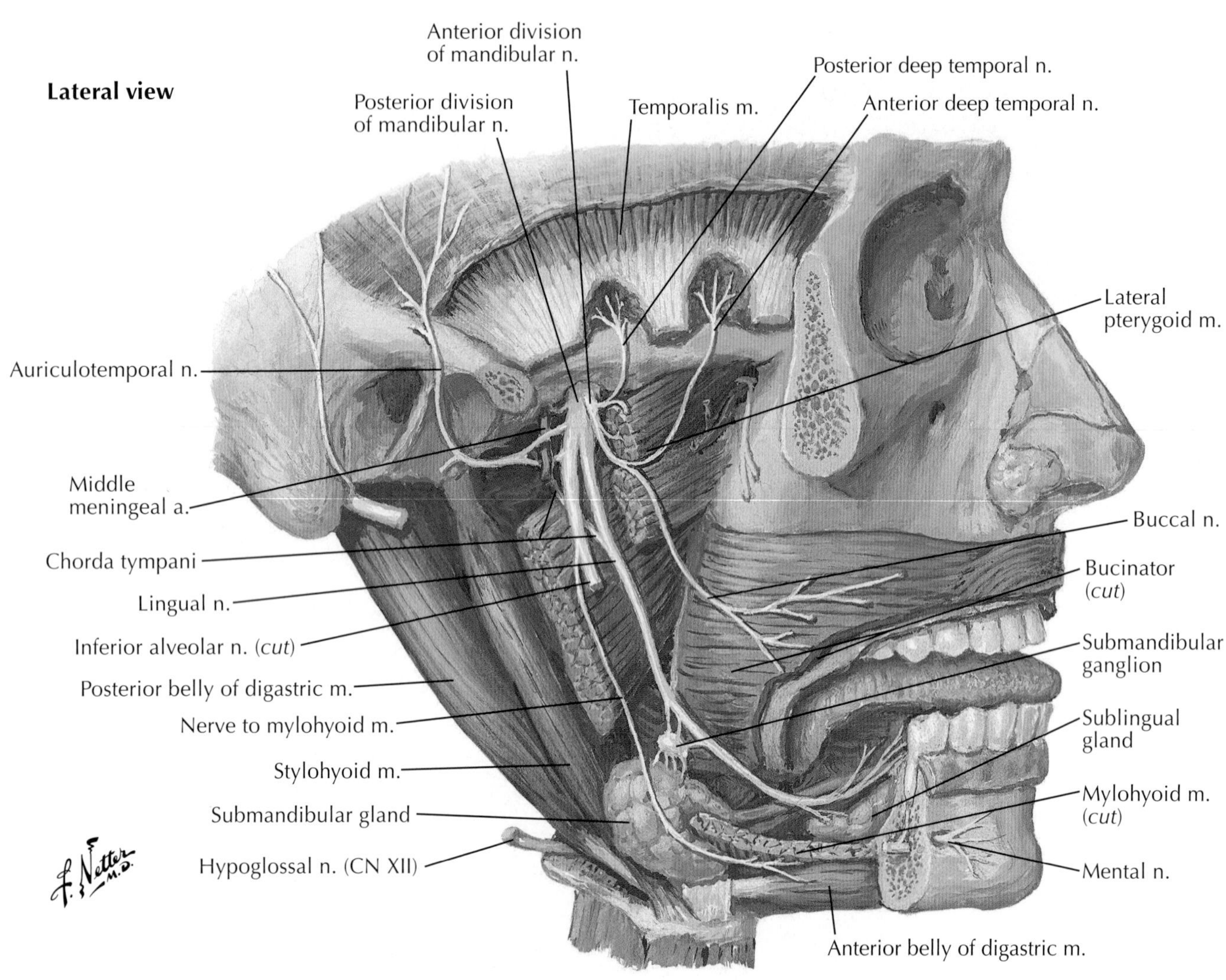
Lateral view
Anterior division of mandibular n.
Posterior division of mandibular n.
Temporalis m.
Posterior deep temporal n.
Anterior deep temporal n.
Lateral pterygoid m.
Auriculotemporal n.
Middle meningeal a.
Buccal n.
Chorda tympani
Bucinator (cut)
Lingual n.
Inferior alveolar n. (cut)
Submandibular ganglion
Posterior belly of digastric m.
Nerve to mylohyoid m.
Sublingual gland
Stylohyoid m.
Mylohyoid m. (cut)
Submandibular gland
Hypoglossal n. (CN XII)
Mental n.
Anterior belly of digastric m.

Fig. 1.17 Mandibular Nerve (CN V_3) (Illustration)

Lateral view

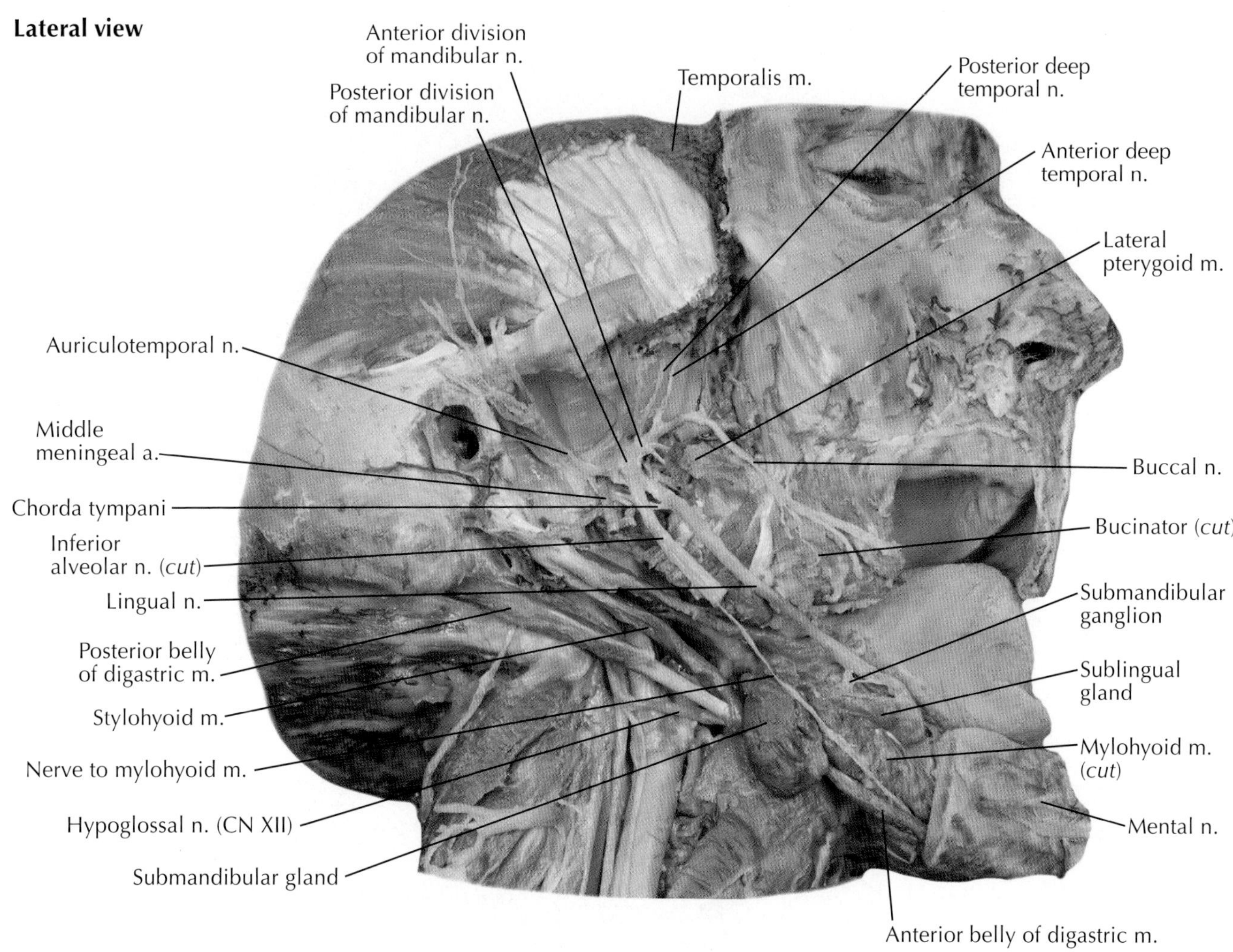
Anterior division of mandibular n.
Posterior division of mandibular n.
Temporalis m.
Posterior deep temporal n.
Anterior deep temporal n.
Lateral pterygoid m.
Auriculotemporal n.
Middle meningeal a.
Buccal n.
Chorda tympani
Bucinator (*cut*)
Inferior alveolar n. (*cut*)
Lingual n.
Submandibular ganglion
Posterior belly of digastric m.
Sublingual gland
Stylohyoid m.
Mylohyoid m. (*cut*)
Nerve to mylohyoid m.
Hypoglossal n. (CN XII)
Mental n.
Submandibular gland
Anterior belly of digastric m.

Fig. 1.18 Mandibular Nerve (CN V_3) (Photograph)

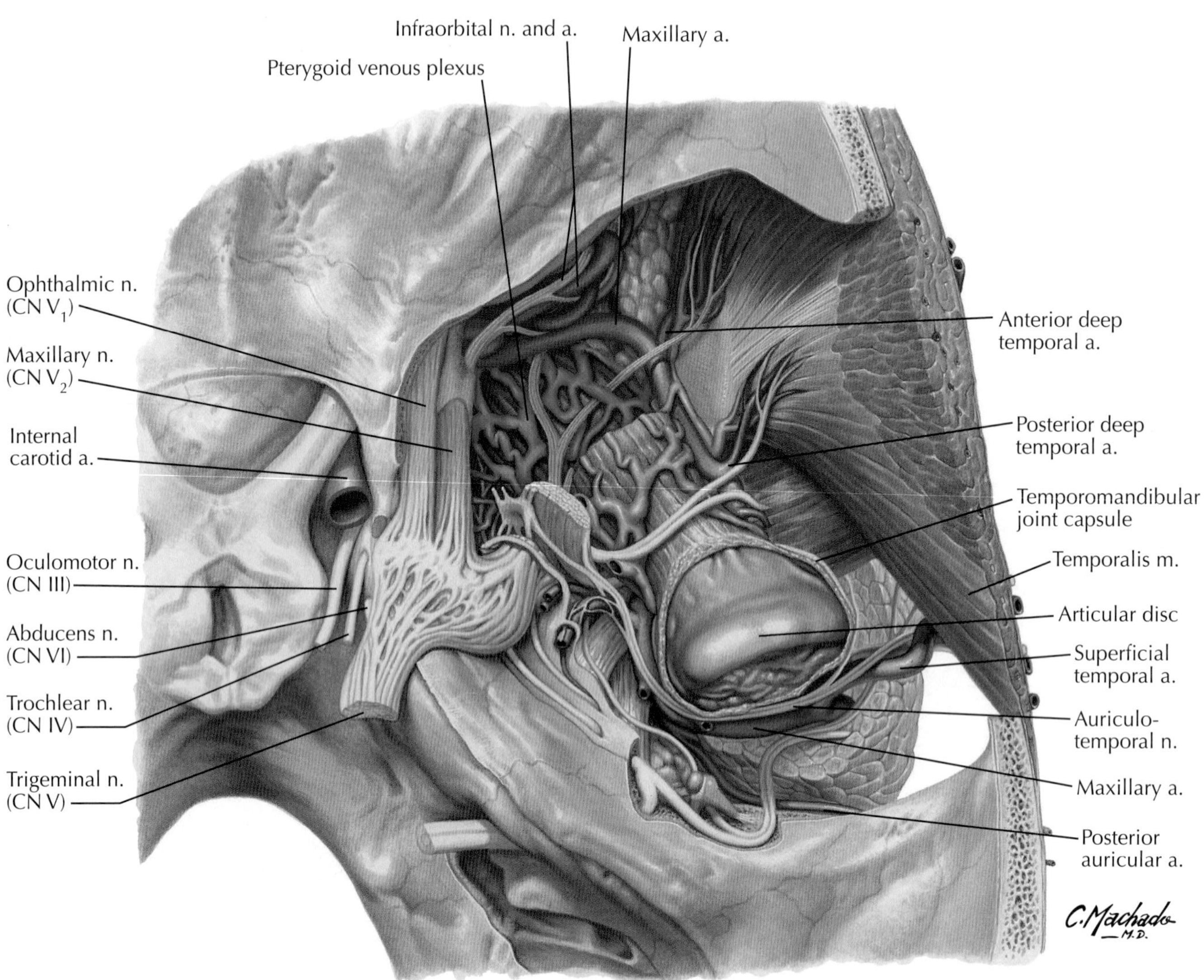
Infraorbital n. and a.
Maxillary a.
Pterygoid venous plexus
Ophthalmic n. (CN V1)
Maxillary n. (CN V2)
Internal carotid a.
Oculomotor n. (CN III)
Abducens n. (CN VI)
Trochlear n. (CN IV)
Trigeminal n. (CN V)
Anterior deep temporal a.
Posterior deep temporal a.
Temporomandibular joint capsule
Temporalis m.
Articular disc
Superficial temporal a.
Auriculo-temporal n.
Maxillary a.
Posterior auricular a.
C.Machado M.D.

Fig. 1.19 Infratemporal Fossa (Illustration)

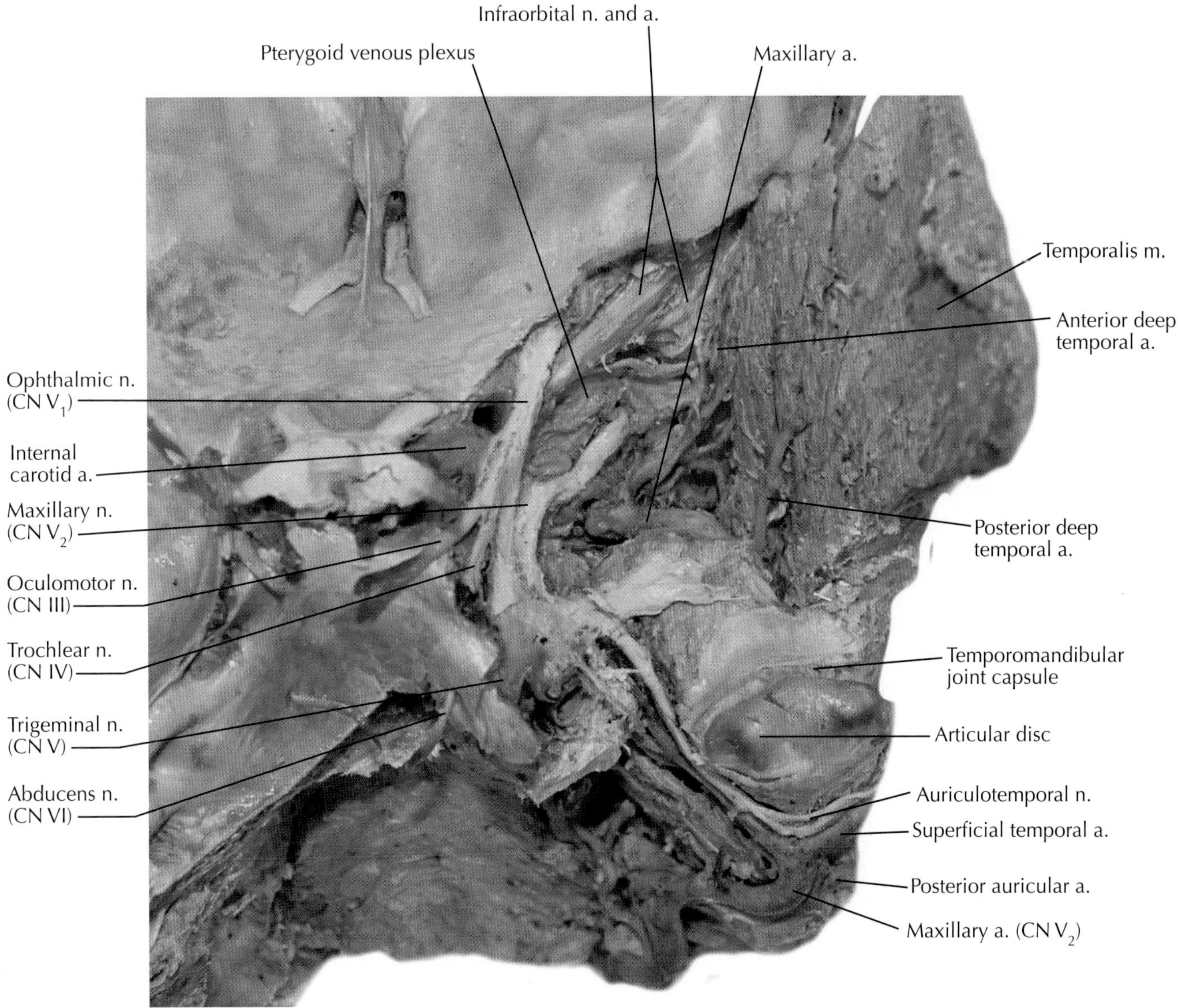
Infraorbital n. and a.
Pterygoid venous plexus
Maxillary a.
Temporalis m.
Anterior deep temporal a.
Ophthalmic n. (CN V$_1$)
Internal carotid a.
Maxillary n. (CN V$_2$)
Oculomotor n. (CN III)
Trochlear n. (CN IV)
Trigeminal n. (CN V)
Abducens n. (CN VI)
Posterior deep temporal a.
Temporomandibular joint capsule
Articular disc
Auriculotemporal n.
Superficial temporal a.
Posterior auricular a.
Maxillary a. (CN V$_2$)

Fig. 1.20 Infratemporal Fossa (Photograph) (see Fig. A.2)

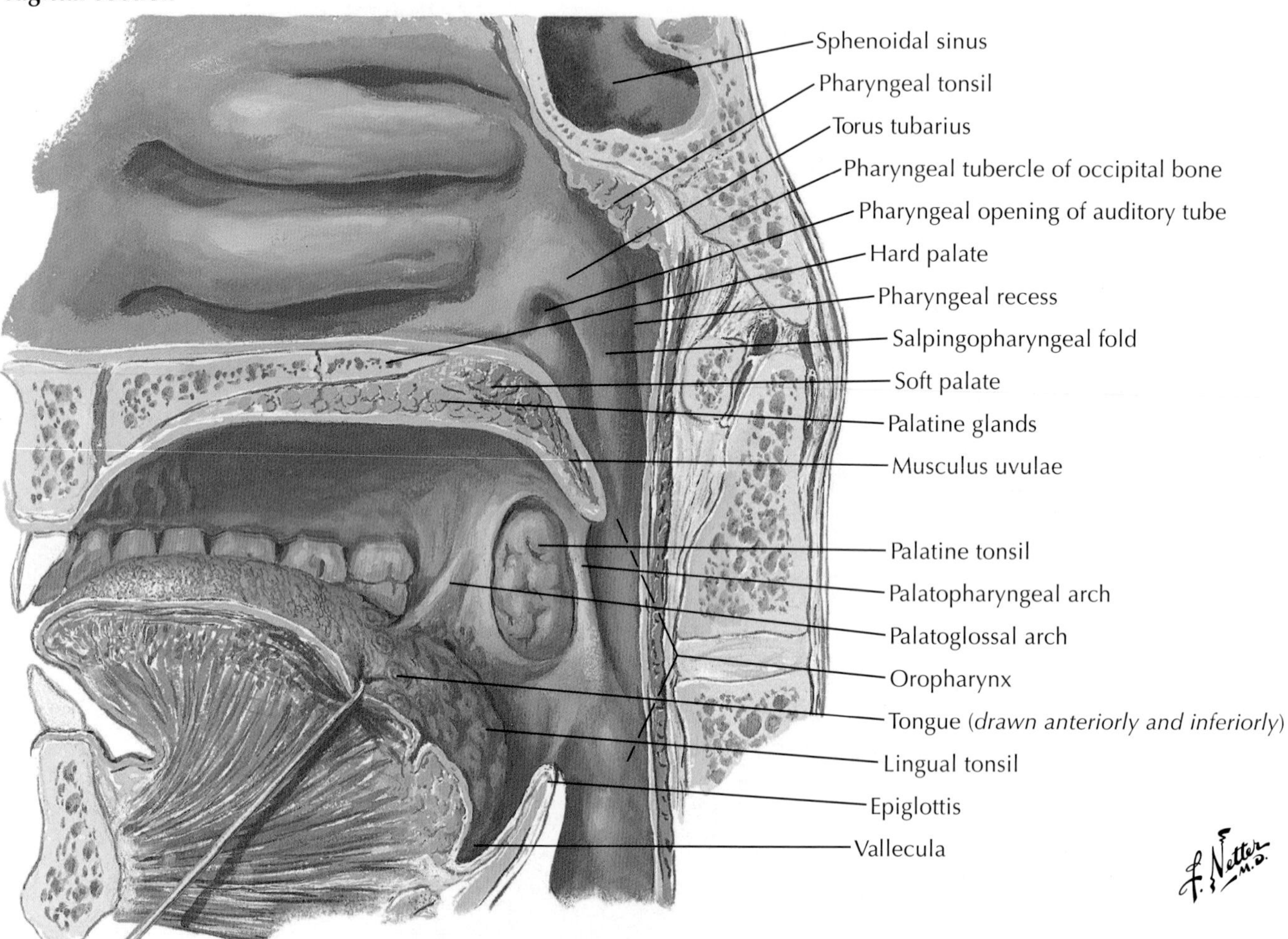
Medial view
sagittal section
Sphenoidal sinus
Pharyngeal tonsil
Torus tubarius
Pharyngeal tubercle of occipital bone
Pharyngeal opening of auditory tube
Hard palate
Pharyngeal recess
Salpingopharyngeal fold
Soft palate
Palatine glands
Musculus uvulae
Palatine tonsil
Palatopharyngeal arch
Palatoglossal arch
Oropharynx
Tongue (*drawn anteriorly and inferiorly*)
Lingual tonsil
Epiglottis
Vallecula

Fig. 1.21 Fauces (Illustration)

Medial view
sagittal section

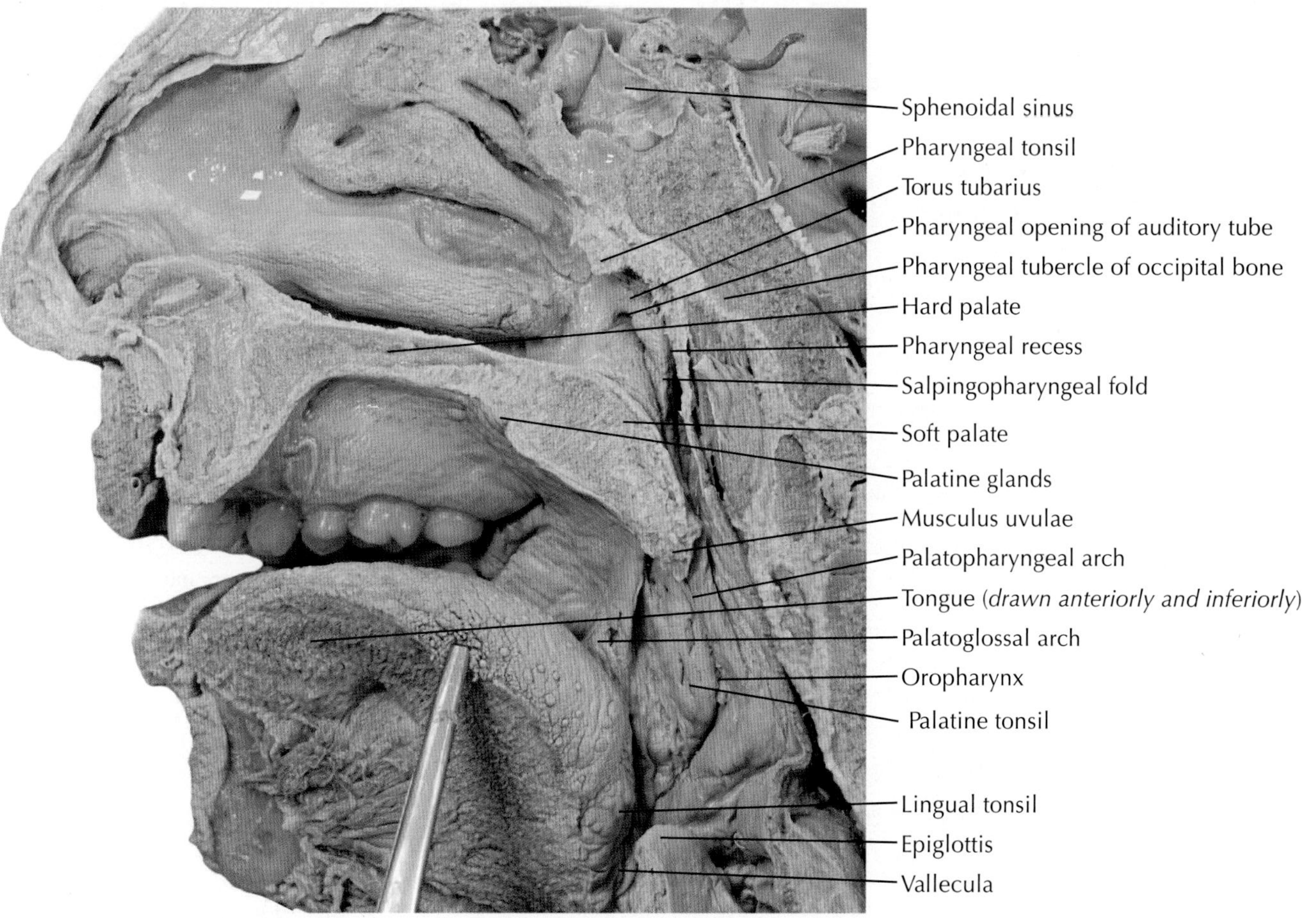
Sphenoidal sinus
Pharyngeal tonsil
Torus tubarius
Pharyngeal opening of auditory tube
Pharyngeal tubercle of occipital bone
Hard palate
Pharyngeal recess
Salpingopharyngeal fold
Soft palate
Palatine glands
Musculus uvulae
Palatopharyngeal arch
Tongue (*drawn anteriorly and inferiorly*)
Palatoglossal arch
Oropharynx
Palatine tonsil
Lingual tonsil
Epiglottis
Vallecula

Fig. 1.22 Fauces (Photograph)

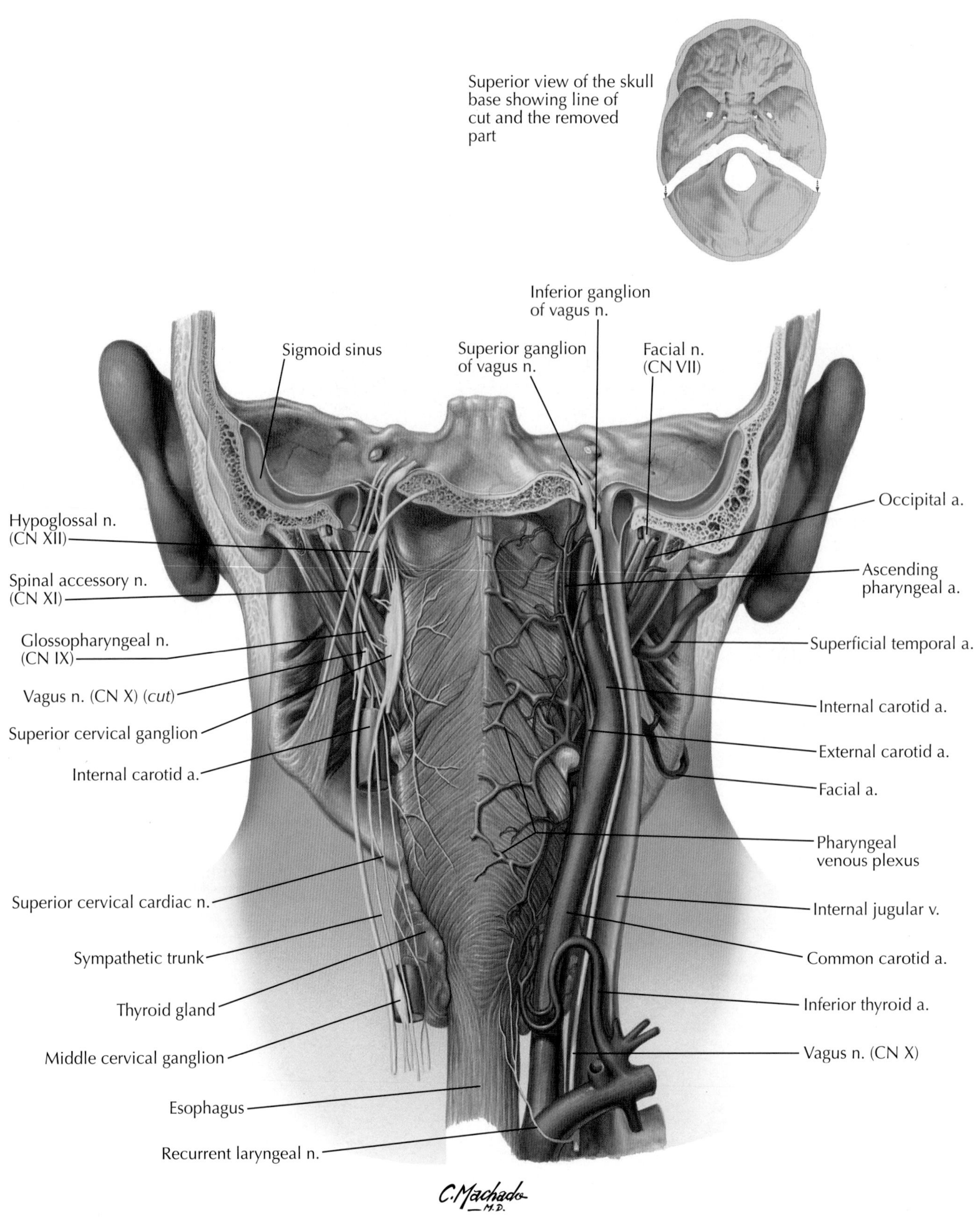

Superior view of the skull base showing line of cut and the removed part
Inferior ganglion of vagus n.
Sigmoid sinus
Superior ganglion of vagus n.
Facial n. (CN VII)
Occipital a.
Hypoglossal n. (CN XII)
Ascending pharyngeal a.
Spinal accessory n. (CN XI)
Superficial temporal a.
Glossopharyngeal n. (CN IX)
Vagus n. (CN X) (cut)
Internal carotid a.
Superior cervical ganglion
External carotid a.
Internal carotid a.
Facial a.
Pharyngeal venous plexus
Superior cervical cardiac n.
Internal jugular v.
Sympathetic trunk
Common carotid a.
Thyroid gland
Inferior thyroid a.
Middle cervical ganglion
Vagus n. (CN X)
Esophagus
Recurrent laryngeal n.
C. Machado M.D.

Fig. 1.23 Posterior View of Pharynx: Nerves and Vessels (Illustration)

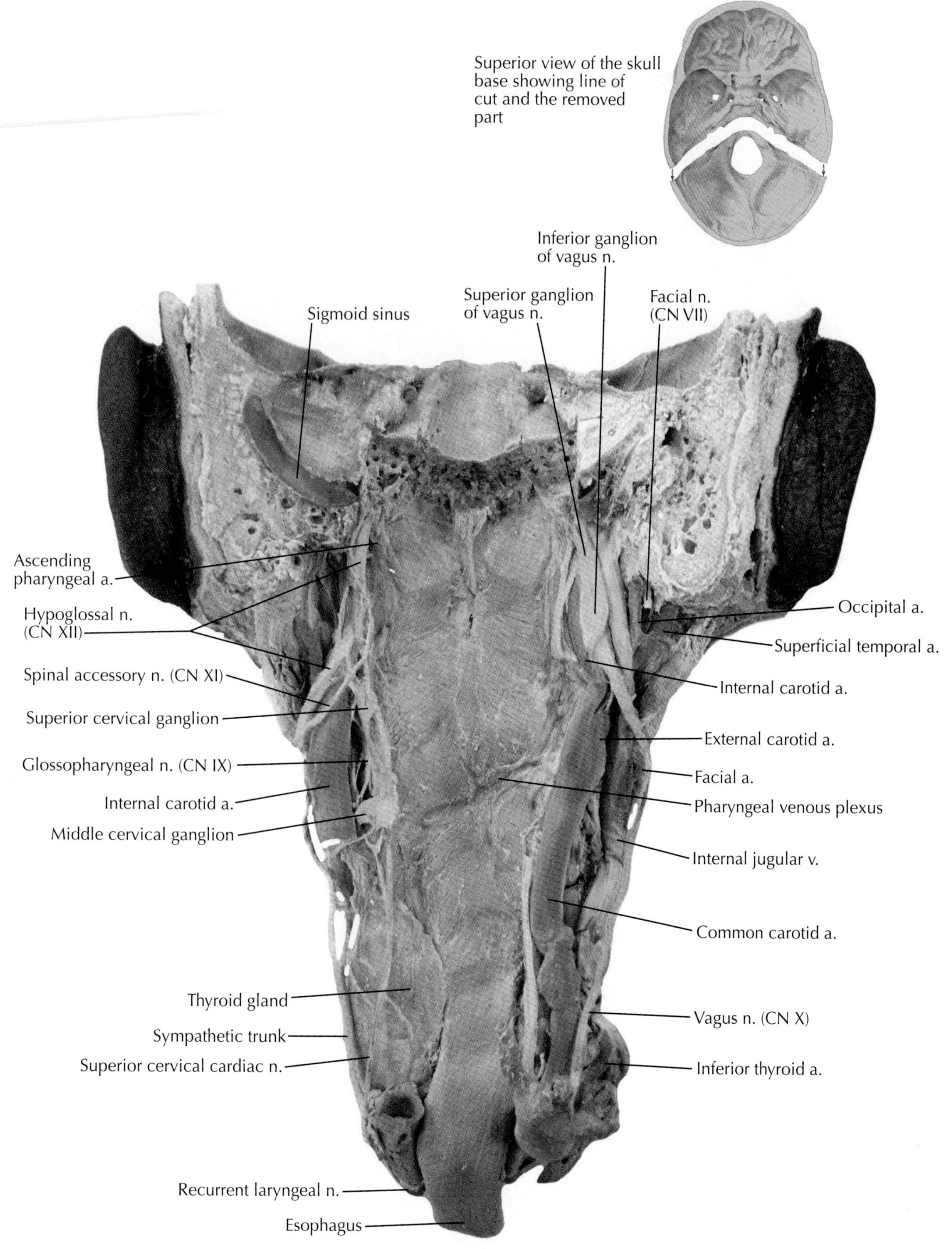
Superior view of the skull base showing line of cut and the removed part
Inferior ganglion of vagus n.
Superior ganglion of vagus n.
Facial n. (CN VII)
Sigmoid sinus
Ascending pharyngeal a.
Hypoglossal n. (CN XII)
Spinal accessory n. (CN XI)
Superior cervical ganglion
Glossopharyngeal n. (CN IX)
Internal carotid a.
Middle cervical ganglion
Thyroid gland
Sympathetic trunk
Superior cervical cardiac n.
Recurrent laryngeal n.
Esophagus
Occipital a.
Superficial temporal a.
Internal carotid a.
External carotid a.
Facial a.
Pharyngeal venous plexus
Internal jugular v.
Common carotid a.
Vagus n. (CN X)
Inferior thyroid a.

Fig. 1.24 Posterior View of Pharynx: Nerves and Vessels (Photograph) (see Fig. A.3)

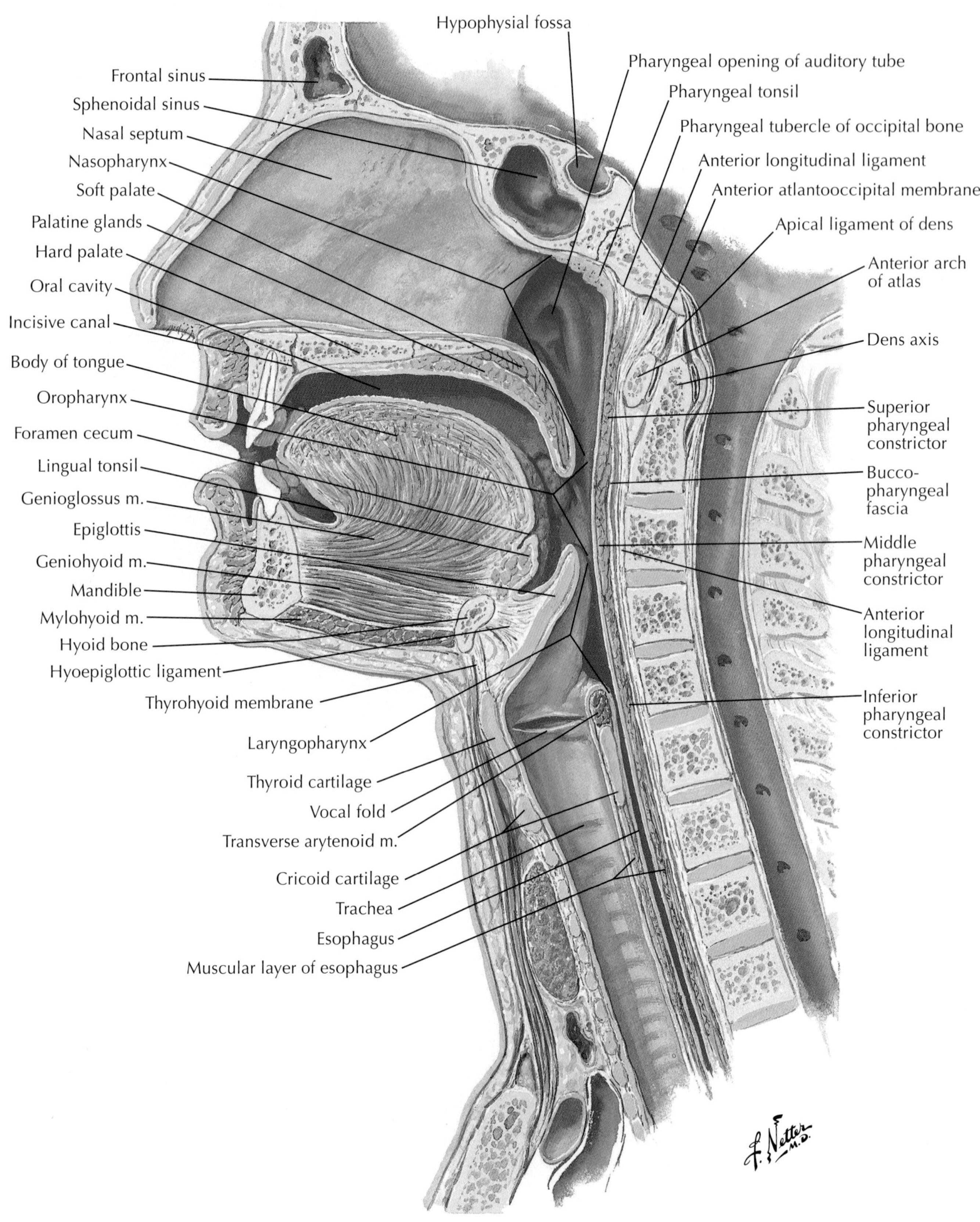
Hypophysial fossa
Pharyngeal opening of auditory tube
Pharyngeal tonsil
Pharyngeal tubercle of occipital bone
Anterior longitudinal ligament
Anterior atlantooccipital membrane
Apical ligament of dens
Anterior arch of atlas
Dens axis
Superior pharyngeal constrictor
Bucco-pharyngeal fascia
Middle pharyngeal constrictor
Anterior longitudinal ligament
Inferior pharyngeal constrictor
Frontal sinus
Sphenoidal sinus
Nasal septum
Nasopharynx
Soft palate
Palatine glands
Hard palate
Oral cavity
Incisive canal
Body of tongue
Oropharynx
Foramen cecum
Lingual tonsil
Genioglossus m.
Epiglottis
Geniohyoid m.
Mandible
Mylohyoid m.
Hyoid bone
Hyoepiglottic ligament
Thyrohyoid membrane
Laryngopharynx
Thyroid cartilage
Vocal fold
Transverse arytenoid m.
Cricoid cartilage
Trachea
Esophagus
Muscular layer of esophagus
F. Netter M.D.

Fig. 1.25 Pharynx: Medial View (Illustration)

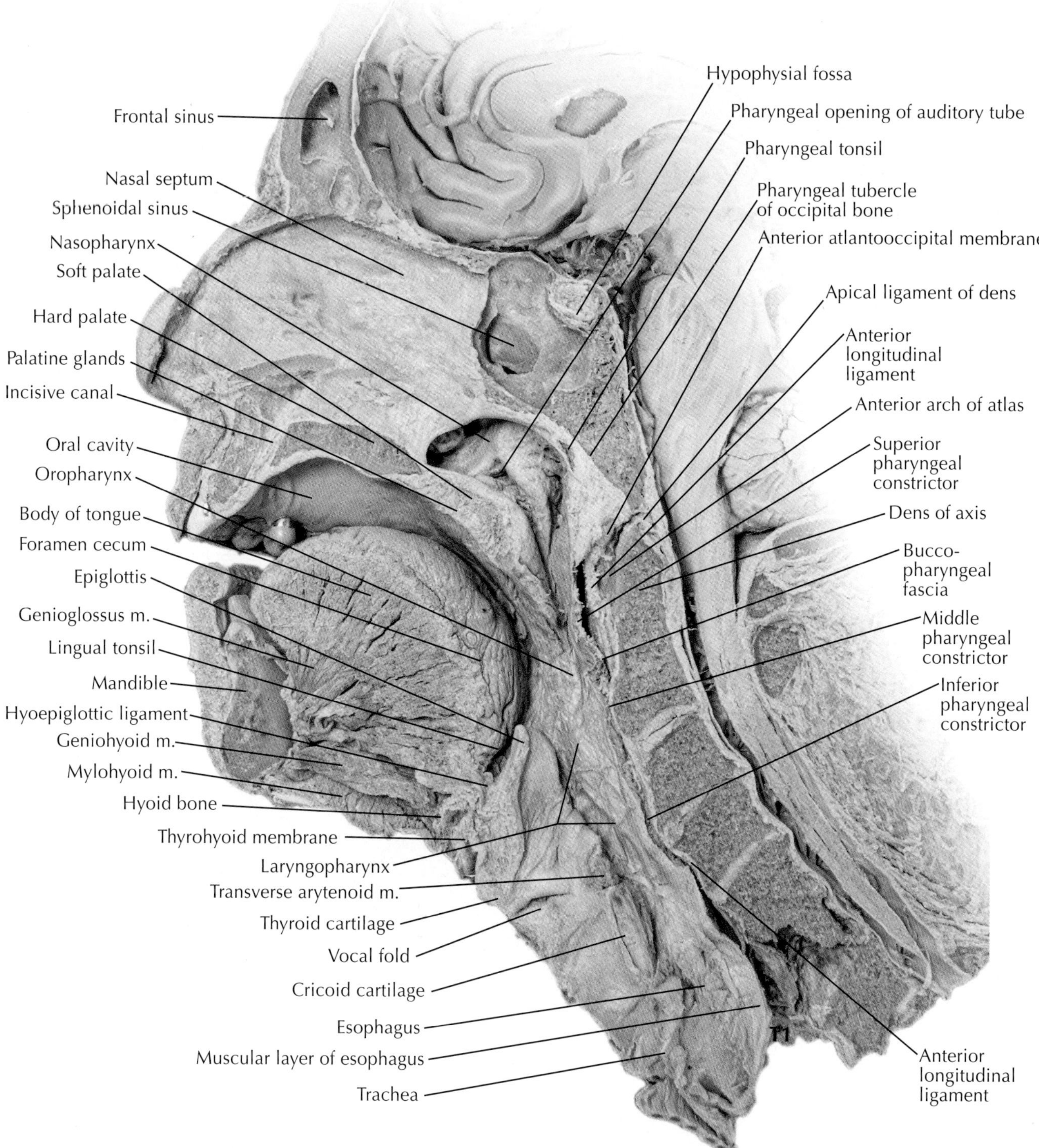

Frontal sinus
Nasal septum
Sphenoidal sinus
Nasopharynx
Soft palate
Hard palate
Palatine glands
Incisive canal
Oral cavity
Oropharynx
Body of tongue
Foramen cecum
Epiglottis
Genioglossus m.
Lingual tonsil
Mandible
Hyoepiglottic ligament
Geniohyoid m.
Mylohyoid m.
Hyoid bone
Thyrohyoid membrane
Laryngopharynx
Transverse arytenoid m.
Thyroid cartilage
Vocal fold
Cricoid cartilage
Esophagus
Muscular layer of esophagus
Trachea
Hypophysial fossa
Pharyngeal opening of auditory tube
Pharyngeal tonsil
Pharyngeal tubercle of occipital bone
Anterior atlantooccipital membrane
Apical ligament of dens
Anterior longitudinal ligament
Anterior arch of atlas
Superior pharyngeal constrictor
Dens of axis
Bucco-pharyngeal fascia
Middle pharyngeal constrictor
Inferior pharyngeal constrictor
Anterior longitudinal ligament

Fig. 1.26 Pharynx: Medial View (Photograph)

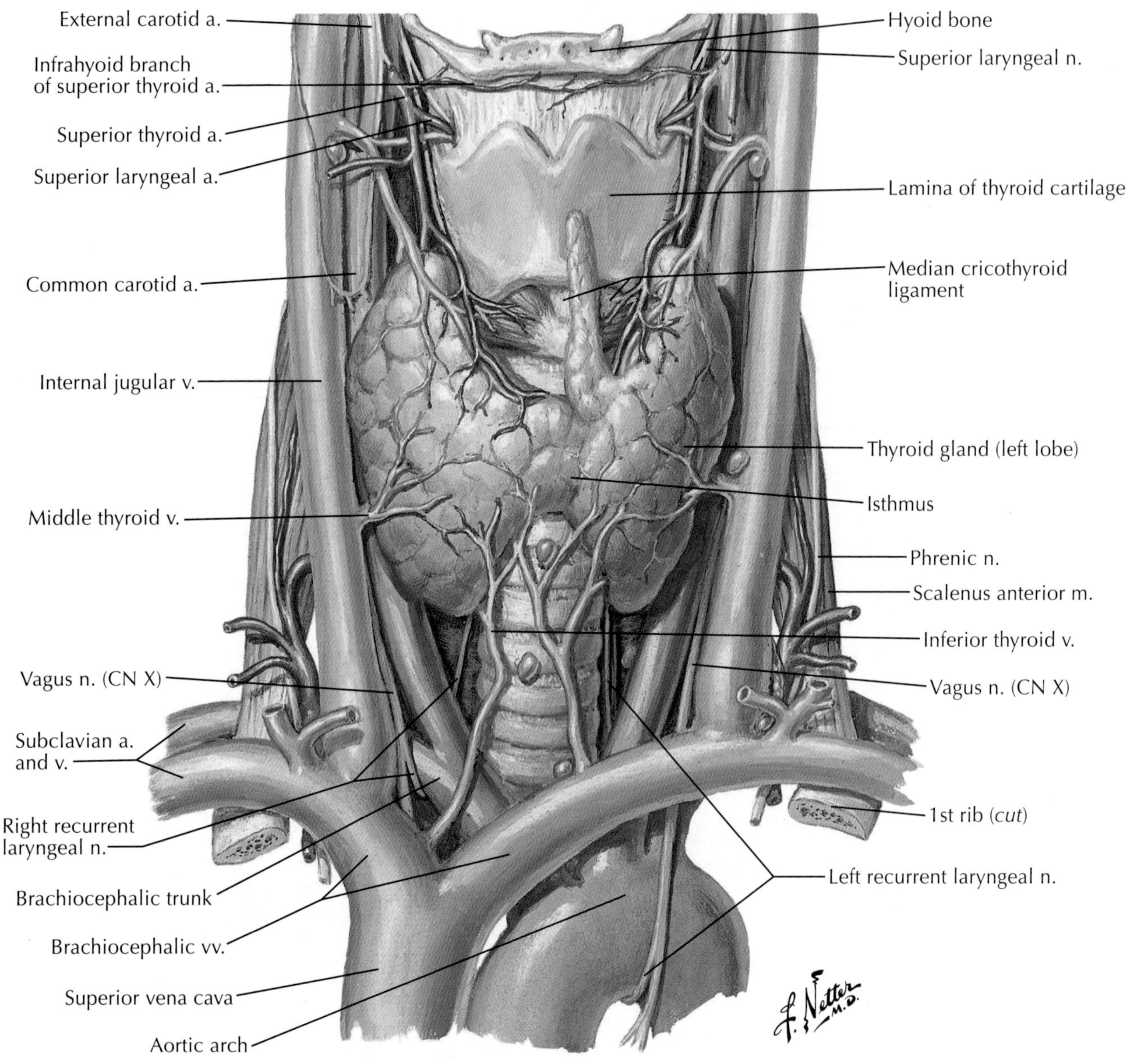
External carotid a.
Infrahyoid branch of superior thyroid a.
Superior thyroid a.
Superior laryngeal a.
Common carotid a.
Internal jugular v.
Middle thyroid v.
Vagus n. (CN X)
Subclavian a. and v.
Right recurrent laryngeal n.
Brachiocephalic trunk
Brachiocephalic vv.
Superior vena cava
Aortic arch
Hyoid bone
Superior laryngeal n.
Lamina of thyroid cartilage
Median cricothyroid ligament
Thyroid gland (left lobe)
Isthmus
Phrenic n.
Scalenus anterior m.
Inferior thyroid v.
Vagus n. (CN X)
1st rib (cut)
Left recurrent laryngeal n.
F. Netter M.D.

Fig. 1.27 Thyroid Gland: Anterior View (Illustration)

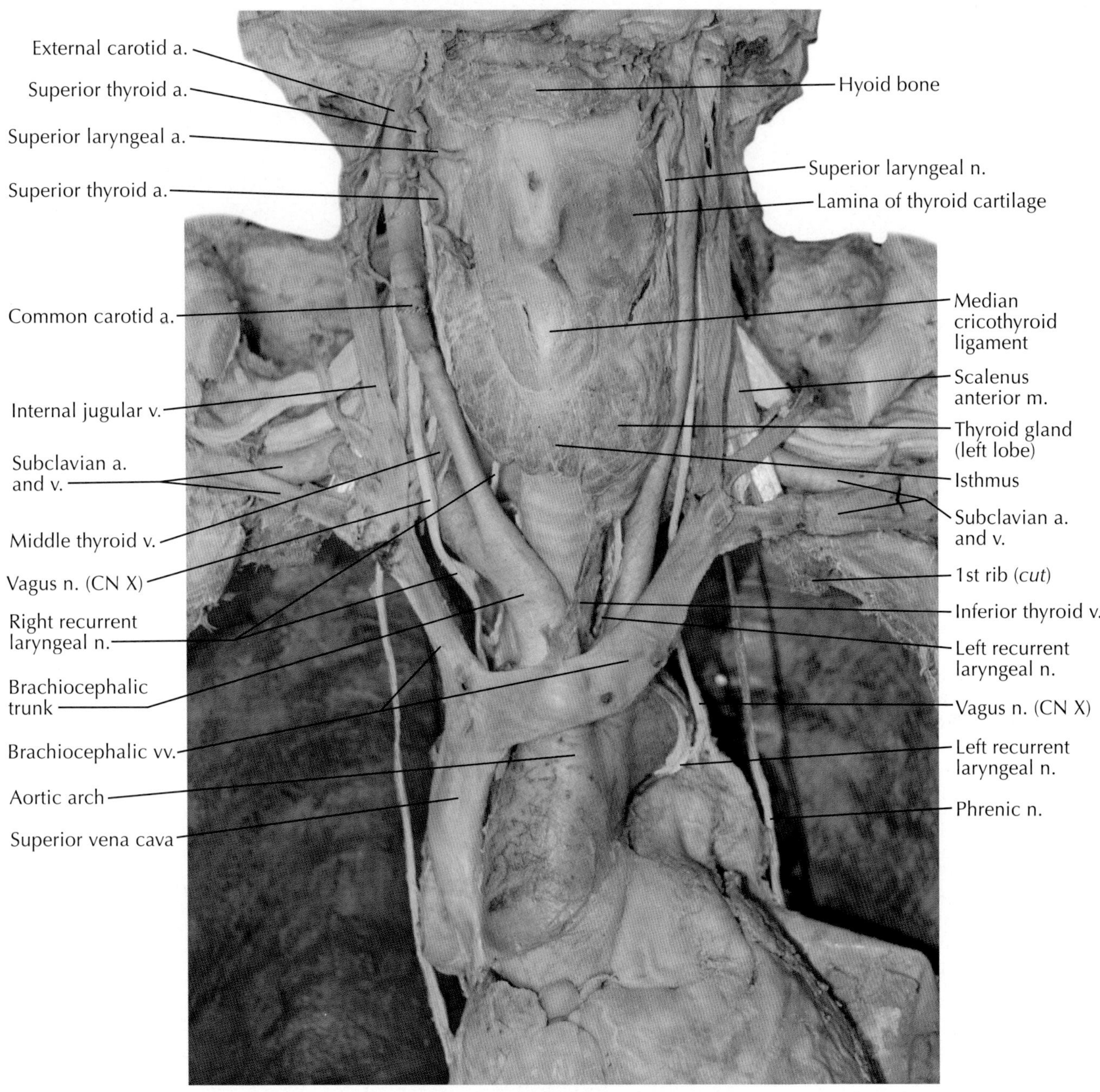
External carotid a.
Superior thyroid a.
Superior laryngeal a.
Superior thyroid a.
Common carotid a.
Internal jugular v.
Subclavian a.
and v.
Middle thyroid v.
Vagus n. (CN X)
Right recurrent
laryngeal n.
Brachiocephalic
trunk
Brachiocephalic vv.
Aortic arch
Superior vena cava
Hyoid bone
Superior laryngeal n.
Lamina of thyroid cartilage
Median
cricothyroid
ligament
Scalenus
anterior m.
Thyroid gland
(left lobe)
Isthmus
Subclavian a.
and v.
1st rib (*cut*)
Inferior thyroid v.
Left recurrent
laryngeal n.
Vagus n. (CN X)
Left recurrent
laryngeal n.
Phrenic n.

Fig. 1.28 Thyroid Gland: Anterior View (Photograph) (see Fig. A.4)

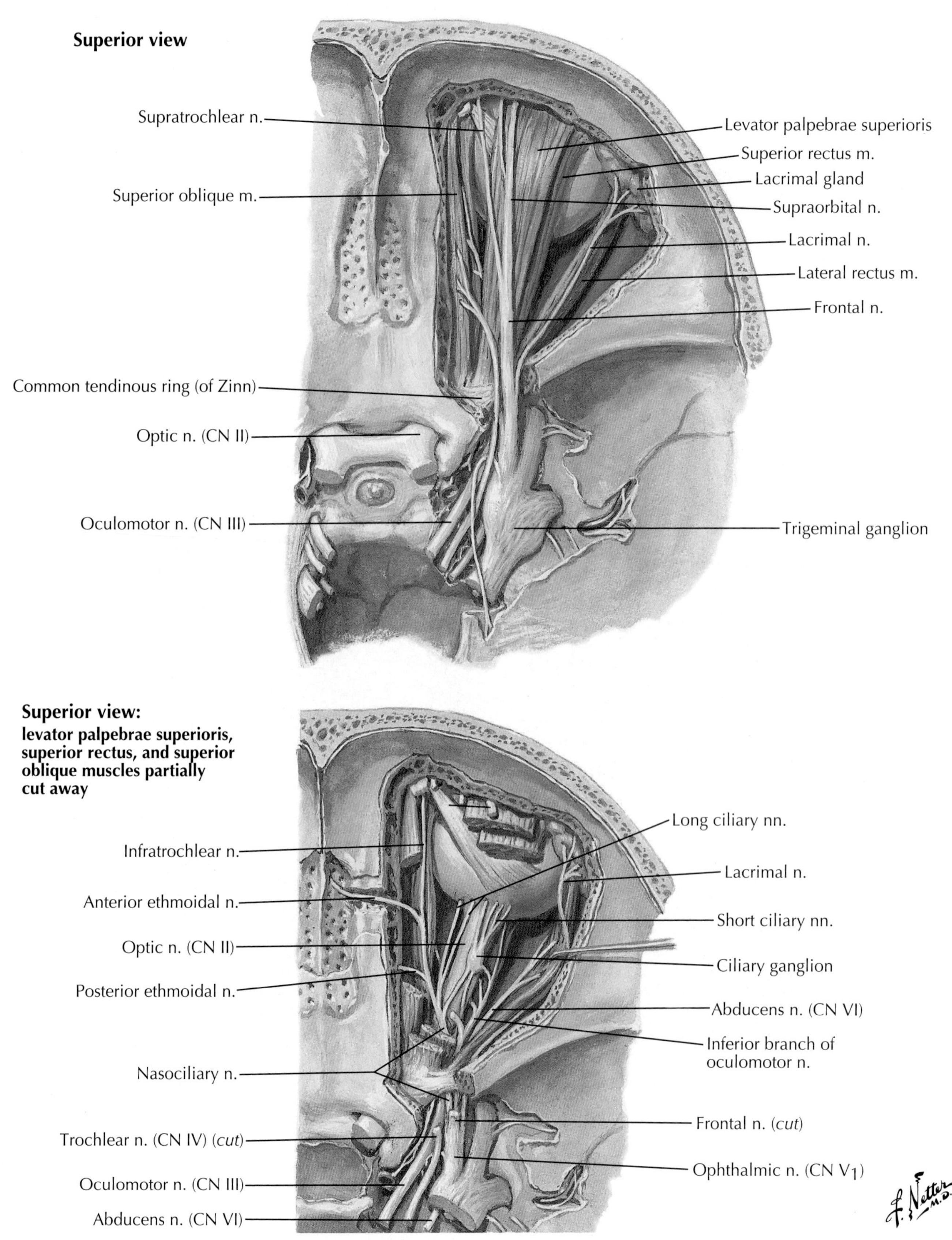
Superior view
Supratrochlear n.
Superior oblique m.
Levator palpebrae superioris
Superior rectus m.
Lacrimal gland
Supraorbital n.
Lacrimal n.
Lateral rectus m.
Frontal n.
Common tendinous ring (of Zinn)
Optic n. (CN II)
Oculomotor n. (CN III)
Trigeminal ganglion
Superior view:
levator palpebrae superioris, superior rectus, and superior oblique muscles partially cut away
Infratrochlear n.
Anterior ethmoidal n.
Optic n. (CN II)
Posterior ethmoidal n.
Nasociliary n.
Trochlear n. (CN IV) (cut)
Oculomotor n. (CN III)
Abducens n. (CN VI)
Long ciliary nn.
Lacrimal n.
Short ciliary nn.
Ciliary ganglion
Abducens n. (CN VI)
Inferior branch of oculomotor n.
Frontal n. (cut)
Ophthalmic n. (CN V1)

Fig. 1.29 Nerves of Orbit (Illustration)

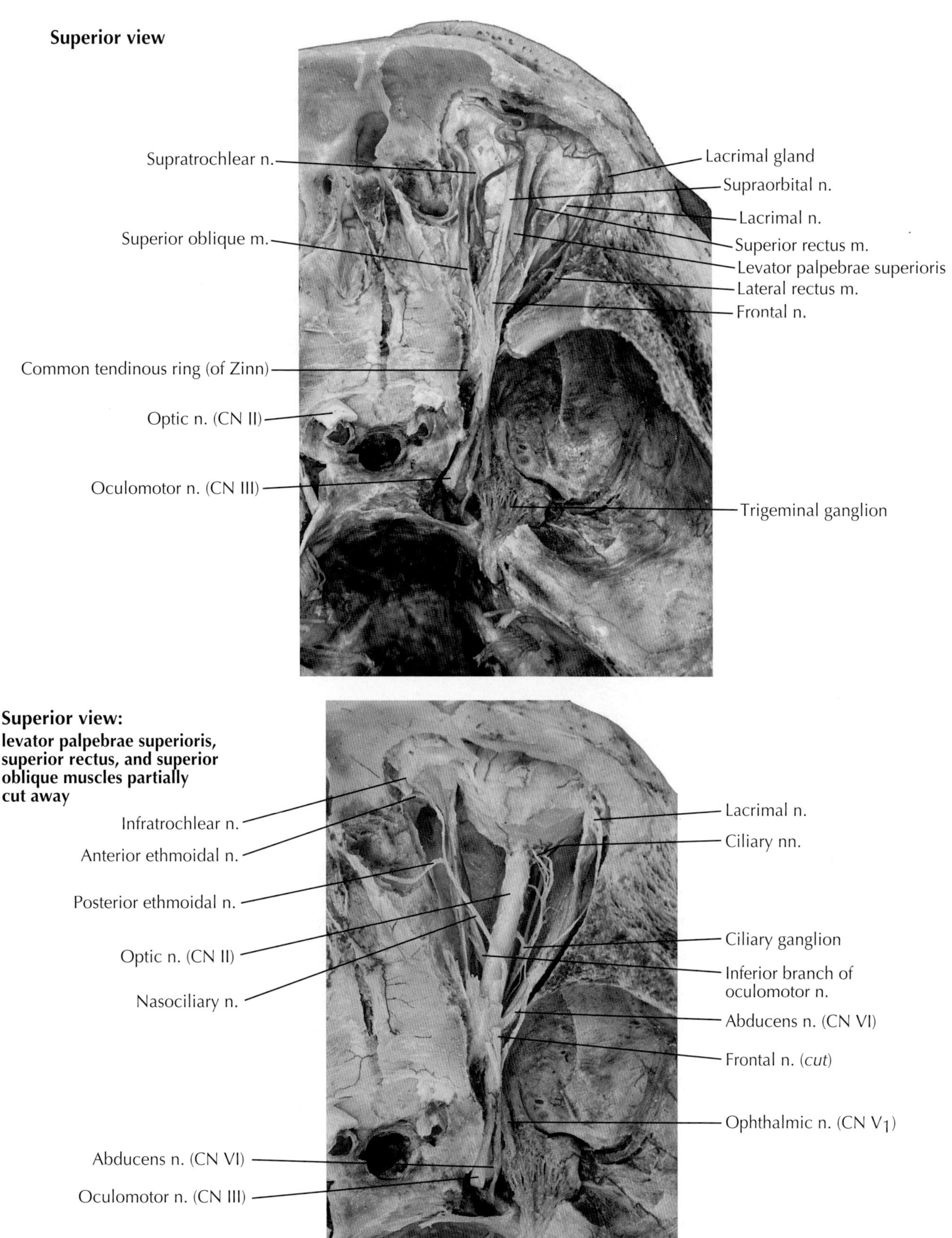
Superior view
Supratrochlear n.
Superior oblique m.
Common tendinous ring (of Zinn)
Optic n. (CN II)
Oculomotor n. (CN III)
Lacrimal gland
Supraorbital n.
Lacrimal n.
Superior rectus m.
Levator palpebrae superioris
Lateral rectus m.
Frontal n.
Trigeminal ganglion
Superior view:
levator palpebrae superioris, superior rectus, and superior oblique muscles partially cut away
Infratrochlear n.
Anterior ethmoidal n.
Posterior ethmoidal n.
Optic n. (CN II)
Nasociliary n.
Abducens n. (CN VI)
Oculomotor n. (CN III)
Lacrimal n.
Ciliary nn.
Ciliary ganglion
Inferior branch of oculomotor n.
Abducens n. (CN VI)
Frontal n. (cut)
Ophthalmic n. (CN V1)

Fig. 1.30 Nerves of Orbit (Photograph)

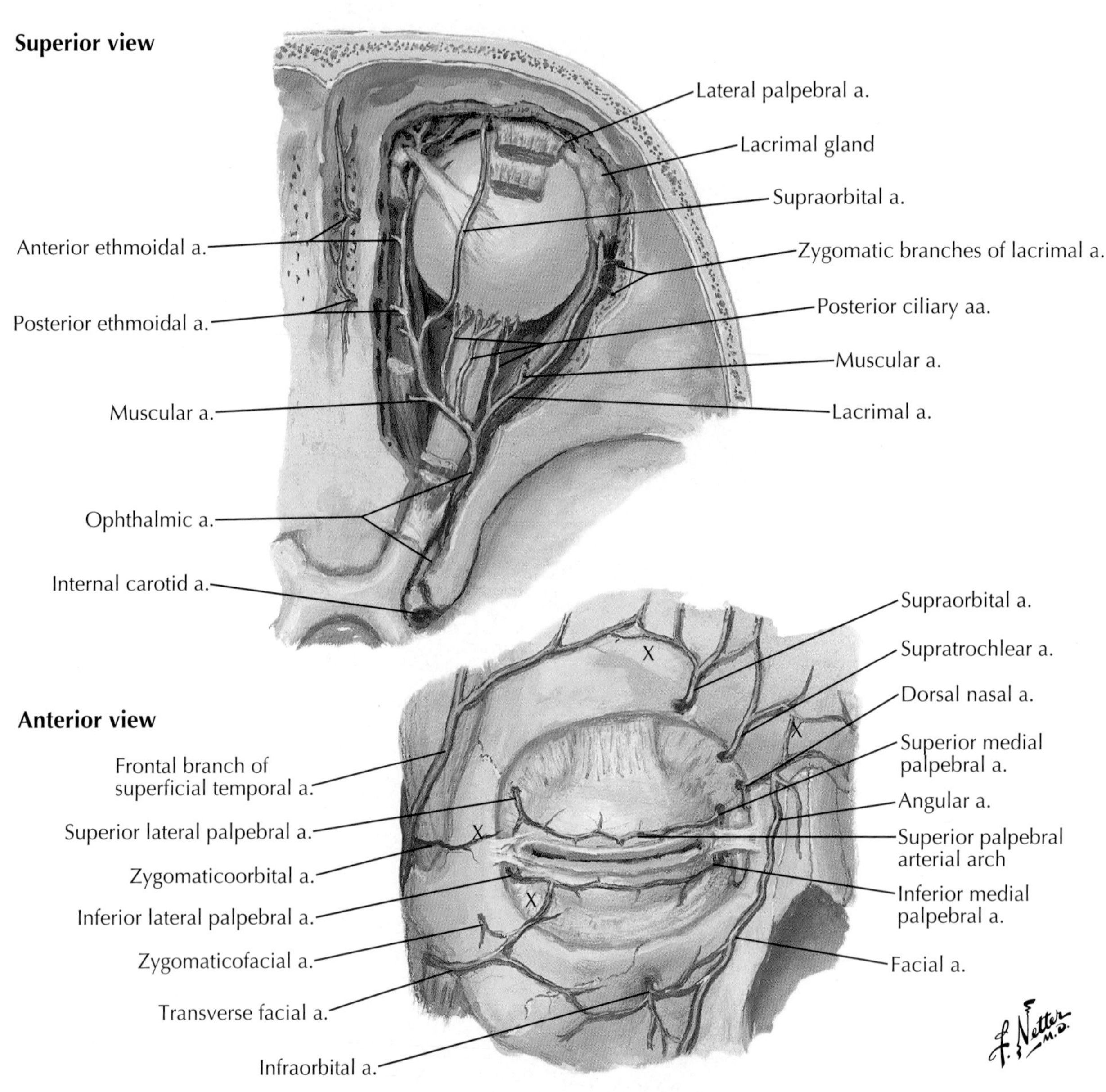
Superior view
Lateral palpebral a.
Lacrimal gland
Supraorbital a.
Anterior ethmoidal a.
Zygomatic branches of lacrimal a.
Posterior ethmoidal a.
Posterior ciliary aa.
Muscular a.
Muscular a.
Lacrimal a.
Ophthalmic a.
Internal carotid a.
Anterior view
Supraorbital a.
Supratrochlear a.
Dorsal nasal a.
Frontal branch of superficial temporal a.
Superior medial palpebral a.
Angular a.
Superior lateral palpebral a.
Superior palpebral arterial arch
Zygomaticoorbital a.
Inferior lateral palpebral a.
Inferior medial palpebral a.
Zygomaticofacial a.
Facial a.
Transverse facial a.
Infraorbital a.
X
X
X
X
F. Netter M.D.

Fig. 1.31 Arteries and Veins of Orbit and Eyelids (Illustration)

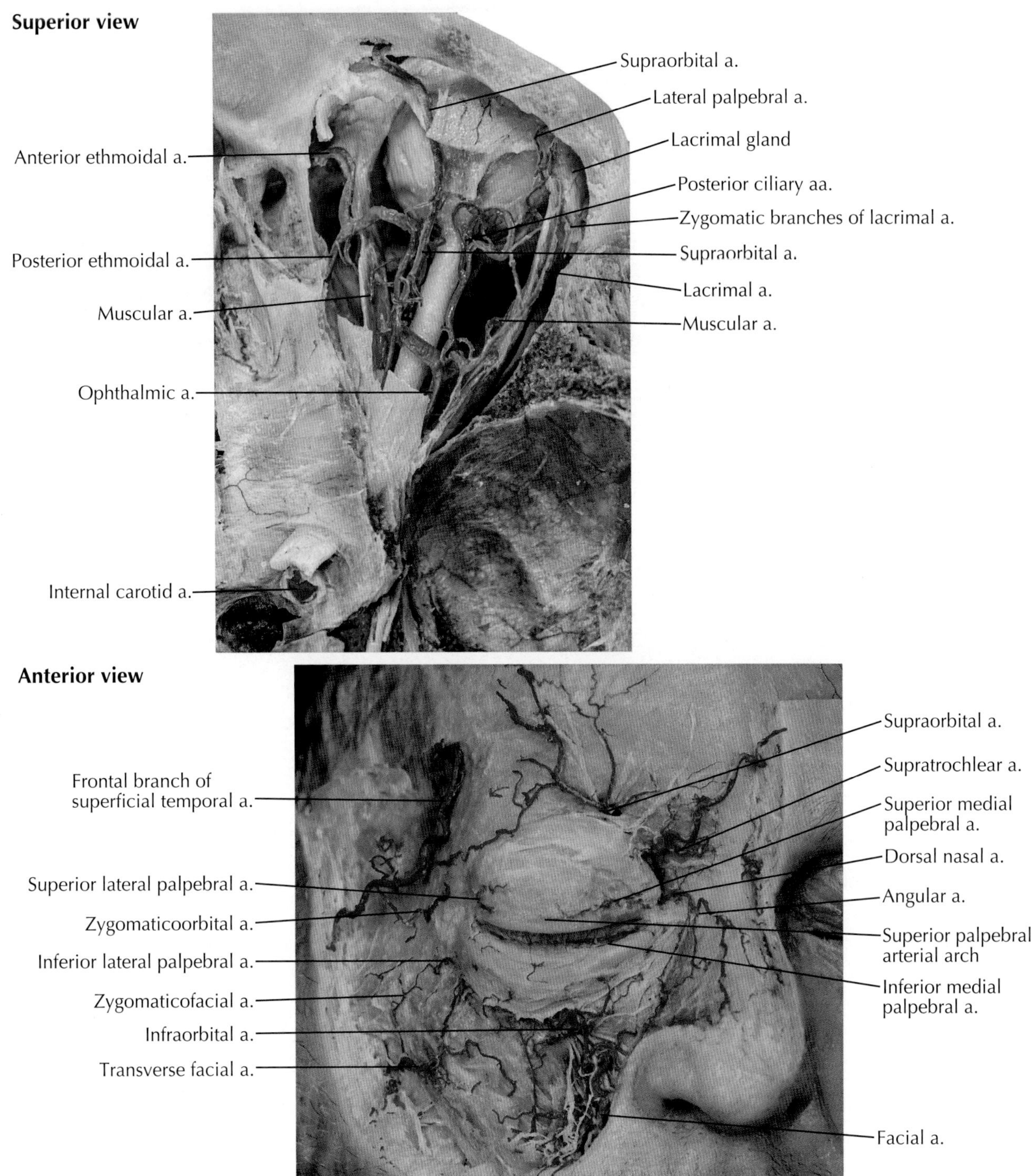
Superior view
Supraorbital a.
Lateral palpebral a.
Anterior ethmoidal a.
Lacrimal gland
Posterior ciliary aa.
Zygomatic branches of lacrimal a.
Posterior ethmoidal a.
Supraorbital a.
Lacrimal a.
Muscular a.
Muscular a.
Ophthalmic a.
Internal carotid a.
Anterior view
Supraorbital a.
Supratrochlear a.
Frontal branch of superficial temporal a.
Superior medial palpebral a.
Dorsal nasal a.
Superior lateral palpebral a.
Angular a.
Zygomaticoorbital a.
Superior palpebral arterial arch
Inferior lateral palpebral a.
Inferior medial palpebral a.
Zygomaticofacial a.
Infraorbital a.
Transverse facial a.
Facial a.

Fig. 1.32 Arteries and Veins of Orbit and Eyelids (Photograph)

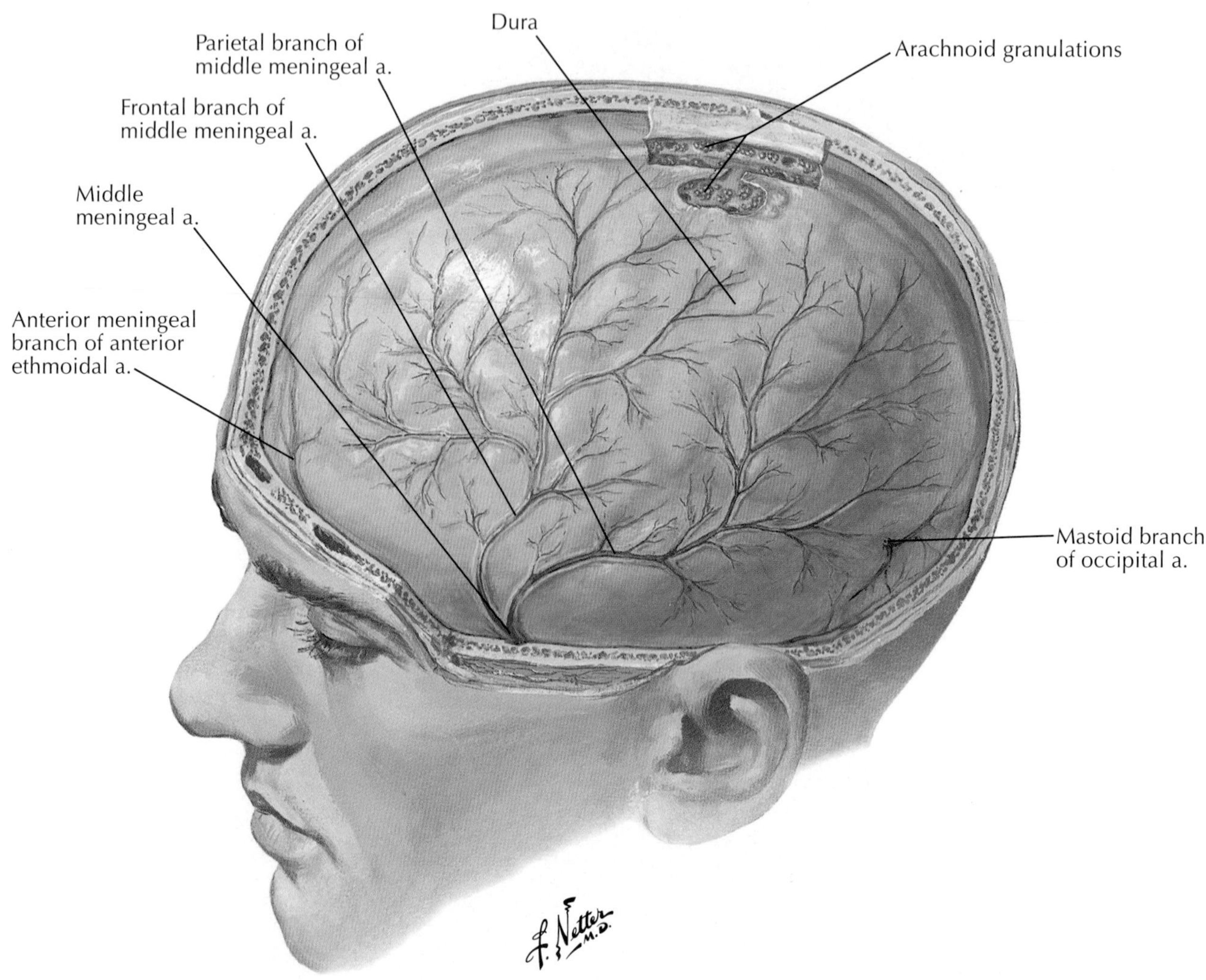
Dura
Parietal branch of middle meningeal a.
Arachnoid granulations
Frontal branch of middle meningeal a.
Middle meningeal a.
Anterior meningeal branch of anterior ethmoidal a.
Mastoid branch of occipital a.
F. Netter M.D.

Fig. 1.33 Meningeal Arteries (Illustration)

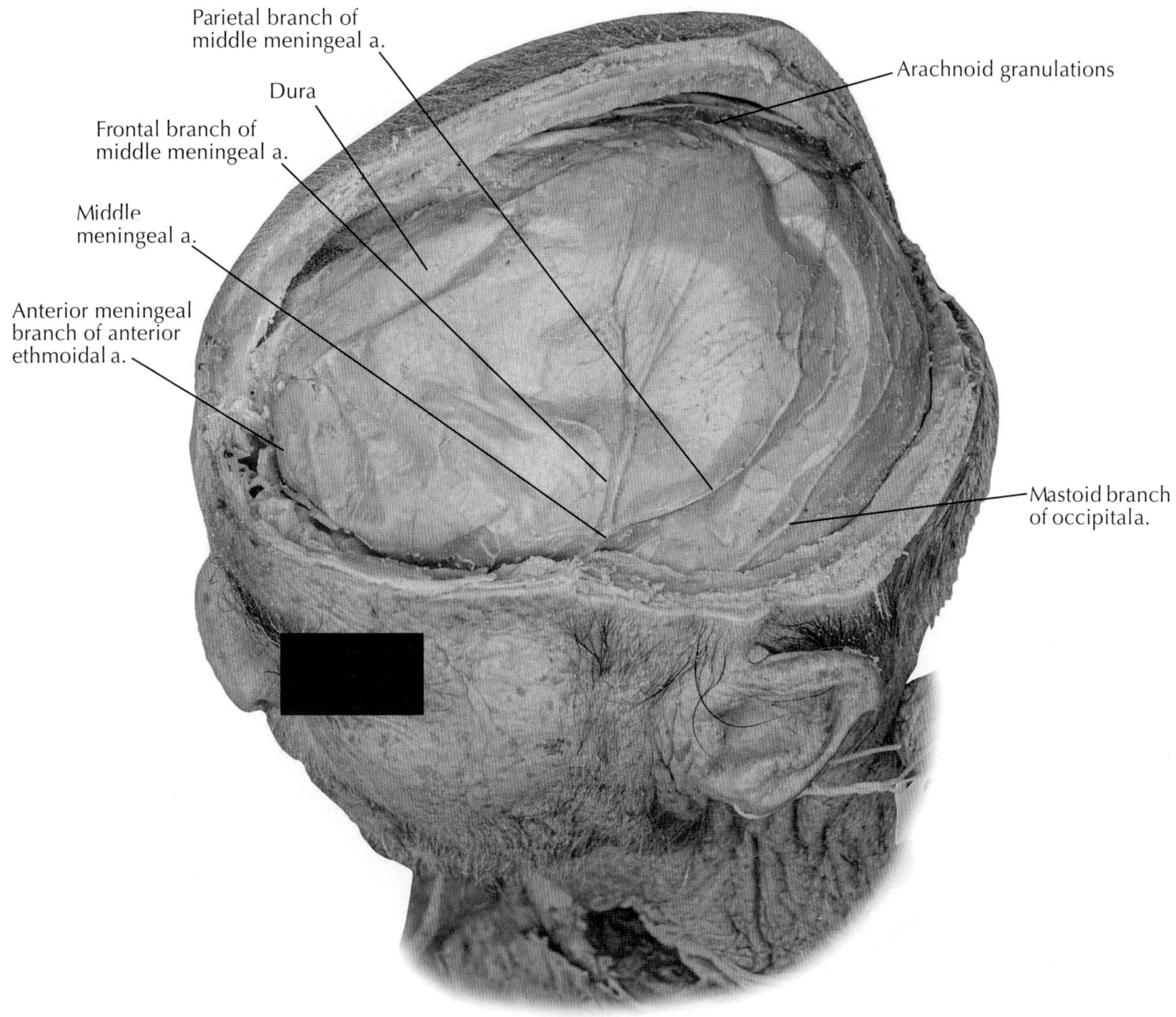
Parietal branch of middle meningeal a.
Dura
Frontal branch of middle meningeal a.
Middle meningeal a.
Anterior meningeal branch of anterior ethmoidal a.
Arachnoid granulations
Mastoid branch of occipitala.

Fig. 1.34 Meningeal Arteries (Photograph)

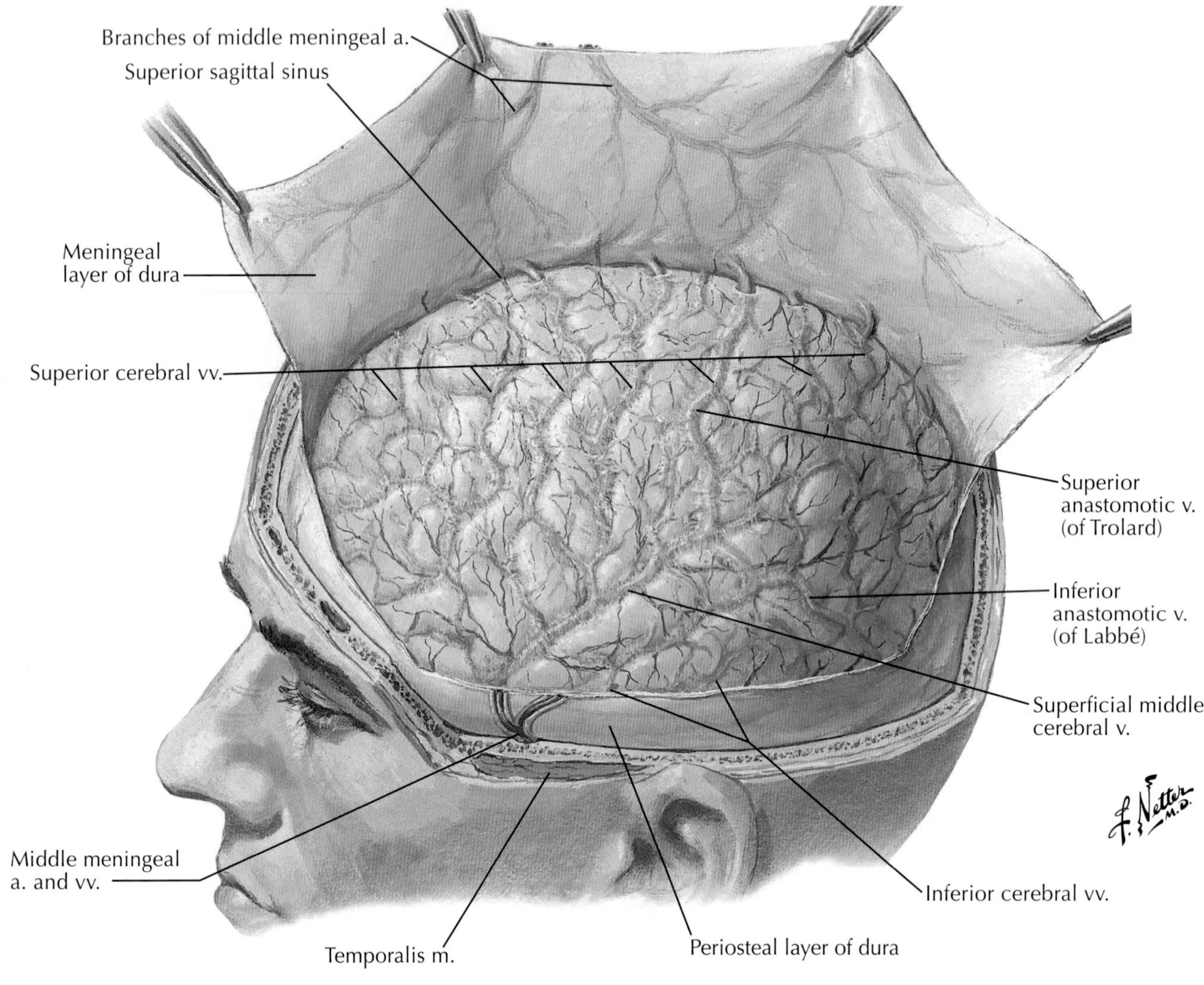
Branches of middle meningeal a.
Superior sagittal sinus
Meningeal layer of dura
Superior cerebral vv.
Superior anastomotic v. (of Trolard)
Inferior anastomotic v. (of Labbé)
Superficial middle cerebral v.
Middle meningeal a. and vv.
Inferior cerebral vv.
Temporalis m.
Periosteal layer of dura

Fig. 1.35 Meninges and Superficial Cerebral Veins (Illustration)

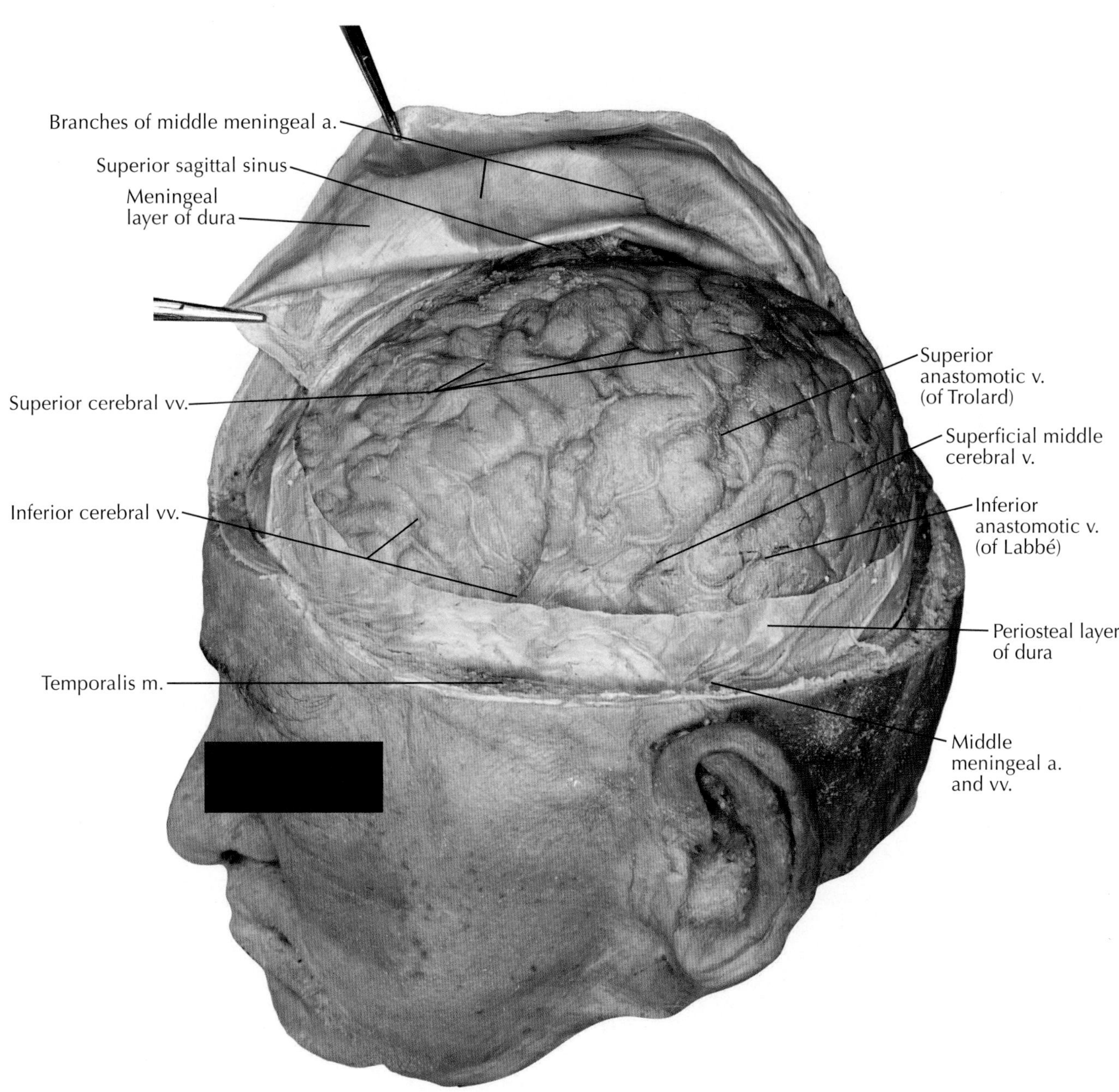
Branches of middle meningeal a.
Superior sagittal sinus
Meningeal layer of dura
Superior cerebral vv.
Inferior cerebral vv.
Temporalis m.
Superior anastomotic v. (of Trolard)
Superficial middle cerebral v.
Inferior anastomotic v. (of Labbé)
Periosteal layer of dura
Middle meningeal a. and vv.

Fig. 1.36 Meninges and Superficial Cerebral Veins (Photograph)

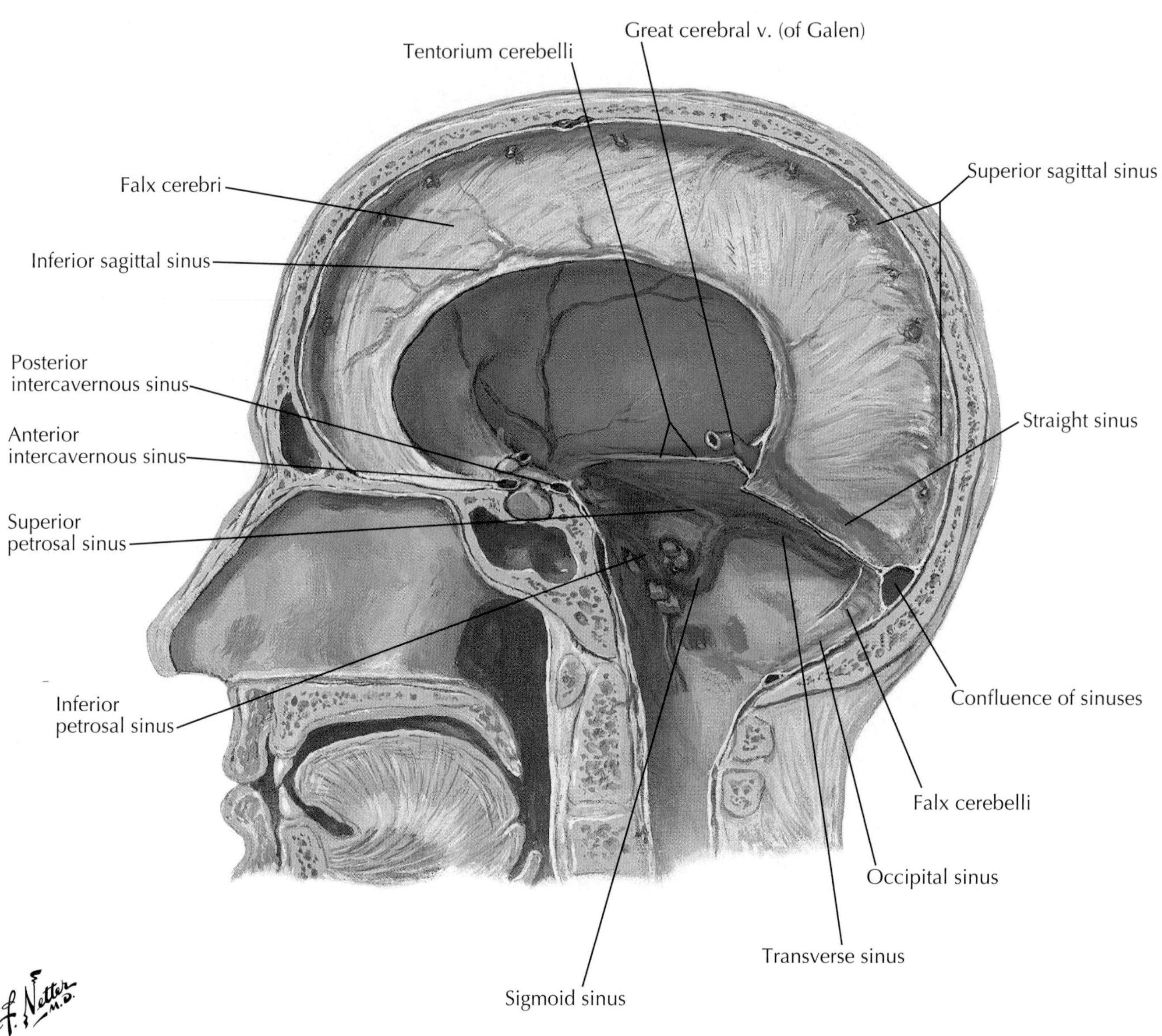
Great cerebral v. (of Galen)
Tentorium cerebelli
Falx cerebri
Superior sagittal sinus
Inferior sagittal sinus
Posterior intercavernous sinus
Straight sinus
Anterior intercavernous sinus
Superior petrosal sinus
Confluence of sinuses
Inferior petrosal sinus
Falx cerebelli
Occipital sinus
Transverse sinus
Sigmoid sinus
F. Netter M.D.

Fig. 1.37 Dural Venous Sinuses: Sagittal Section (Illustration)

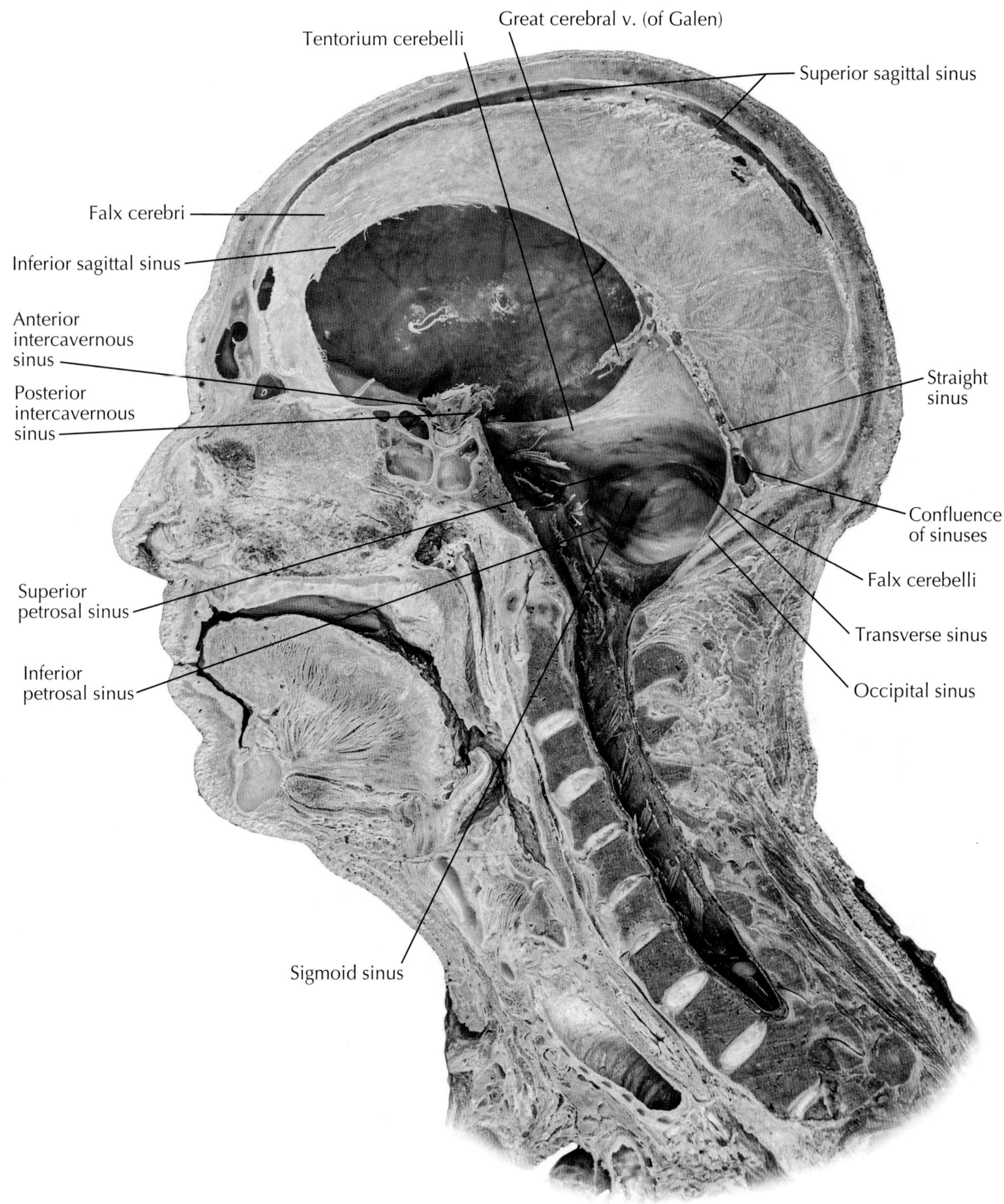
Great cerebral v. (of Galen)
Tentorium cerebelli
Superior sagittal sinus
Falx cerebri
Inferior sagittal sinus
Anterior intercavernous sinus
Posterior intercavernous sinus
Straight sinus
Confluence of sinuses
Falx cerebelli
Superior petrosal sinus
Transverse sinus
Inferior petrosal sinus
Occipital sinus
Sigmoid sinus

Fig. 1.38 Dural Venous Sinuses: Sagittal Section (Photograph)

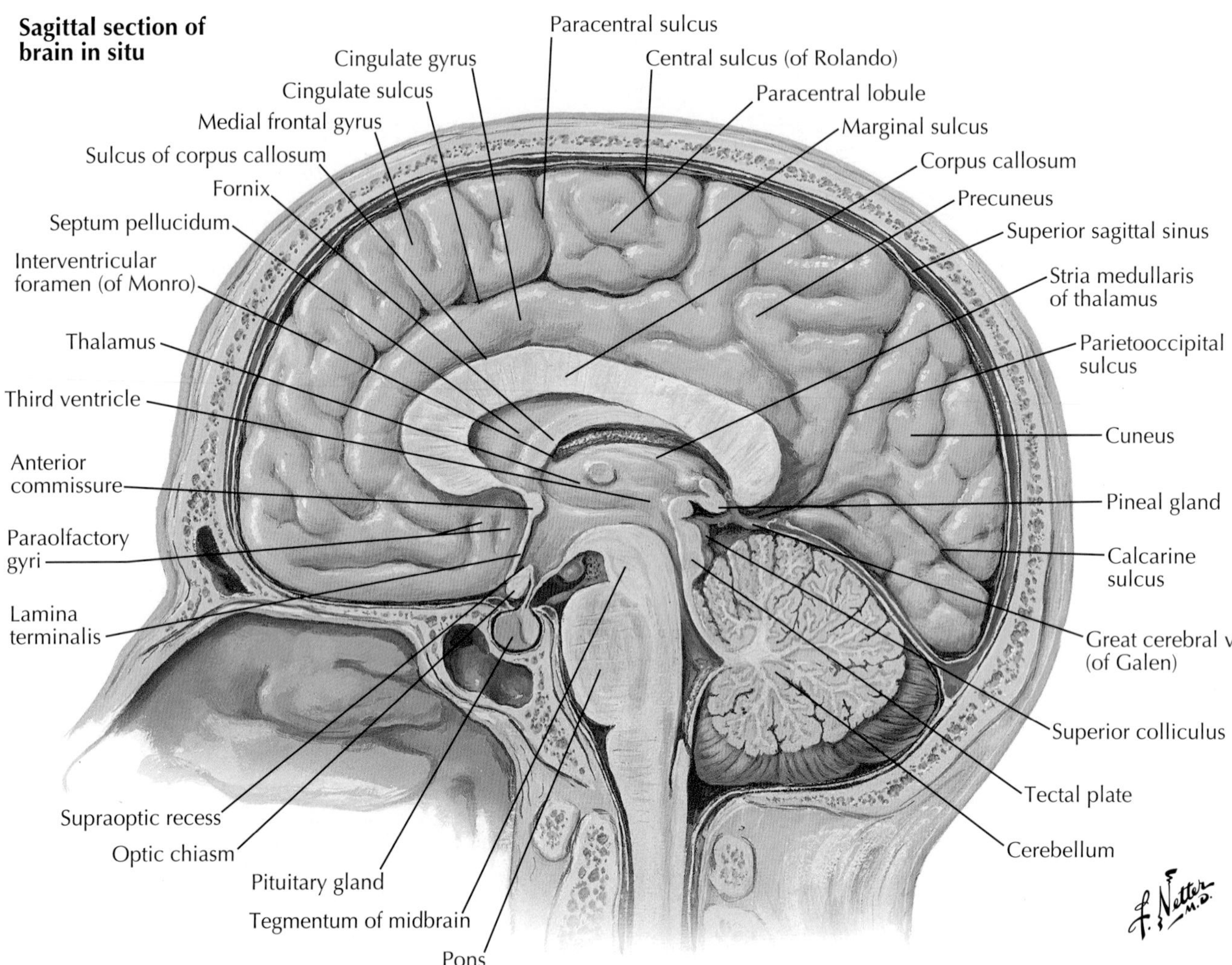
Sagittal section of brain in situ
Paracentral sulcus
Cingulate gyrus
Central sulcus (of Rolando)
Cingulate sulcus
Paracentral lobule
Medial frontal gyrus
Marginal sulcus
Sulcus of corpus callosum
Corpus callosum
Fornix
Precuneus
Septum pellucidum
Superior sagittal sinus
Interventricular foramen (of Monro)
Stria medullaris of thalamus
Thalamus
Parietooccipital sulcus
Third ventricle
Cuneus
Anterior commissure
Pineal gland
Paraolfactory gyri
Calcarine sulcus
Lamina terminalis
Great cerebral v. (of Galen)
Superior colliculus
Tectal plate
Supraoptic recess
Cerebellum
Optic chiasm
Pituitary gland
Tegmentum of midbrain
Pons

Fig. 1.39 Brain: Medial Views (Illustration)

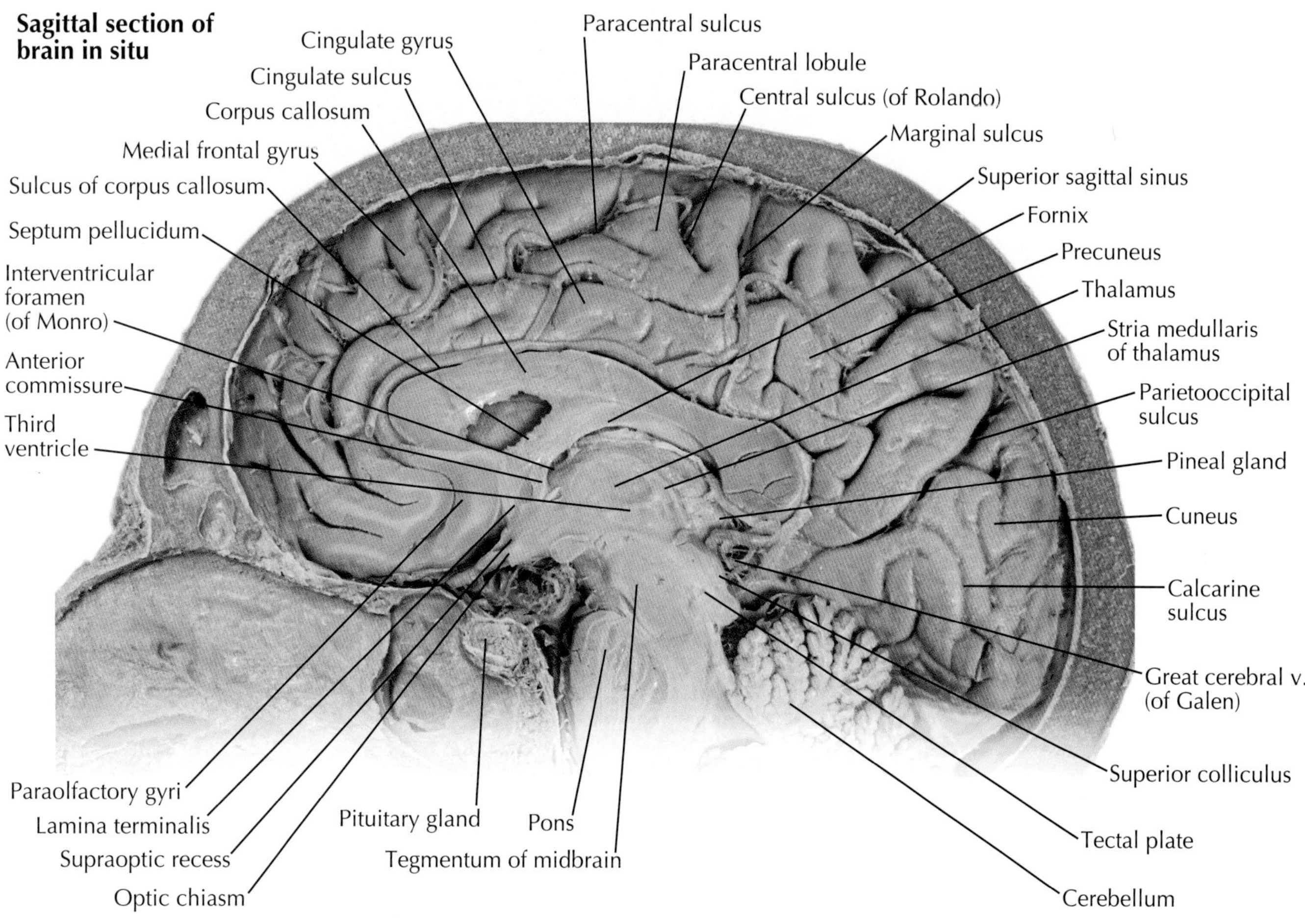
Sagittal section of brain in situ
Cingulate gyrus
Cingulate sulcus
Corpus callosum
Medial frontal gyrus
Sulcus of corpus callosum
Septum pellucidum
Interventricular foramen (of Monro)
Anterior commissure
Third ventricle
Paracentral sulcus
Paracentral lobule
Central sulcus (of Rolando)
Marginal sulcus
Superior sagittal sinus
Fornix
Precuneus
Thalamus
Stria medullaris of thalamus
Parietooccipital sulcus
Pineal gland
Cuneus
Calcarine sulcus
Great cerebral v. (of Galen)
Superior colliculus
Tectal plate
Cerebellum
Paraolfactory gyri
Lamina terminalis
Supraoptic recess
Optic chiasm
Pituitary gland
Pons
Tegmentum of midbrain

Fig. 1.40 Brain: Medial Views (Photograph)

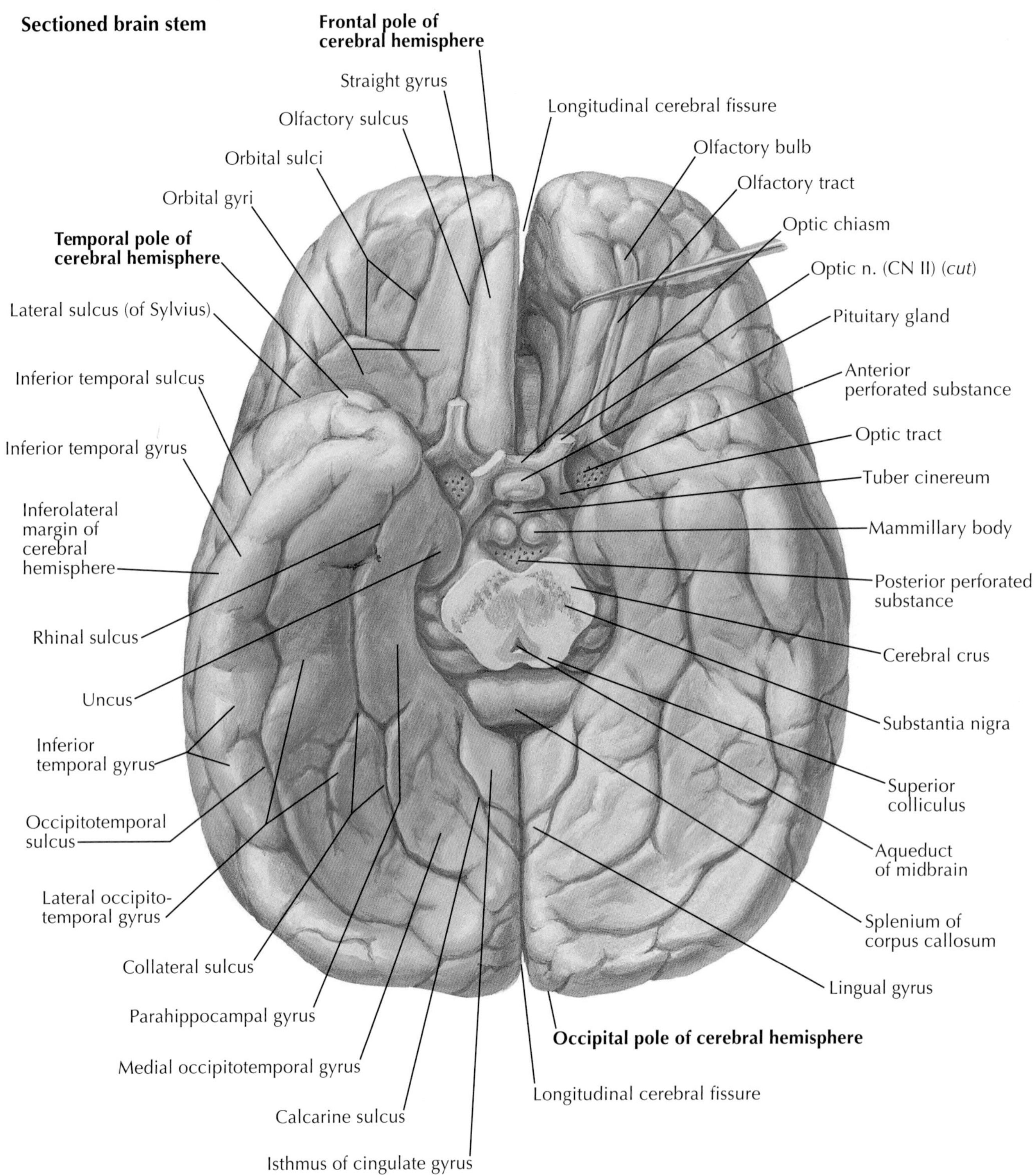
Sectioned brain stem
Frontal pole of cerebral hemisphere
Straight gyrus
Olfactory sulcus
Orbital sulci
Orbital gyri
Temporal pole of cerebral hemisphere
Lateral sulcus (of Sylvius)
Inferior temporal sulcus
Inferior temporal gyrus
Inferolateral margin of cerebral hemisphere
Rhinal sulcus
Uncus
Inferior temporal gyrus
Occipitotemporal sulcus
Lateral occipito-temporal gyrus
Collateral sulcus
Parahippocampal gyrus
Medial occipitotemporal gyrus
Calcarine sulcus
Isthmus of cingulate gyrus
Longitudinal cerebral fissure
Olfactory bulb
Olfactory tract
Optic chiasm
Optic n. (CN II) (cut)
Pituitary gland
Anterior perforated substance
Optic tract
Tuber cinereum
Mammillary body
Posterior perforated substance
Cerebral crus
Substantia nigra
Superior colliculus
Aqueduct of midbrain
Splenium of corpus callosum
Lingual gyrus
Occipital pole of cerebral hemisphere
Longitudinal cerebral fissure

Fig. 1.41 Brain: Inferior View (Illustration)

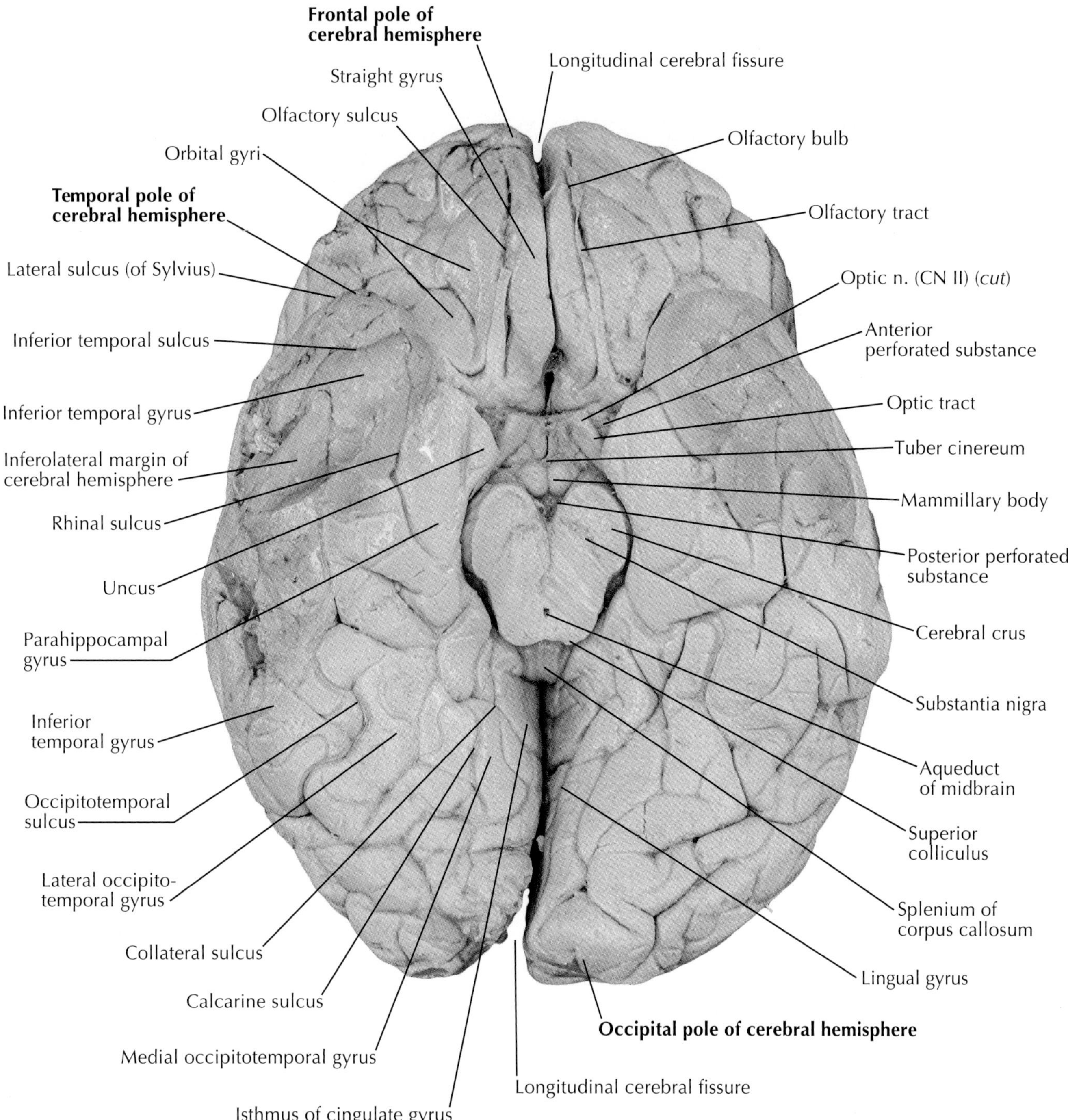
Sectioned brain stem
Frontal pole of cerebral hemisphere
Longitudinal cerebral fissure
Straight gyrus
Olfactory sulcus
Orbital gyri
Olfactory bulb
Temporal pole of cerebral hemisphere
Olfactory tract
Lateral sulcus (of Sylvius)
Optic n. (CN II) (cut)
Inferior temporal sulcus
Anterior perforated substance
Inferior temporal gyrus
Optic tract
Tuber cinereum
Inferolateral margin of cerebral hemisphere
Mammillary body
Rhinal sulcus
Posterior perforated substance
Uncus
Cerebral crus
Parahippocampal gyrus
Substantia nigra
Inferior temporal gyrus
Aqueduct of midbrain
Occipitotemporal sulcus
Superior colliculus
Lateral occipito-temporal gyrus
Splenium of corpus callosum
Collateral sulcus
Lingual gyrus
Calcarine sulcus
Occipital pole of cerebral hemisphere
Medial occipitotemporal gyrus
Longitudinal cerebral fissure
Isthmus of cingulate gyrus

Fig. 1.42 Brain: Inferior View (Photograph)

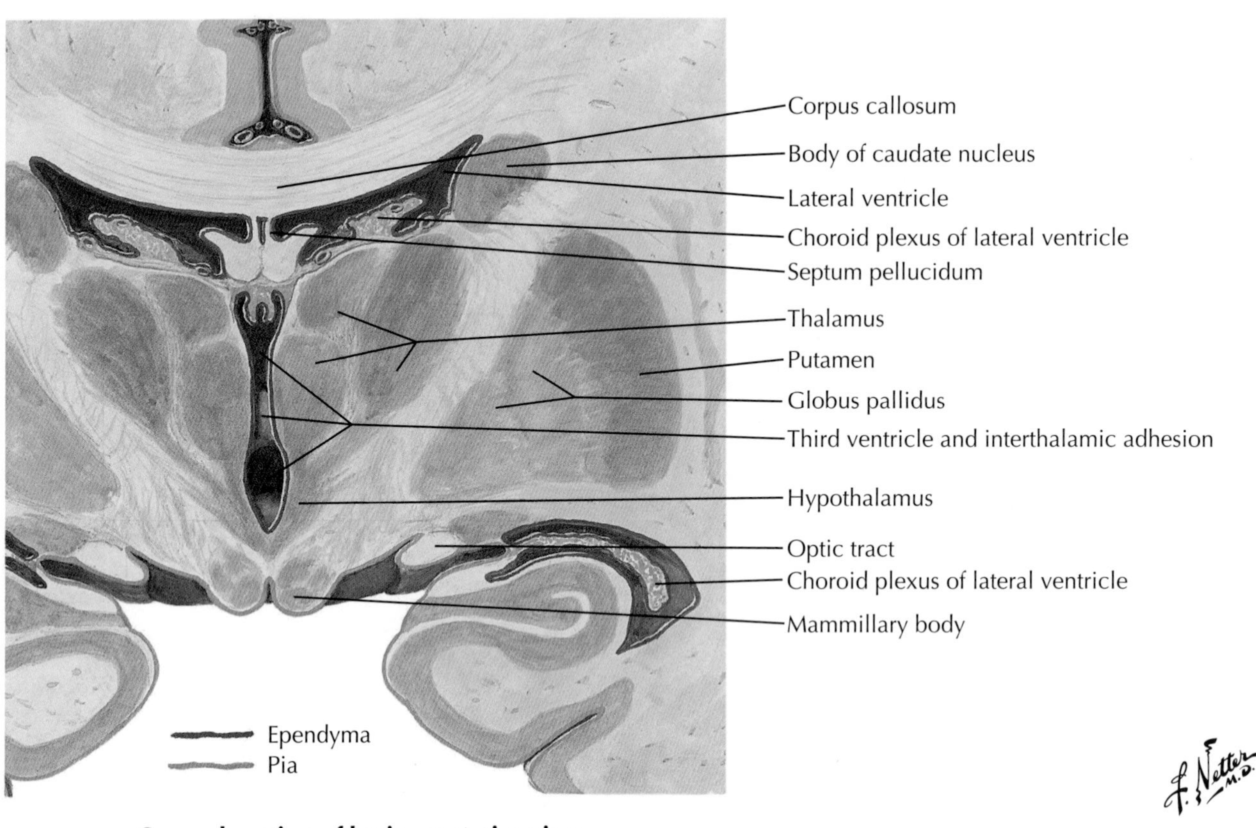
Corpus callosum
Body of caudate nucleus
Lateral ventricle
Choroid plexus of lateral ventricle
Septum pellucidum
Thalamus
Putamen
Globus pallidus
Third ventricle and interthalamic adhesion
Hypothalamus
Optic tract
Choroid plexus of lateral ventricle
Mammillary body
Ependyma
Pia

Coronal section of brain: posterior view

Fig. 1.43 Ventricles of Brain (Illustration)

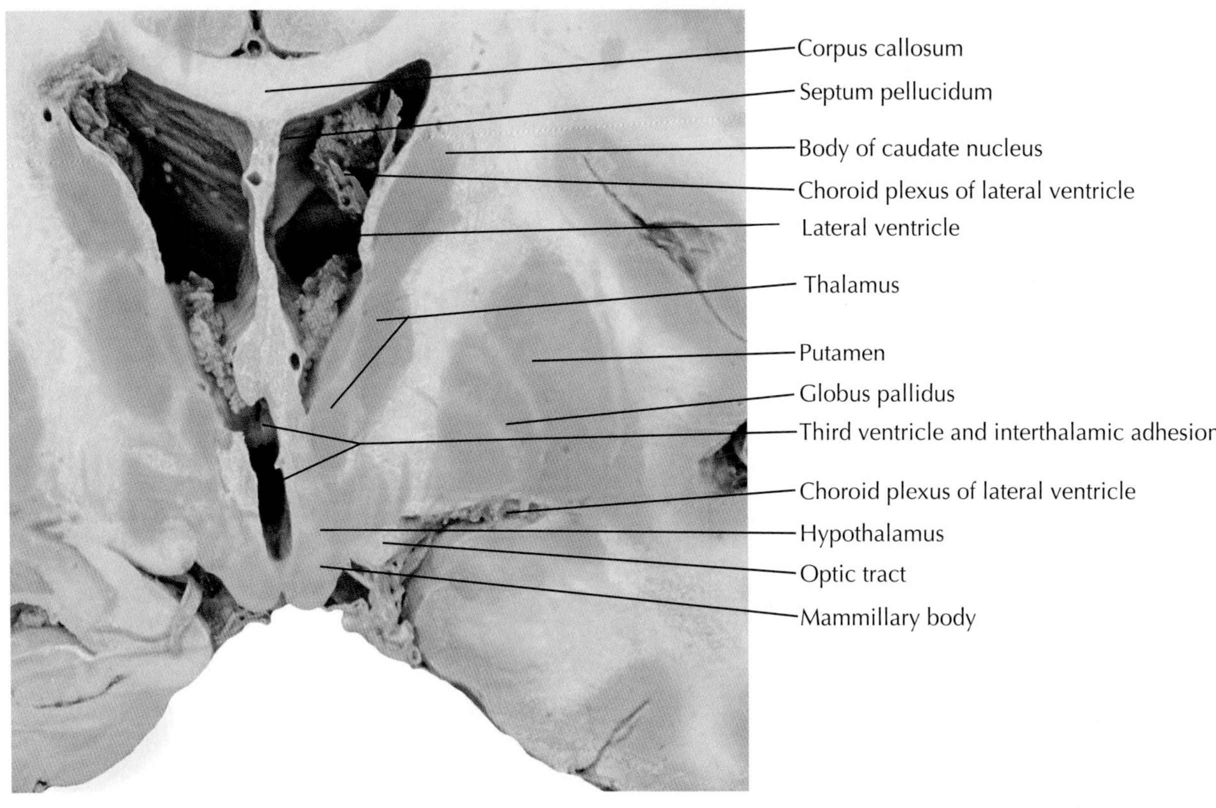
Corpus callosum
Septum pellucidum
Body of caudate nucleus
Choroid plexus of lateral ventricle
Lateral ventricle
Thalamus
Putamen
Globus pallidus
Third ventricle and interthalamic adhesion
Choroid plexus of lateral ventricle
Hypothalamus
Optic tract
Mammillary body

Coronal section of brain: posterior view

Fig. 1.44 Ventricles of Brain (Photograph)

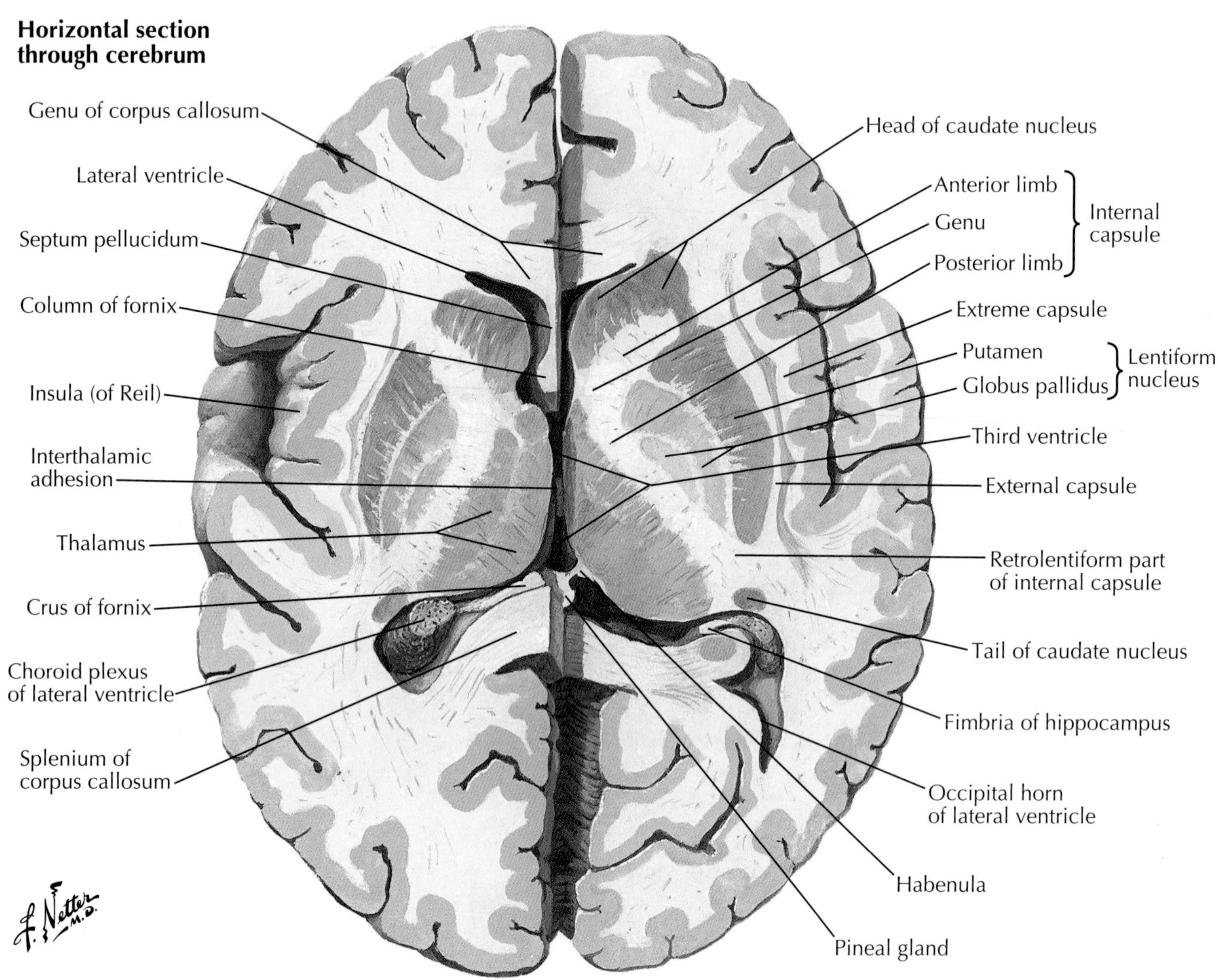
Horizontal section through cerebrum
Genu of corpus callosum
Lateral ventricle
Septum pellucidum
Column of fornix
Insula (of Reil)
Interthalamic adhesion
Thalamus
Crus of fornix
Choroid plexus of lateral ventricle
Splenium of corpus callosum
Head of caudate nucleus
Anterior limb
Genu
Posterior limb
Internal capsule
Extreme capsule
Putamen
Globus pallidus
Lentiform nucleus
Third ventricle
External capsule
Retrolentiform part of internal capsule
Tail of caudate nucleus
Fimbria of hippocampus
Occipital horn of lateral ventricle
Habenula
Pineal gland
F. Netter M.D.

Fig. 1.45 Basal Nuclei (Illustration)

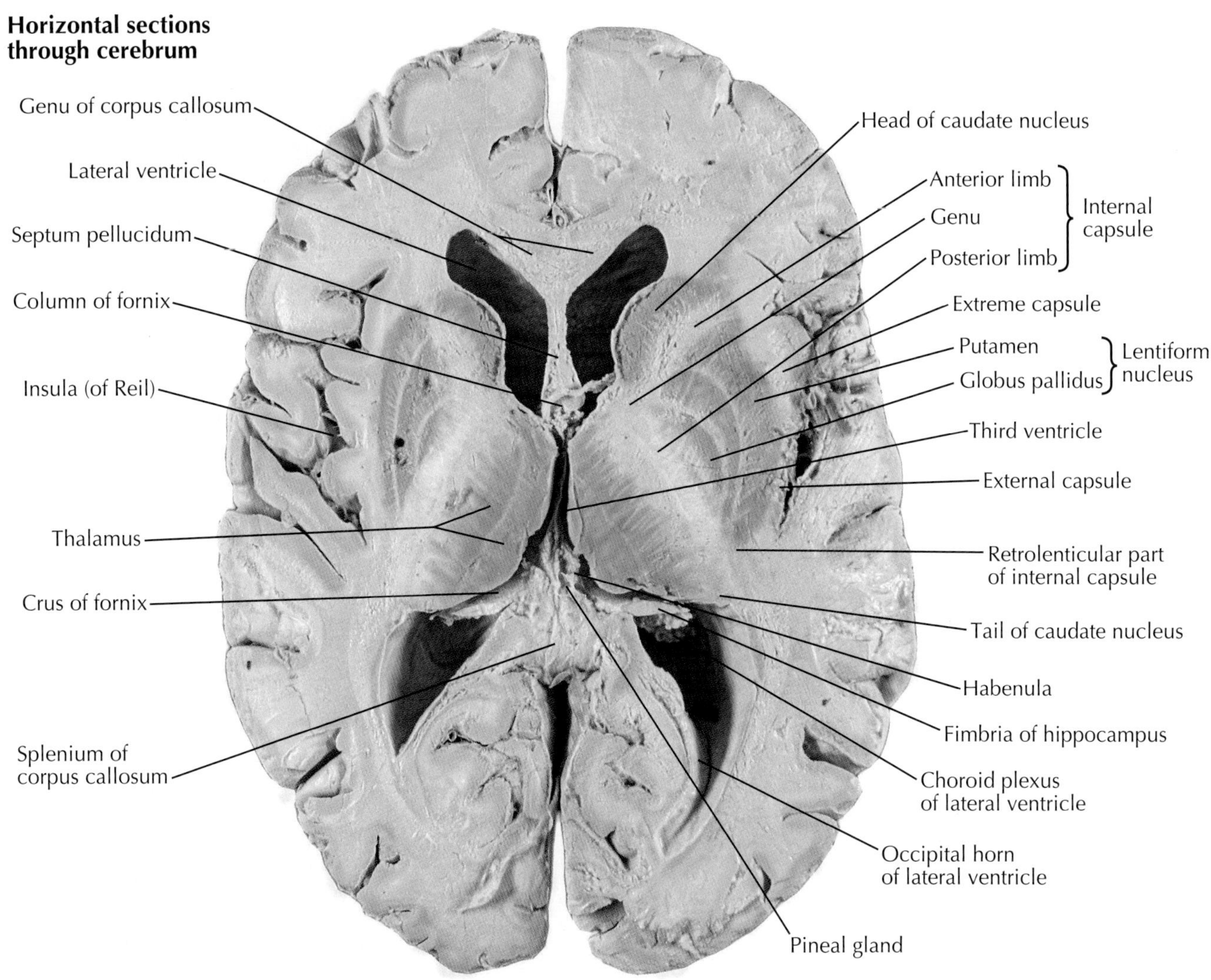
Horizontal sections through cerebrum
Genu of corpus callosum
Lateral ventricle
Septum pellucidum
Column of fornix
Insula (of Reil)
Thalamus
Crus of fornix
Splenium of corpus callosum
Head of caudate nucleus
Anterior limb
Genu
Posterior limb
Internal capsule
Extreme capsule
Putamen
Globus pallidus
Lentiform nucleus
Third ventricle
External capsule
Retrolenticular part of internal capsule
Tail of caudate nucleus
Habenula
Fimbria of hippocampus
Choroid plexus of lateral ventricle
Occipital horn of lateral ventricle
Pineal gland

Fig. 1.46 Basal Nuclei (Photograph)

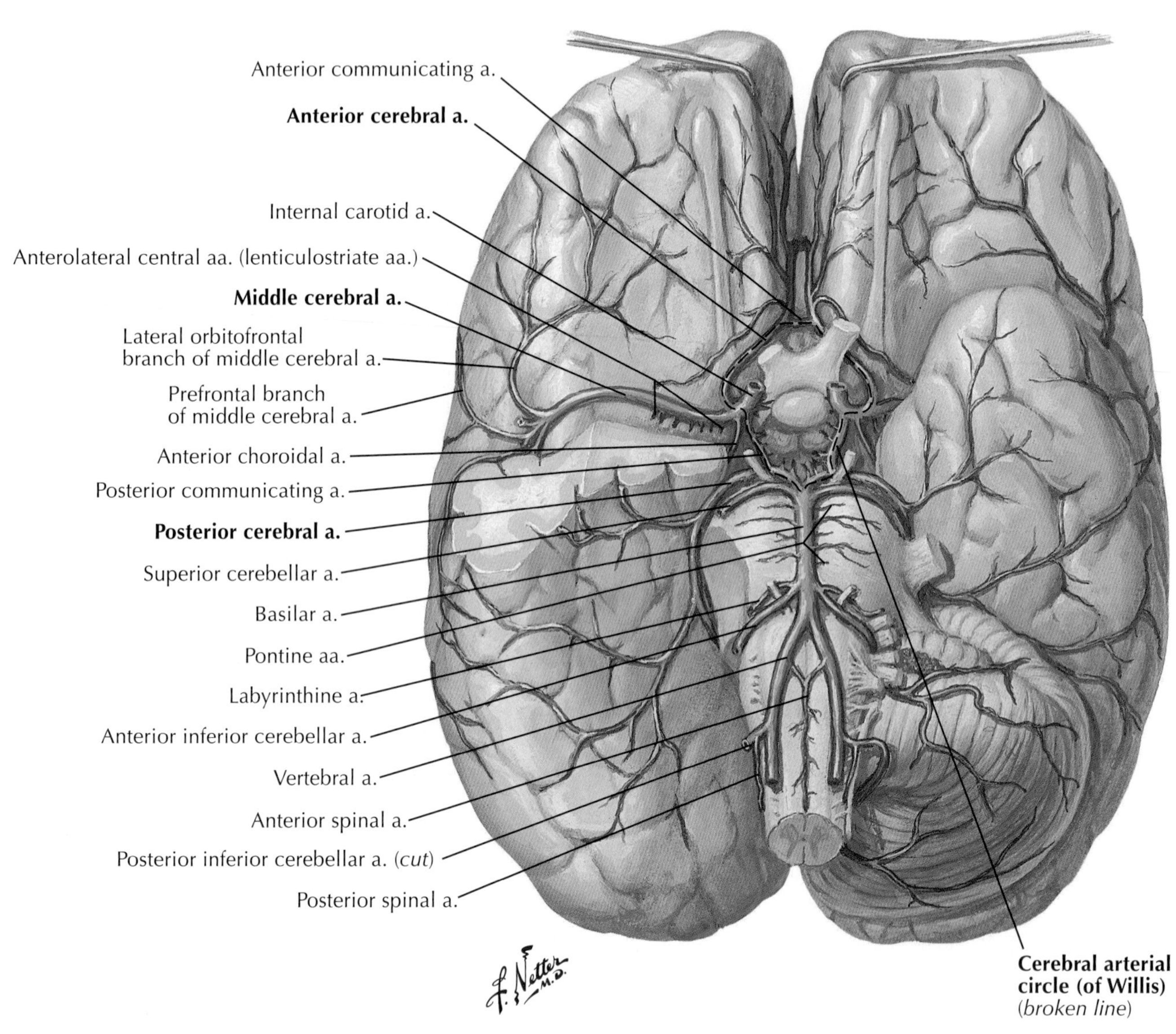
Anterior communicating a.
Anterior cerebral a.
Internal carotid a.
Anterolateral central aa. (lenticulostriate aa.)
Middle cerebral a.
Lateral orbitofrontal branch of middle cerebral a.
Prefrontal branch of middle cerebral a.
Anterior choroidal a.
Posterior communicating a.
Posterior cerebral a.
Superior cerebellar a.
Basilar a.
Pontine aa.
Labyrinthine a.
Anterior inferior cerebellar a.
Vertebral a.
Anterior spinal a.
Posterior inferior cerebellar a. (cut)
Posterior spinal a.
Cerebral arterial circle (of Willis) (broken line)
F. Netter M.D.

Fig. 1.47 Arteries of Brain: Inferior Views (Illustration)

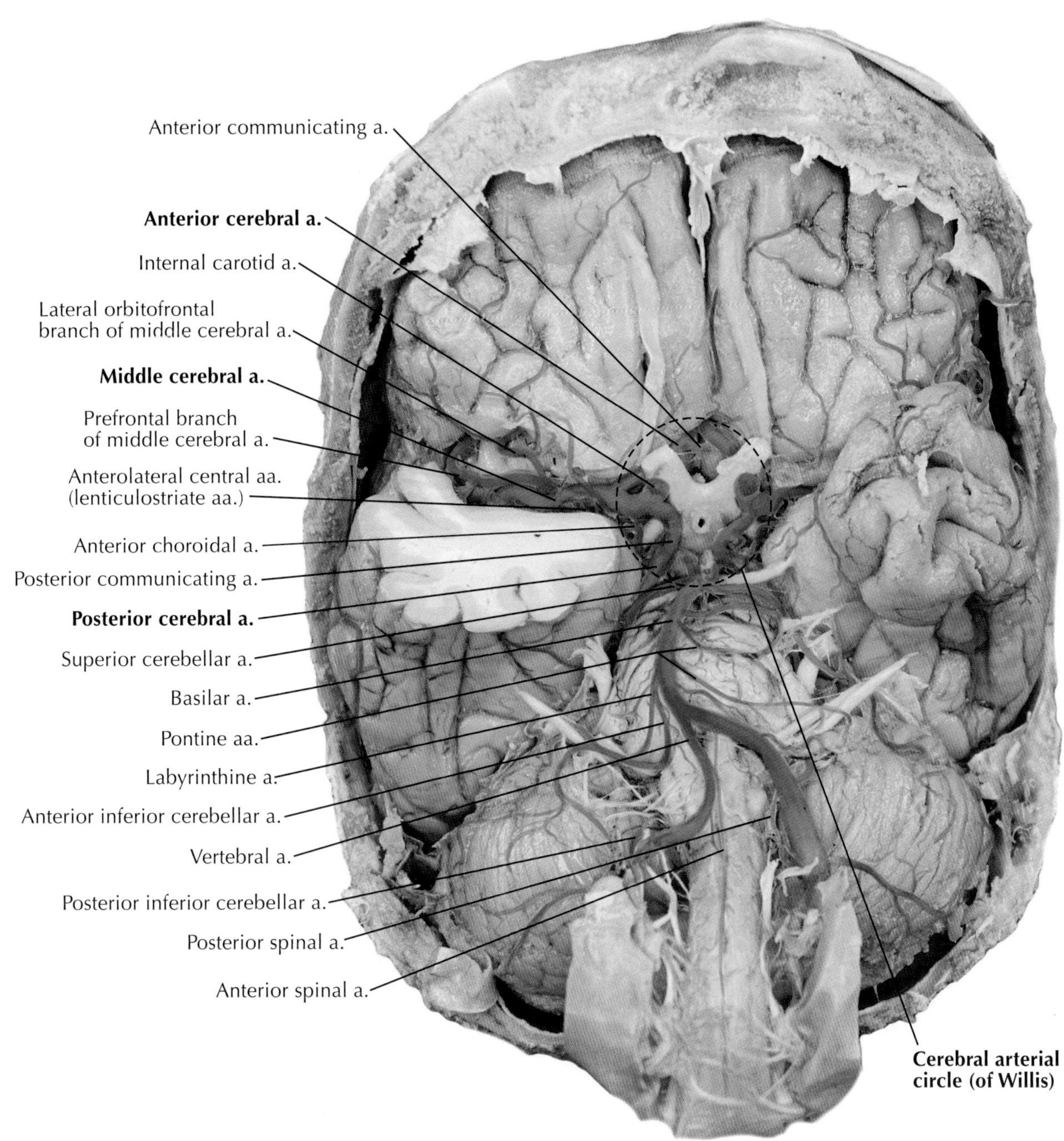
Anterior communicating a.
Anterior cerebral a.
Internal carotid a.
Lateral orbitofrontal branch of middle cerebral a.
Middle cerebral a.
Prefrontal branch of middle cerebral a.
Anterolateral central aa. (lenticulostriate aa.)
Anterior choroidal a.
Posterior communicating a.
Posterior cerebral a.
Superior cerebellar a.
Basilar a.
Pontine aa.
Labyrinthine a.
Anterior inferior cerebellar a.
Vertebral a.
Posterior inferior cerebellar a.
Posterior spinal a.
Anterior spinal a.
Cerebral arterial circle (of Willis)

Fig. 1.48 Arteries of Brain: Inferior Views (Photograph) (see Fig. A.5)

BACK

CHAPTER 2

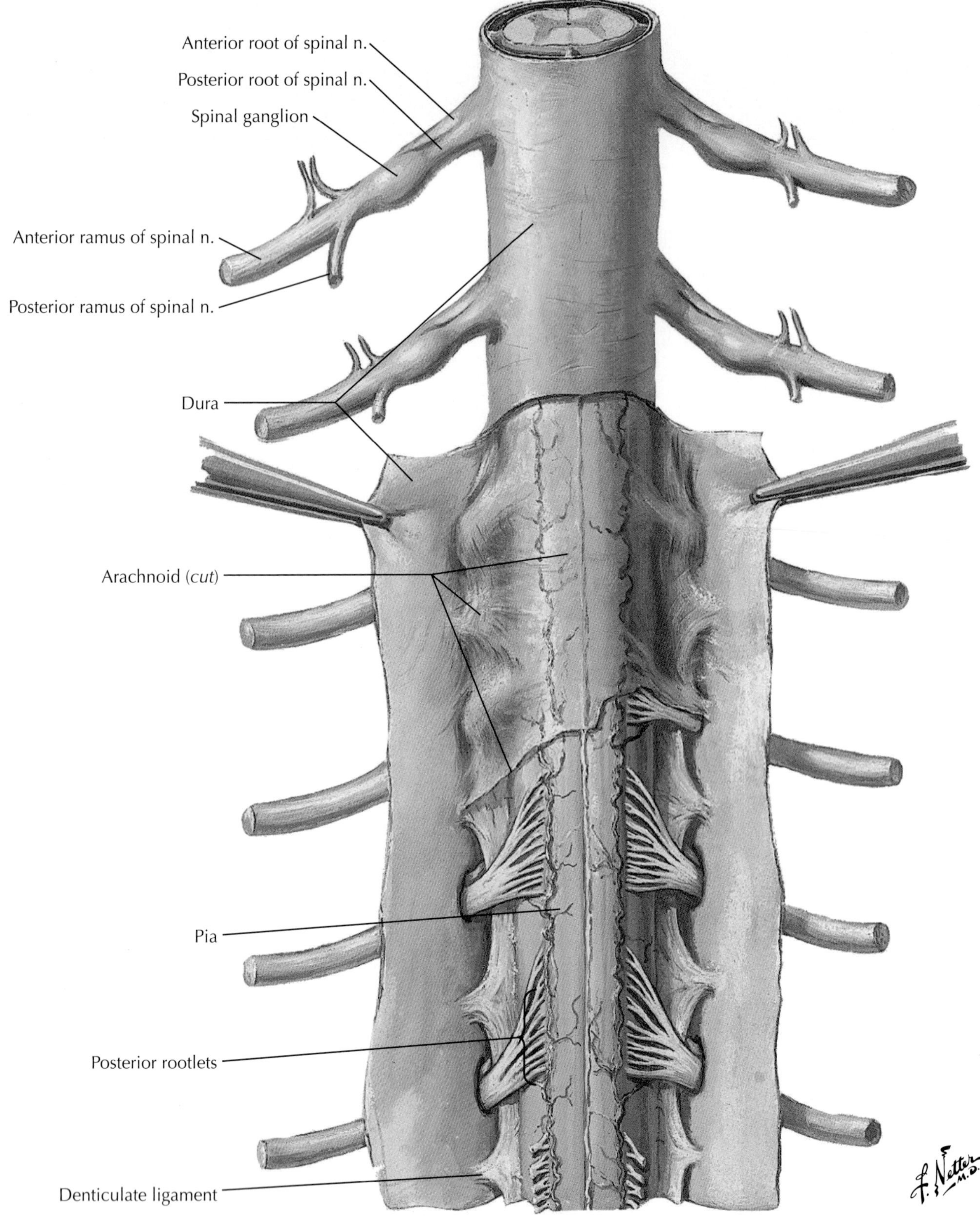
Posterior view
Anterior root of spinal n.
Posterior root of spinal n.
Spinal ganglion
Anterior ramus of spinal n.
Posterior ramus of spinal n.
Dura
Arachnoid (*cut*)
Pia
Posterior rootlets
Denticulate ligament

Fig. 2.1 Spinal Meninges and Nerve Roots (Illustration)

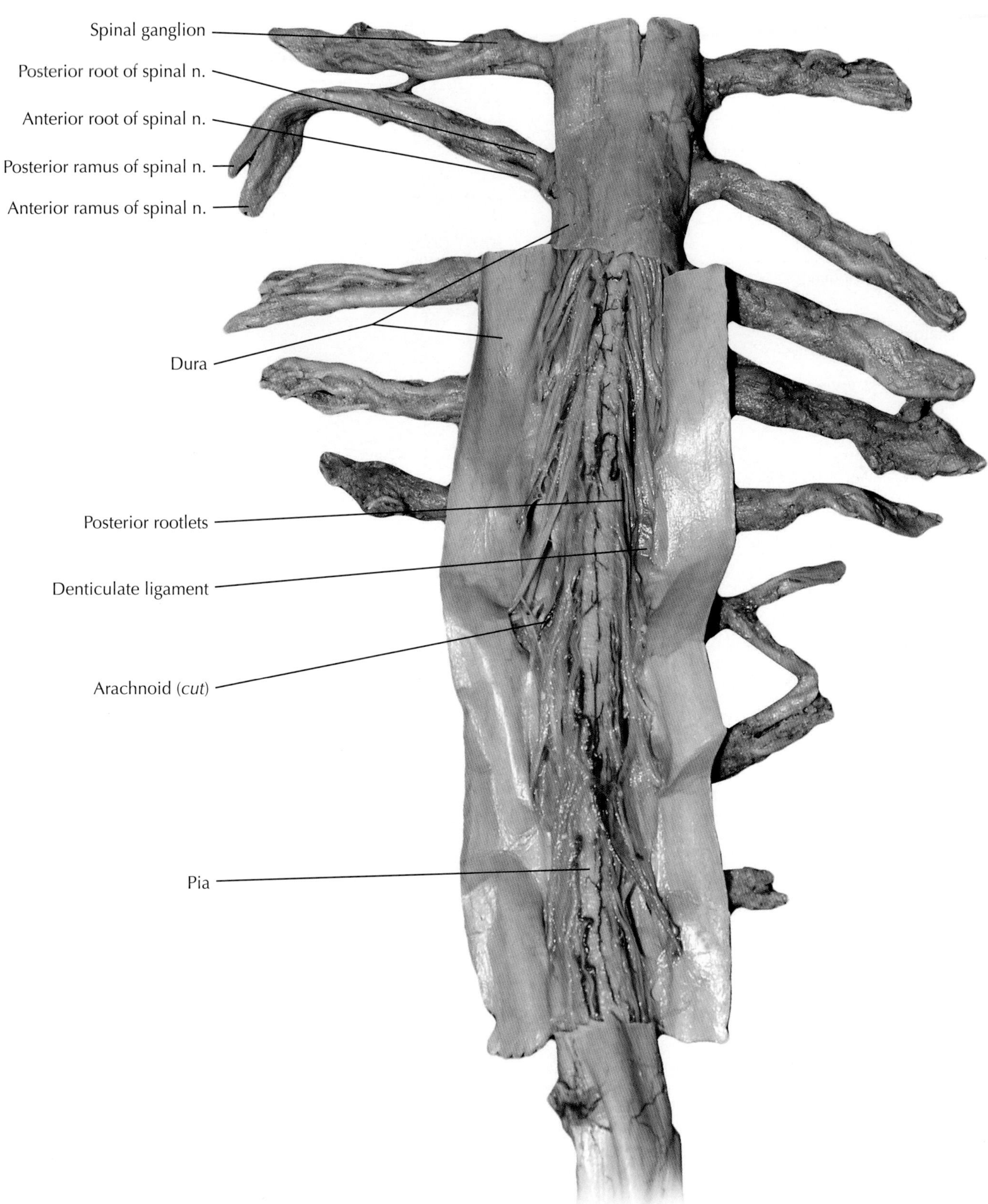
Posterior view
Spinal ganglion
Posterior root of spinal n.
Anterior root of spinal n.
Posterior ramus of spinal n.
Anterior ramus of spinal n.
Dura
Posterior rootlets
Denticulate ligament
Arachnoid (*cut*)
Pia

Fig. 2.2 Spinal Meninges and Nerve Roots (Photograph)

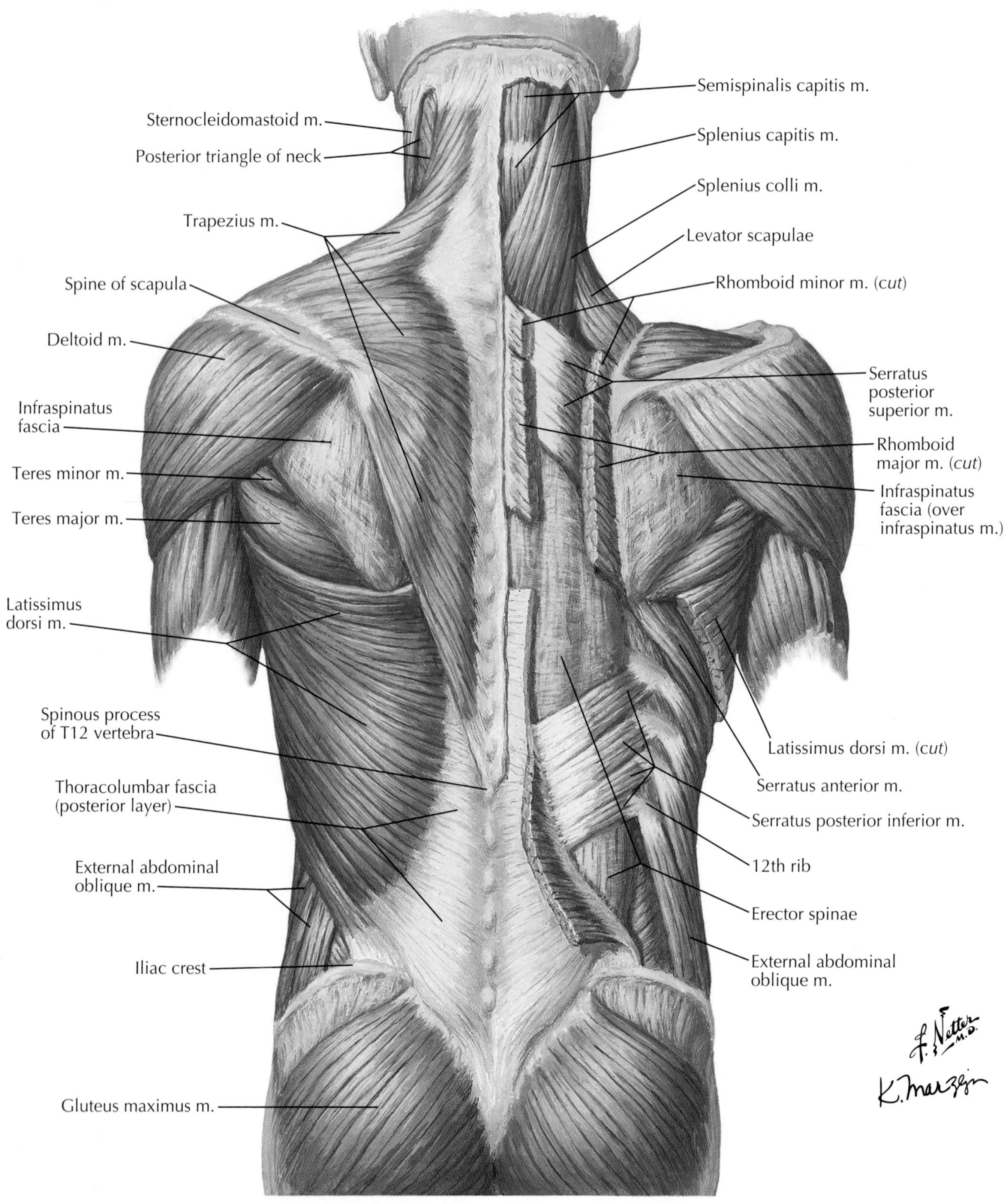

Semispinalis capitis m.
Sternocleidomastoid m.
Splenius capitis m.
Posterior triangle of neck
Splenius colli m.
Trapezius m.
Levator scapulae
Spine of scapula
Rhomboid minor m. (*cut*)
Deltoid m.
Serratus posterior superior m.
Infraspinatus fascia
Rhomboid major m. (*cut*)
Teres minor m.
Infraspinatus fascia (over infraspinatus m.)
Teres major m.
Latissimus dorsi m.
Spinous process of T12 vertebra
Latissimus dorsi m. (*cut*)
Thoracolumbar fascia (posterior layer)
Serratus anterior m.
Serratus posterior inferior m.
12th rib
External abdominal oblique m.
Erector spinae
Iliac crest
External abdominal oblique m.
Gluteus maximus m.
F. Netter M.D.
K. Marzejon

Fig. 2.3 Muscles of Back: Superficial Layer (Illustration)

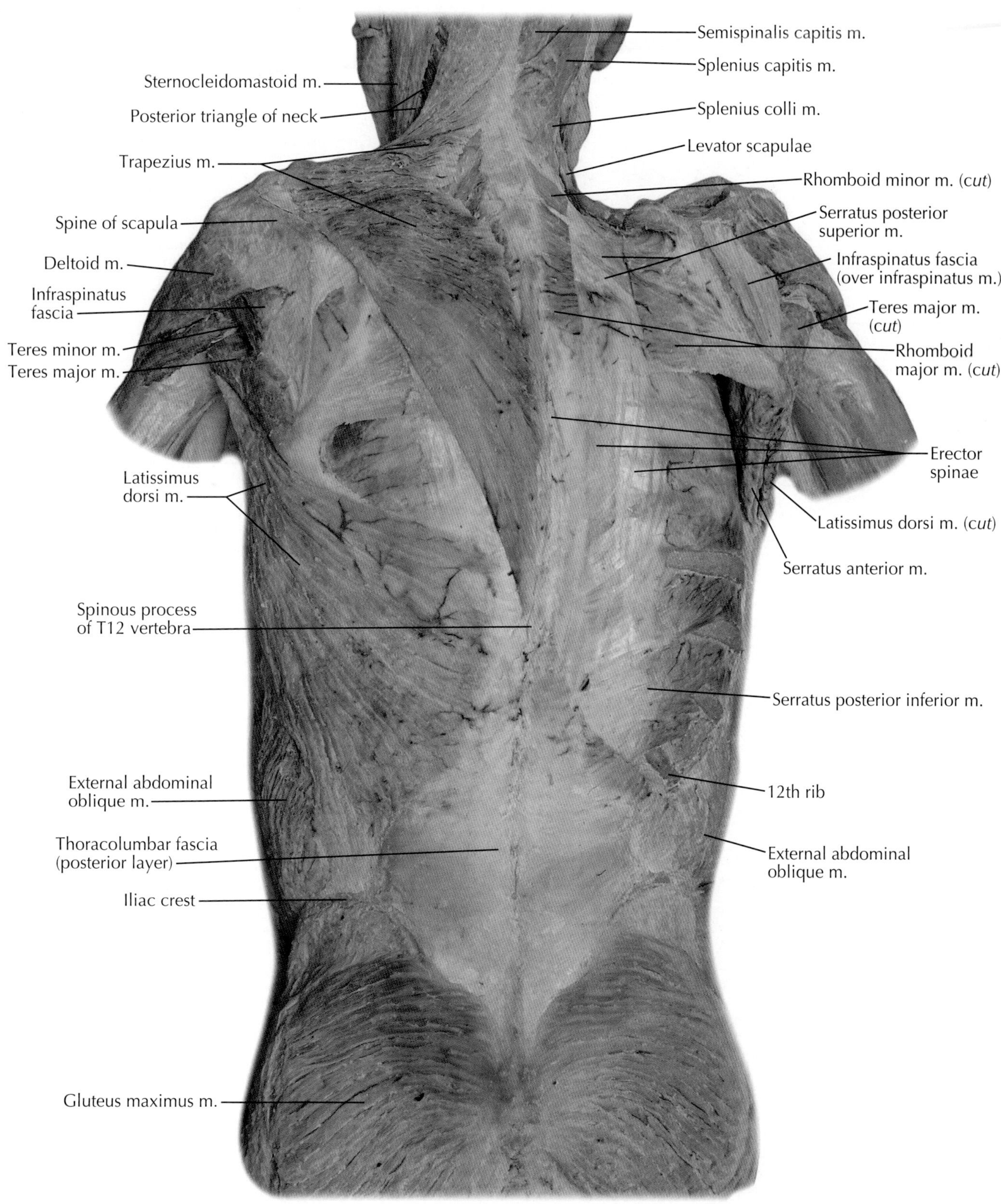
Semispinalis capitis m.
Splenius capitis m.
Sternocleidomastoid m.
Posterior triangle of neck
Splenius colli m.
Levator scapulae
Trapezius m.
Rhomboid minor m. (cut)
Spine of scapula
Serratus posterior superior m.
Deltoid m.
Infraspinatus fascia (over infraspinatus m.)
Infraspinatus fascia
Teres major m. (cut)
Teres minor m.
Teres major m.
Rhomboid major m. (cut)
Erector spinae
Latissimus dorsi m.
Latissimus dorsi m. (cut)
Serratus anterior m.
Spinous process of T12 vertebra
Serratus posterior inferior m.
12th rib
External abdominal oblique m.
Thoracolumbar fascia (posterior layer)
External abdominal oblique m.
Iliac crest
Gluteus maximus m.

Fig. 2.4 Muscles of Back: Superficial Layer (Photograph)

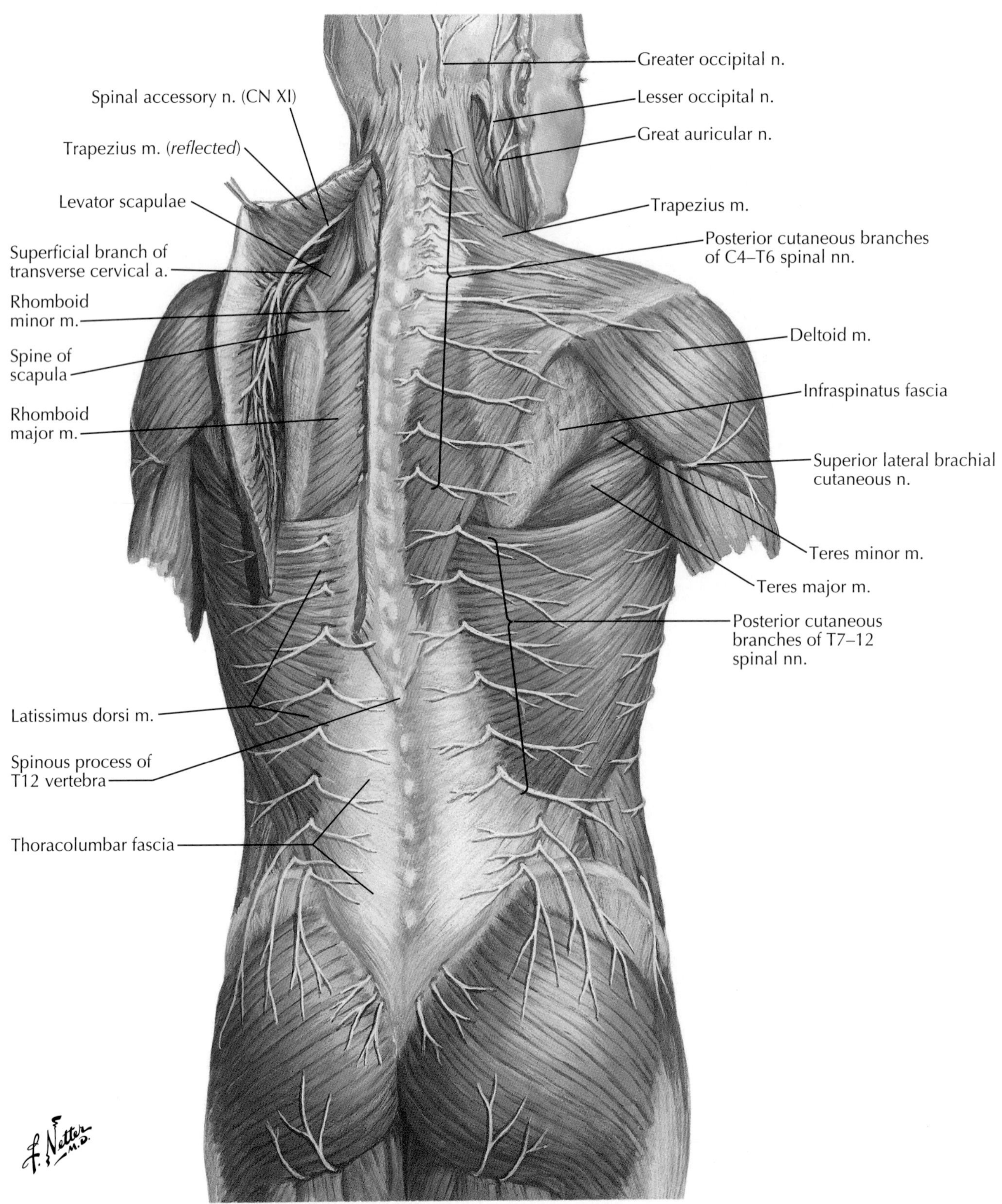
Greater occipital n.
Spinal accessory n. (CN XI)
Lesser occipital n.
Great auricular n.
Trapezius m. (reflected)
Levator scapulae
Trapezius m.
Posterior cutaneous branches of C4–T6 spinal nn.
Superficial branch of transverse cervical a.
Rhomboid minor m.
Deltoid m.
Spine of scapula
Infraspinatus fascia
Rhomboid major m.
Superior lateral brachial cutaneous n.
Teres minor m.
Teres major m.
Posterior cutaneous branches of T7–12 spinal nn.
Latissimus dorsi m.
Spinous process of T12 vertebra
Thoracolumbar fascia
F. Netter M.D.

Fig. 2.5 Nerves of Back (Illustration)

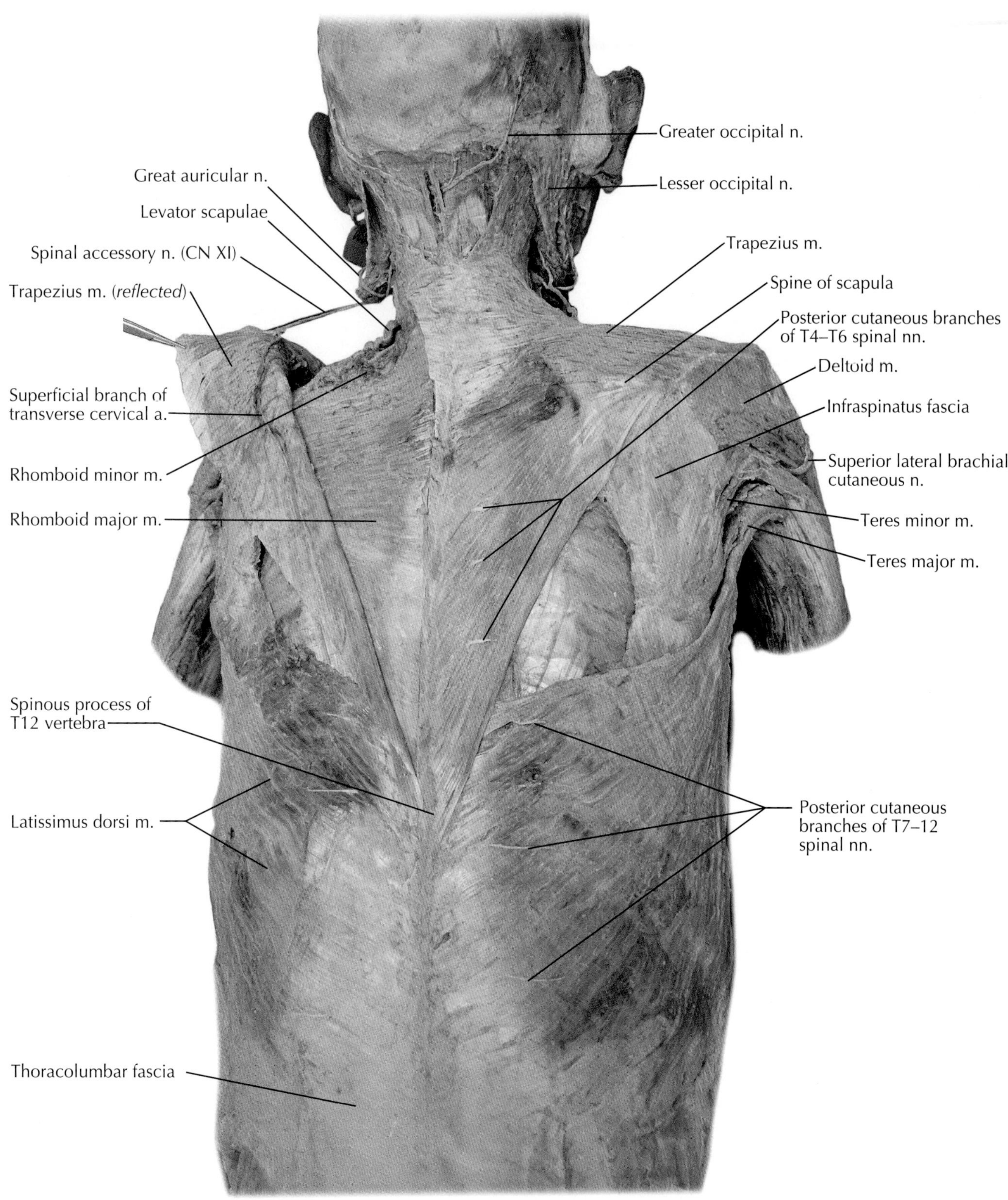
Greater occipital n.
Lesser occipital n.
Great auricular n.
Levator scapulae
Spinal accessory n. (CN XI)
Trapezius m. (*reflected*)
Trapezius m.
Spine of scapula
Posterior cutaneous branches of T4–T6 spinal nn.
Deltoid m.
Superficial branch of transverse cervical a.
Infraspinatus fascia
Rhomboid minor m.
Superior lateral brachial cutaneous n.
Rhomboid major m.
Teres minor m.
Teres major m.
Spinous process of T12 vertebra
Latissimus dorsi m.
Posterior cutaneous branches of T7–12 spinal nn.
Thoracolumbar fascia

Fig. 2.6 Nerves of Back (Photograph)

Thorax

CHAPTER 3

Alternate Version Available in Appendix

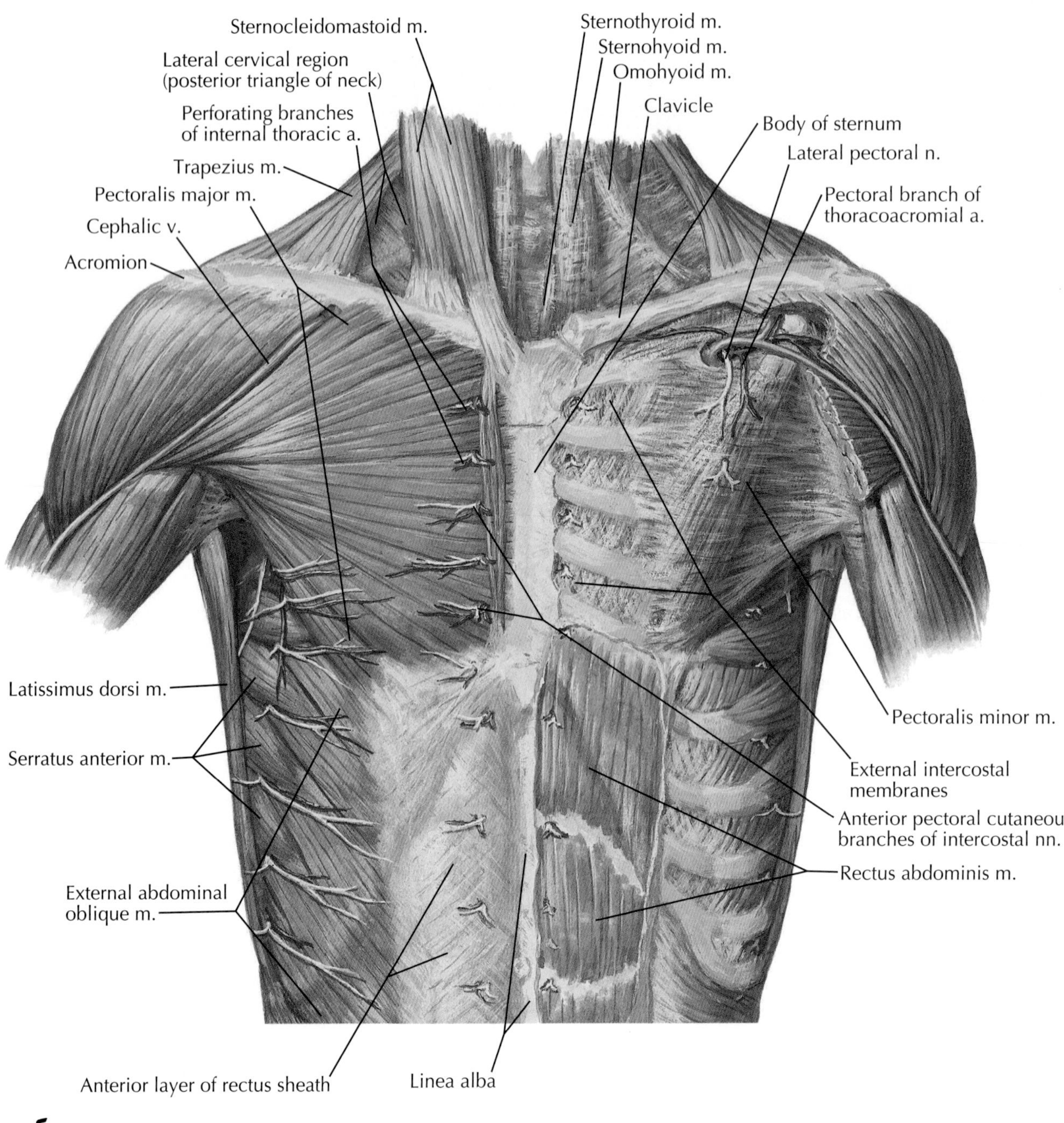
Sternocleidomastoid m.
Lateral cervical region (posterior triangle of neck)
Perforating branches of internal thoracic a.
Trapezius m.
Pectoralis major m.
Cephalic v.
Acromion
Sternothyroid m.
Sternohyoid m.
Omohyoid m.
Clavicle
Body of sternum
Lateral pectoral n.
Pectoral branch of thoracoacromial a.
Latissimus dorsi m.
Serratus anterior m.
Pectoralis minor m.
External intercostal membranes
Anterior pectoral cutaneous branches of intercostal nn.
Rectus abdominis m.
External abdominal oblique m.
Anterior layer of rectus sheath
Linea alba
F. Netter M.D.
C. Machado M.D.

Fig. 3.1 Anterior Thoracic Wall: Superficial Dissection (Illustration)

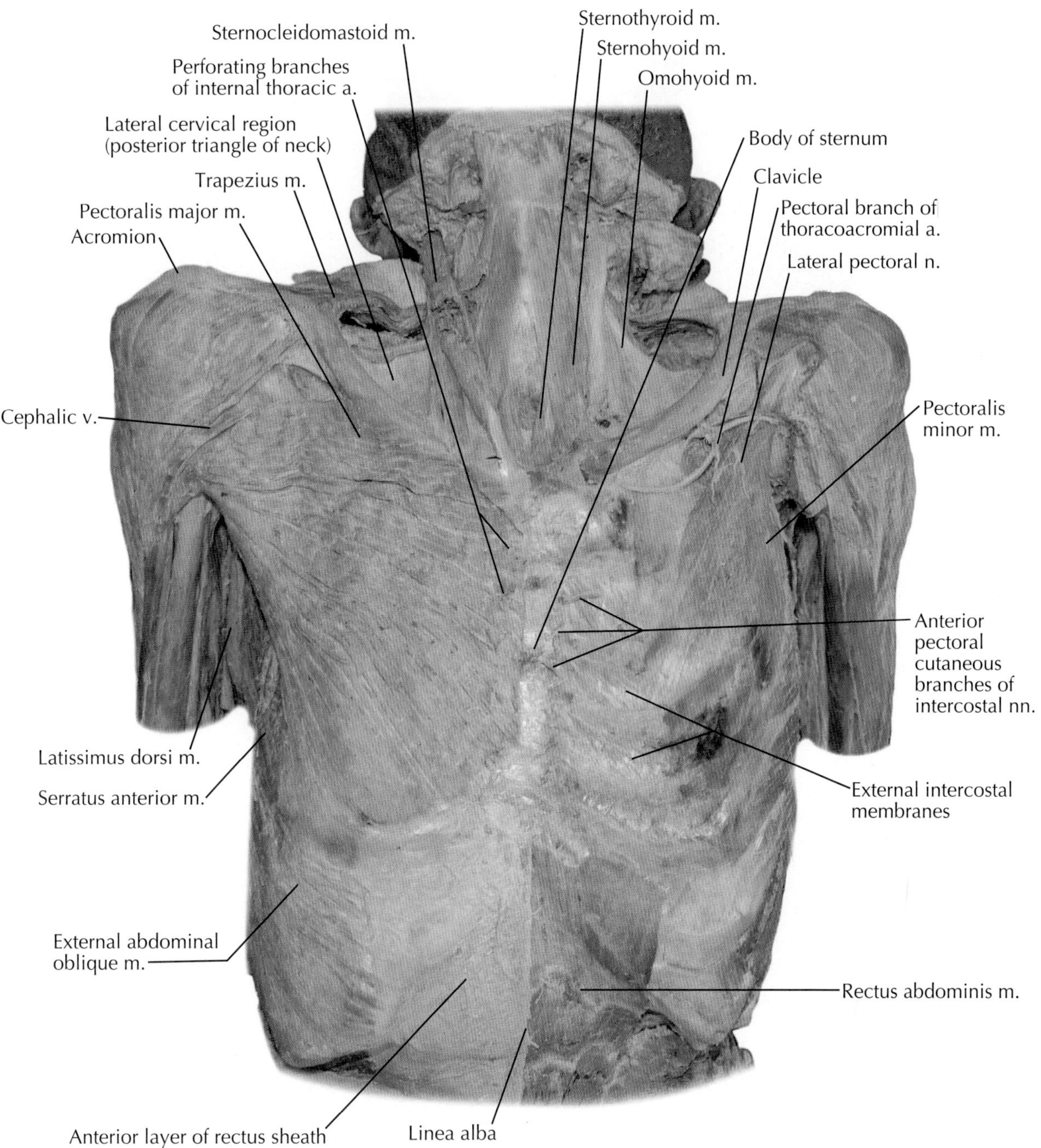
Sternocleidomastoid m.
Perforating branches of internal thoracic a.
Lateral cervical region (posterior triangle of neck)
Trapezius m.
Pectoralis major m.
Acromion
Cephalic v.
Latissimus dorsi m.
Serratus anterior m.
External abdominal oblique m.
Anterior layer of rectus sheath
Linea alba
Sternothyroid m.
Sternohyoid m.
Omohyoid m.
Body of sternum
Clavicle
Pectoral branch of thoracoacromial a.
Lateral pectoral n.
Pectoralis minor m.
Anterior pectoral cutaneous branches of intercostal nn.
External intercostal membranes
Rectus abdominis m.

Fig. 3.2 Anterior Thoracic Wall: Superficial Dissection (Photograph)

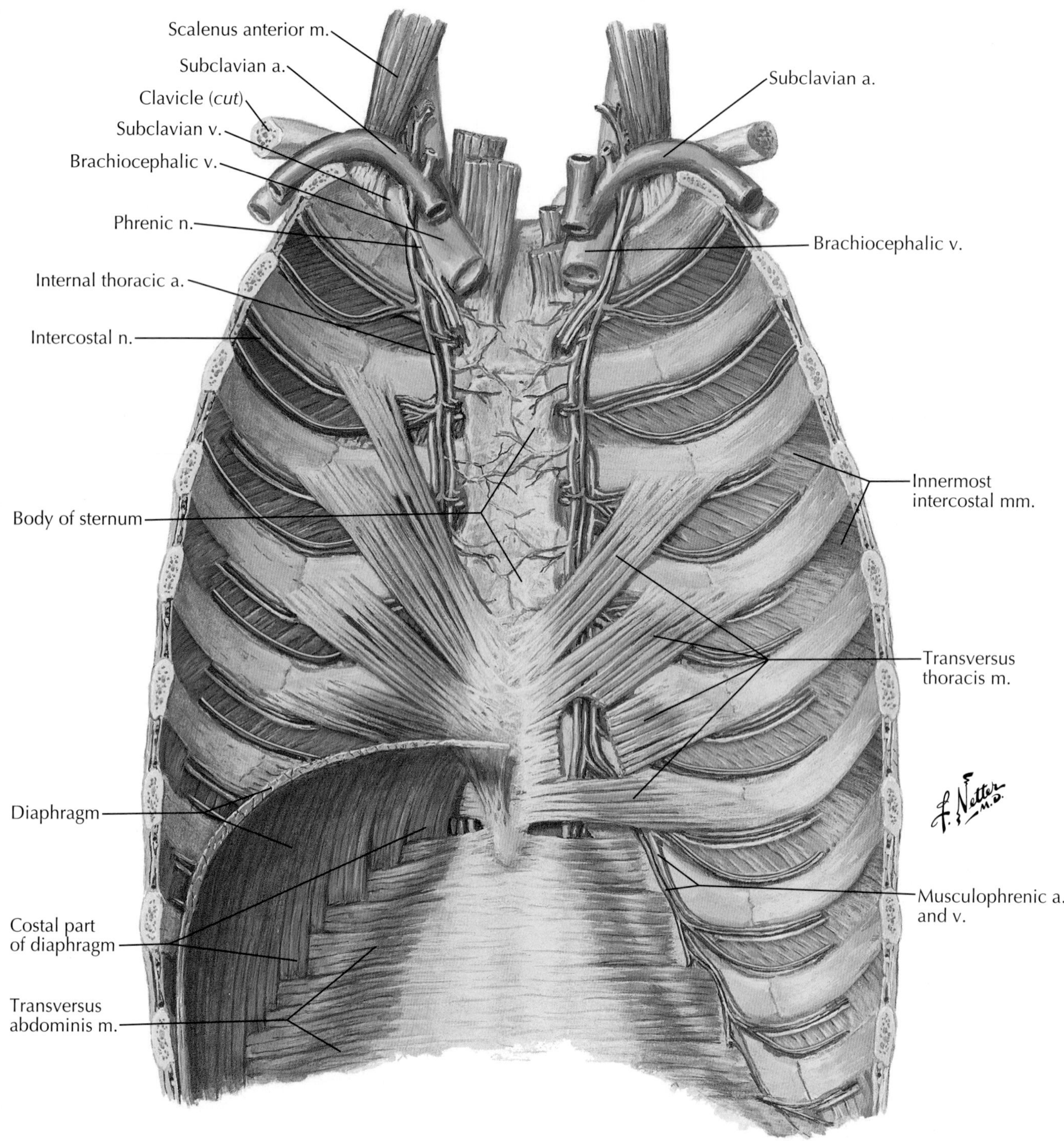
Scalenus anterior m.
Subclavian a.
Clavicle (cut)
Subclavian v.
Brachiocephalic v.
Phrenic n.
Internal thoracic a.
Intercostal n.
Body of sternum
Diaphragm
Costal part of diaphragm
Transversus abdominis m.
Subclavian a.
Brachiocephalic v.
Innermost intercostal mm.
Transversus thoracis m.
Musculophrenic a. and v.
F. Netter M.D.

Fig. 3.3 Anterior Thoracic Wall: Internal View (Illustration)

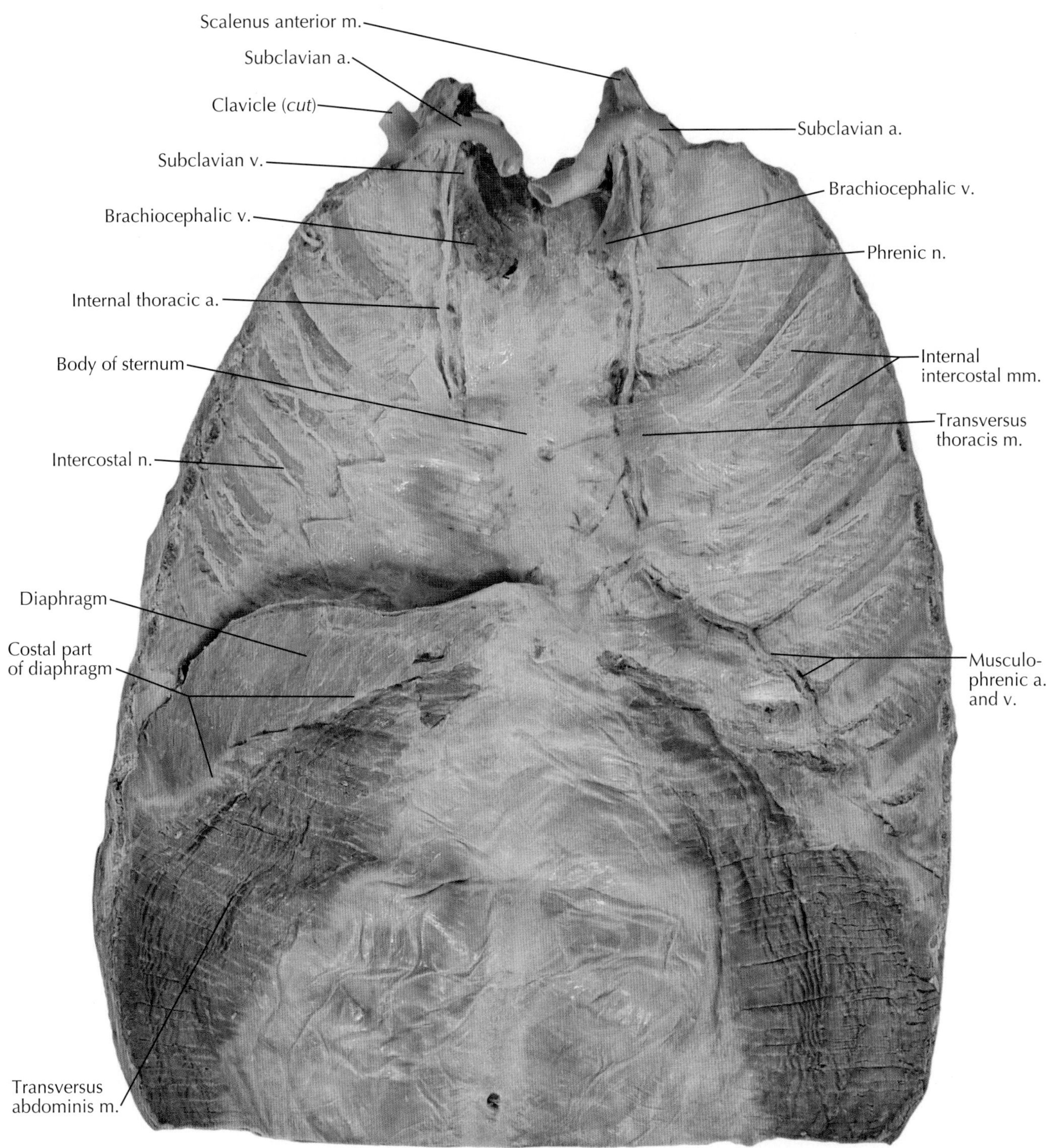
Scalenus anterior m.
Subclavian a.
Clavicle (cut)
Subclavian v.
Brachiocephalic v.
Internal thoracic a.
Body of sternum
Intercostal n.
Diaphragm
Costal part of diaphragm
Transversus abdominis m.
Subclavian a.
Brachiocephalic v.
Phrenic n.
Internal intercostal mm.
Transversus thoracis m.
Musculo-phrenic a. and v.

Fig. 3.4 Anterior Thoracic Wall: Internal View (Photograph)

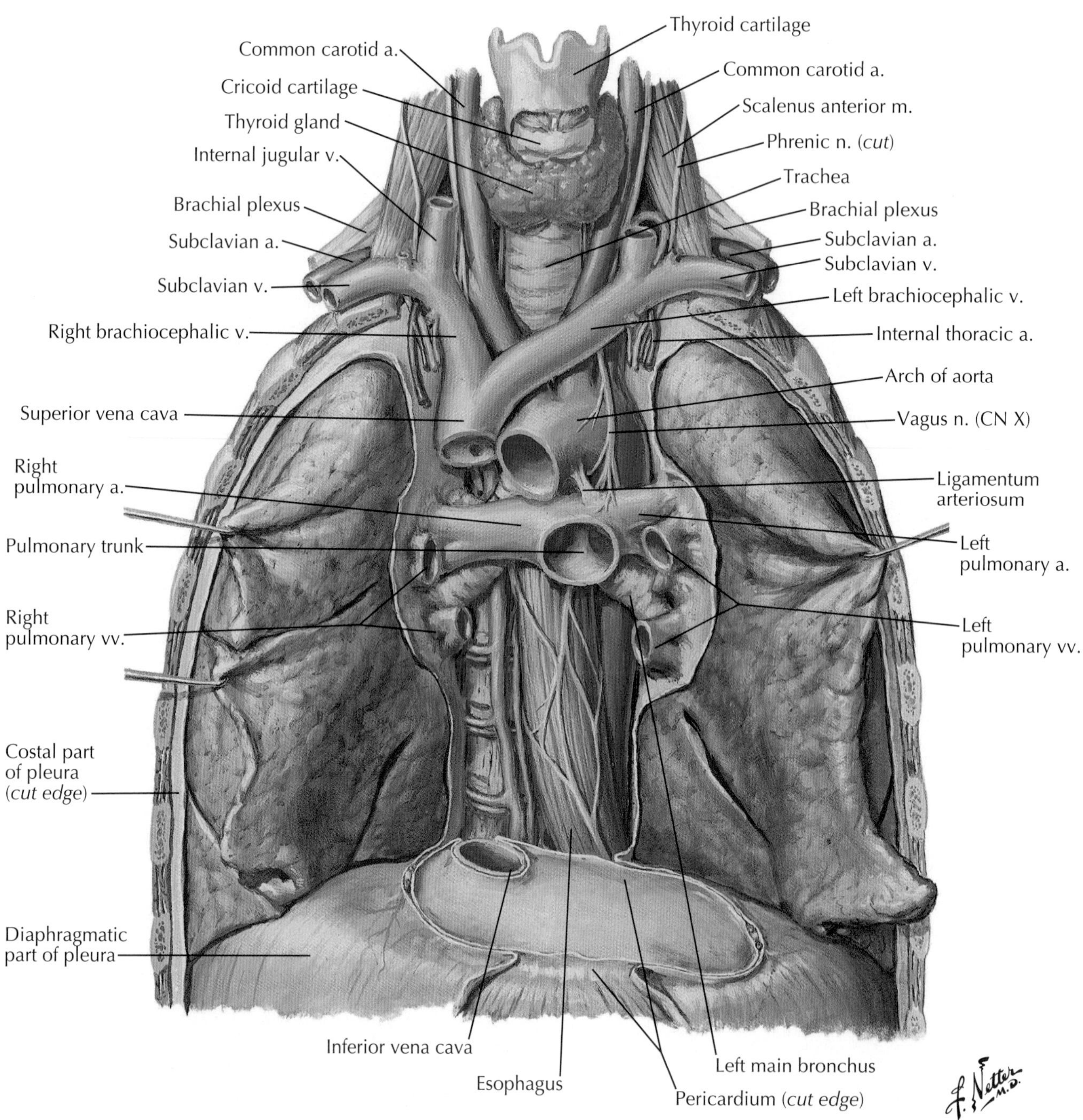
Common carotid a.
Cricoid cartilage
Thyroid gland
Internal jugular v.
Brachial plexus
Subclavian a.
Subclavian v.
Right brachiocephalic v.
Superior vena cava
Right pulmonary a.
Pulmonary trunk
Right pulmonary vv.
Costal part of pleura (*cut edge*)
Diaphragmatic part of pleura
Thyroid cartilage
Common carotid a.
Scalenus anterior m.
Phrenic n. (*cut*)
Trachea
Brachial plexus
Subclavian a.
Subclavian v.
Left brachiocephalic v.
Internal thoracic a.
Arch of aorta
Vagus n. (CN X)
Ligamentum arteriosum
Left pulmonary a.
Left pulmonary vv.
Inferior vena cava
Esophagus
Left main bronchus
Pericardium (*cut edge*)

Fig. 3.5 Great Vessels of Mediastinum (Illustration)

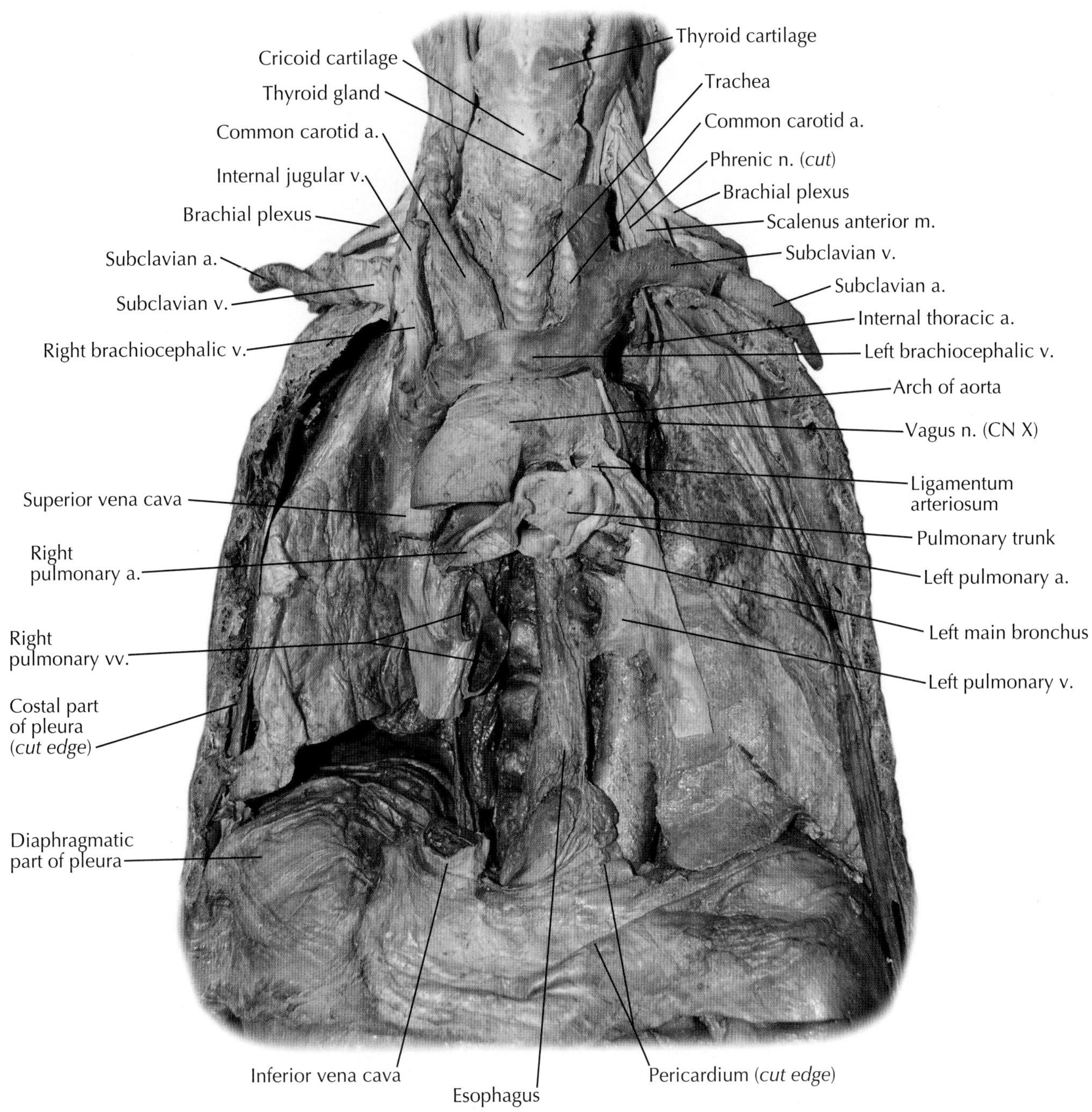
Thyroid cartilage
Cricoid cartilage
Thyroid gland
Trachea
Common carotid a.
Common carotid a.
Phrenic n. (cut)
Internal jugular v.
Brachial plexus
Brachial plexus
Scalenus anterior m.
Subclavian v.
Subclavian a.
Subclavian a.
Subclavian v.
Internal thoracic a.
Right brachiocephalic v.
Left brachiocephalic v.
Arch of aorta
Vagus n. (CN X)
Ligamentum arteriosum
Superior vena cava
Pulmonary trunk
Right pulmonary a.
Left pulmonary a.
Left main bronchus
Right pulmonary vv.
Left pulmonary v.
Costal part of pleura (cut edge)
Diaphragmatic part of pleura
Inferior vena cava
Pericardium (cut edge)
Esophagus

Fig. 3.6 Great Vessels of Mediastinum (Photograph)

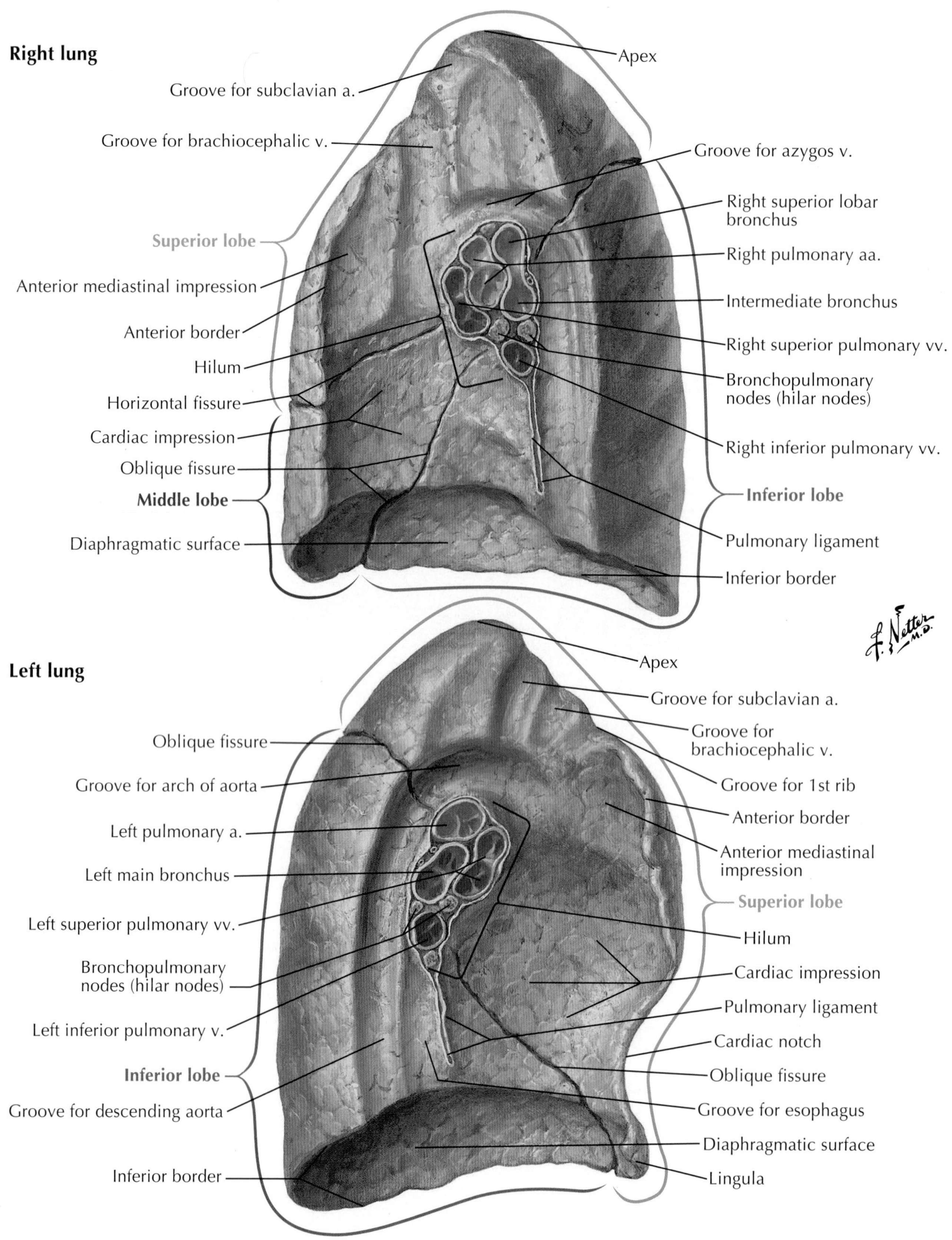
Right lung
Apex
Groove for subclavian a.
Groove for brachiocephalic v.
Groove for azygos v.
Right superior lobar bronchus
Superior lobe
Right pulmonary aa.
Anterior mediastinal impression
Intermediate bronchus
Anterior border
Right superior pulmonary vv.
Hilum
Bronchopulmonary nodes (hilar nodes)
Horizontal fissure
Cardiac impression
Right inferior pulmonary vv.
Oblique fissure
Middle lobe
Inferior lobe
Diaphragmatic surface
Pulmonary ligament
Inferior border
F. Netter M.D.
Left lung
Apex
Groove for subclavian a.
Oblique fissure
Groove for brachiocephalic v.
Groove for arch of aorta
Groove for 1st rib
Anterior border
Left pulmonary a.
Anterior mediastinal impression
Left main bronchus
Superior lobe
Left superior pulmonary vv.
Hilum
Bronchopulmonary nodes (hilar nodes)
Cardiac impression
Pulmonary ligament
Left inferior pulmonary v.
Cardiac notch
Inferior lobe
Oblique fissure
Groove for descending aorta
Groove for esophagus
Diaphragmatic surface
Inferior border
Lingula

Fig. 3.7 Lungs: Medial Views (Illustration)

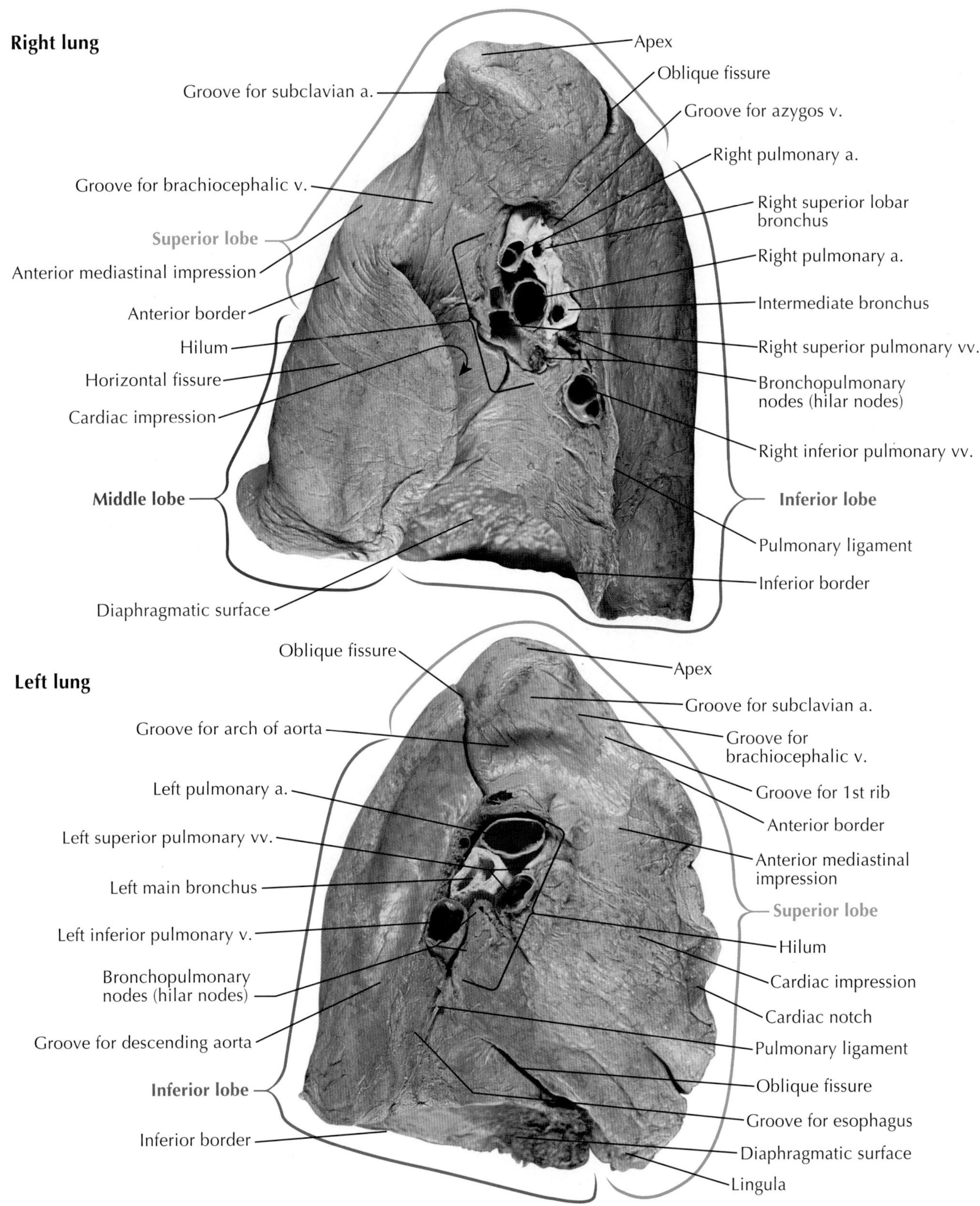
Right lung
Apex
Oblique fissure
Groove for subclavian a.
Groove for azygos v.
Right pulmonary a.
Groove for brachiocephalic v.
Right superior lobar bronchus
Superior lobe
Anterior mediastinal impression
Right pulmonary a.
Intermediate bronchus
Anterior border
Hilum
Right superior pulmonary vv.
Horizontal fissure
Bronchopulmonary nodes (hilar nodes)
Cardiac impression
Right inferior pulmonary vv.
Middle lobe
Inferior lobe
Pulmonary ligament
Inferior border
Diaphragmatic surface
Left lung
Oblique fissure
Apex
Groove for subclavian a.
Groove for arch of aorta
Groove for brachiocephalic v.
Left pulmonary a.
Groove for 1st rib
Anterior border
Left superior pulmonary vv.
Anterior mediastinal impression
Left main bronchus
Superior lobe
Left inferior pulmonary v.
Hilum
Bronchopulmonary nodes (hilar nodes)
Cardiac impression
Cardiac notch
Groove for descending aorta
Pulmonary ligament
Oblique fissure
Inferior lobe
Groove for esophagus
Inferior border
Diaphragmatic surface
Lingula

Fig. 3.8 Lungs: Medial Views (Photograph) (see Fig. A.6)

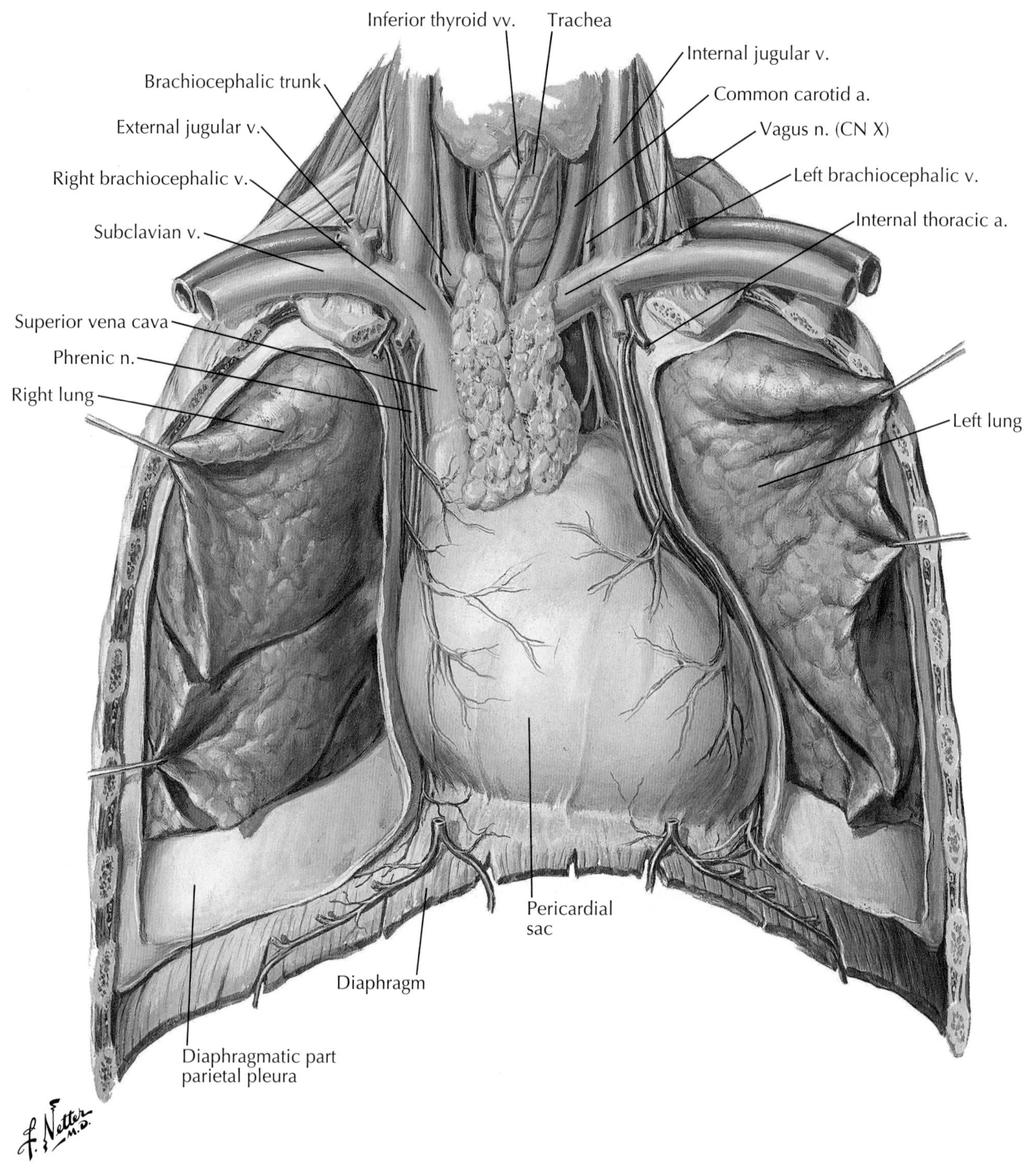
Inferior thyroid vv.
Trachea
Internal jugular v.
Brachiocephalic trunk
Common carotid a.
External jugular v.
Vagus n. (CN X)
Right brachiocephalic v.
Left brachiocephalic v.
Subclavian v.
Internal thoracic a.
Superior vena cava
Phrenic n.
Right lung
Left lung
Pericardial sac
Diaphragm
Diaphragmatic part parietal pleura
F. Netter M.D.

Fig. 3.9 Heart In situ (Illustration)

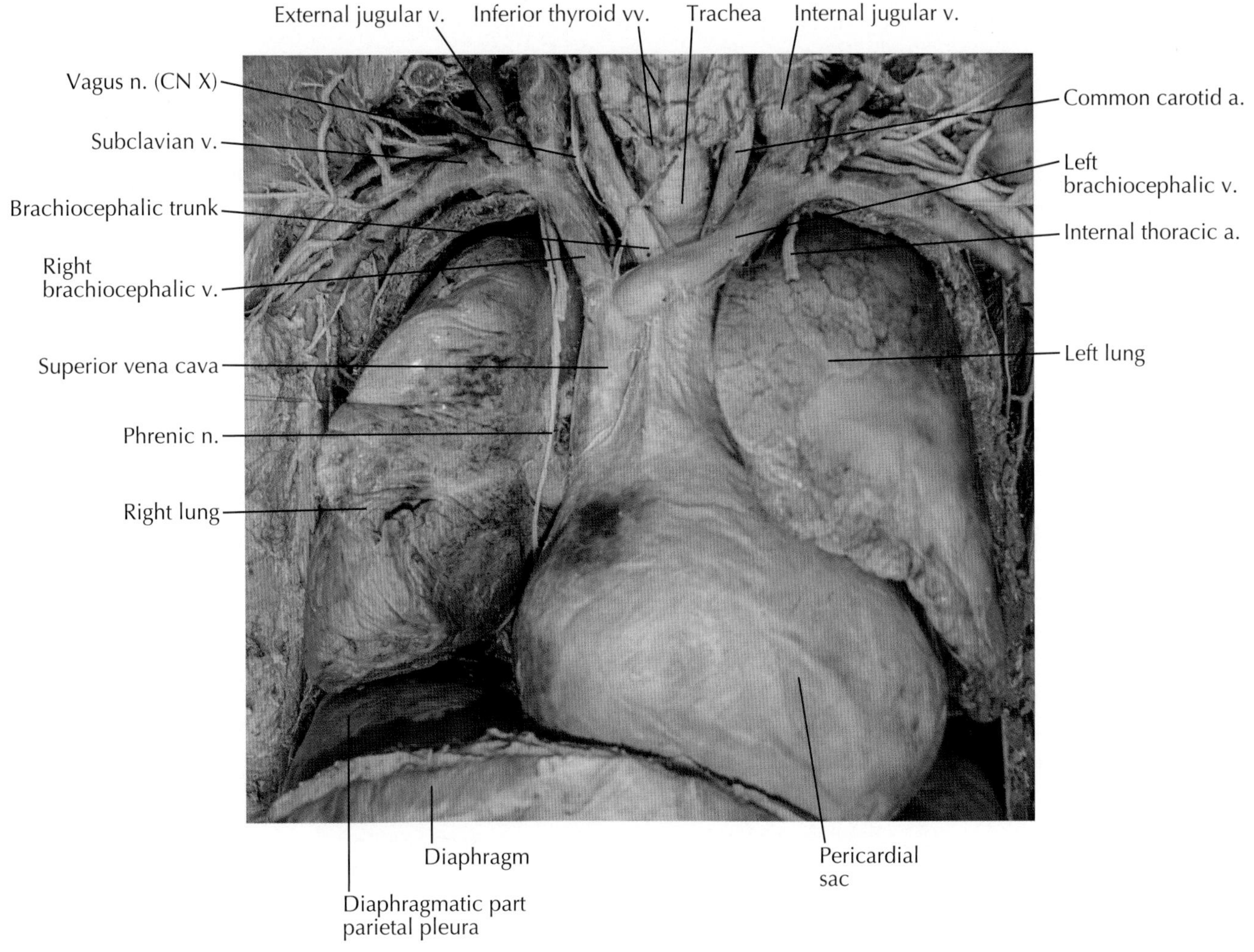
External jugular v.
Inferior thyroid vv.
Trachea
Internal jugular v.
Vagus n. (CN X)
Common carotid a.
Subclavian v.
Left brachiocephalic v.
Brachiocephalic trunk
Internal thoracic a.
Right brachiocephalic v.
Superior vena cava
Left lung
Phrenic n.
Right lung
Diaphragm
Pericardial sac
Diaphragmatic part parietal pleura

Fig. 3.10 Heart In situ (Photograph)

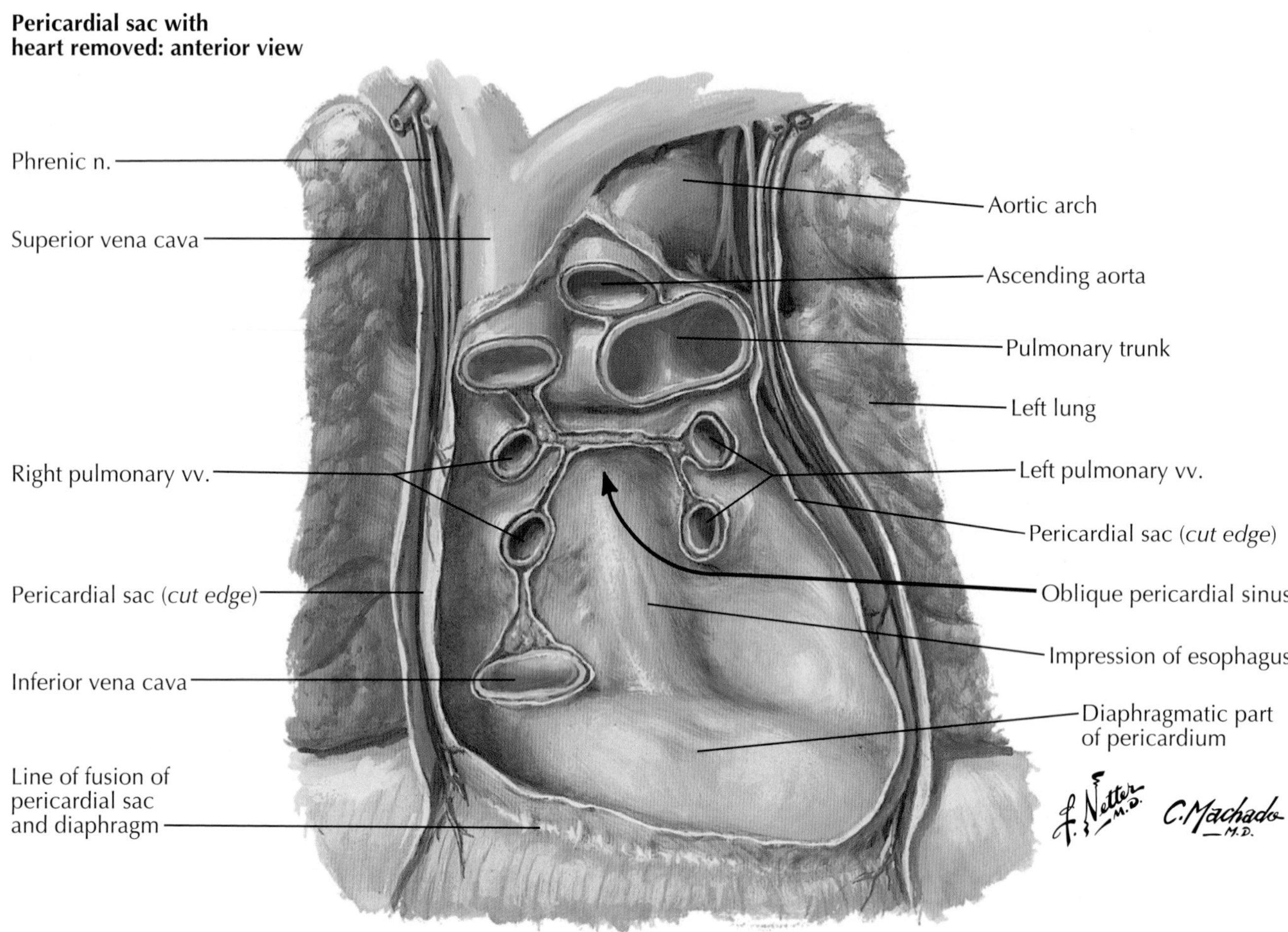
Pericardial sac with
heart removed: anterior view
Phrenic n.
Superior vena cava
Right pulmonary vv.
Pericardial sac (cut edge)
Inferior vena cava
Line of fusion of
pericardial sac
and diaphragm
Aortic arch
Ascending aorta
Pulmonary trunk
Left lung
Left pulmonary vv.
Pericardial sac (cut edge)
Oblique pericardial sinus
Impression of esophagus
Diaphragmatic part
of pericardium

Fig. 3.11 Pericardial Sac and Pericardial Cavity (Illustration)

Pericardial sac with heart removed: anterior view

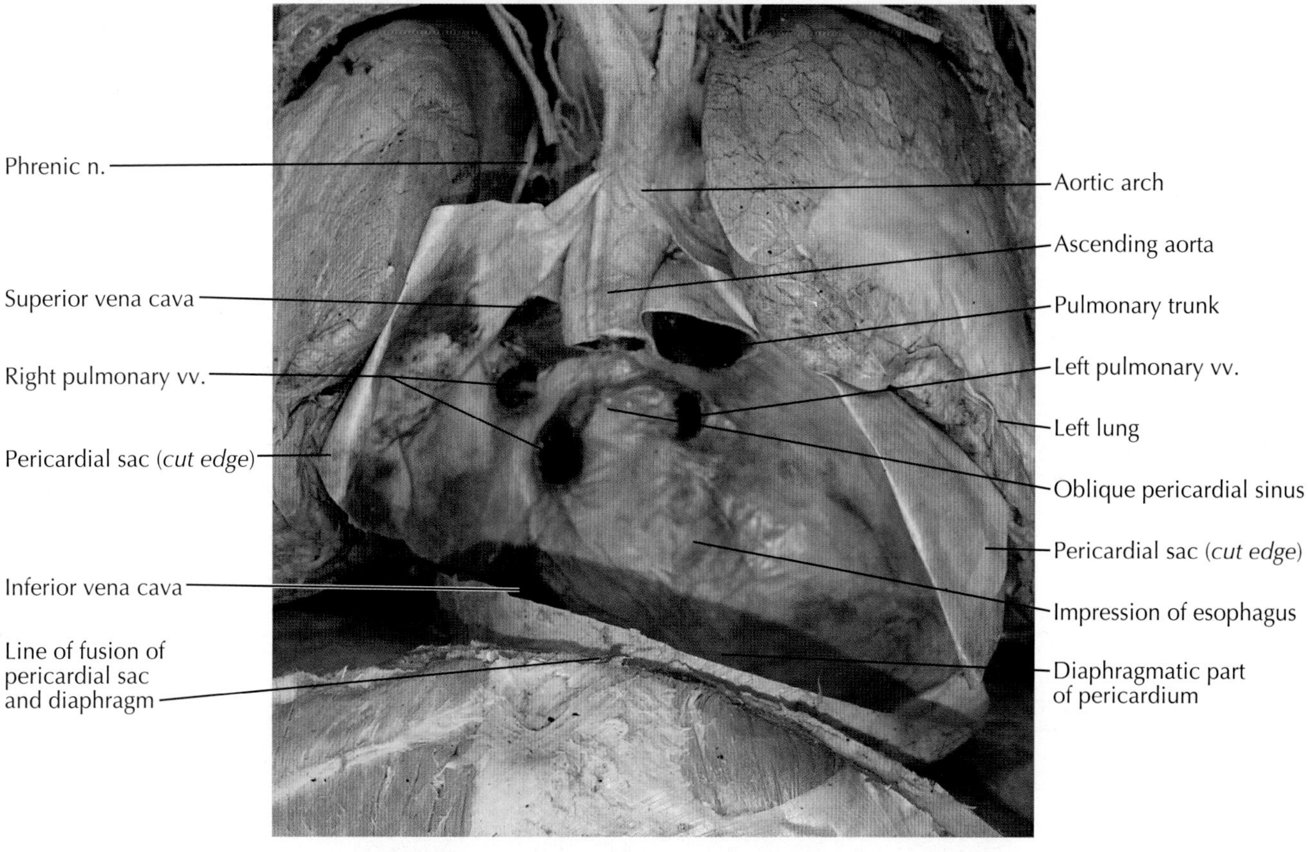
Phrenic n.
Superior vena cava
Right pulmonary vv.
Pericardial sac (*cut edge*)
Inferior vena cava
Line of fusion of pericardial sac and diaphragm
Aortic arch
Ascending aorta
Pulmonary trunk
Left pulmonary vv.
Left lung
Oblique pericardial sinus
Pericardial sac (*cut edge*)
Impression of esophagus
Diaphragmatic part of pericardium

Fig. 3.12 Pericardial Sac and Pericardial Cavity (Photograph)

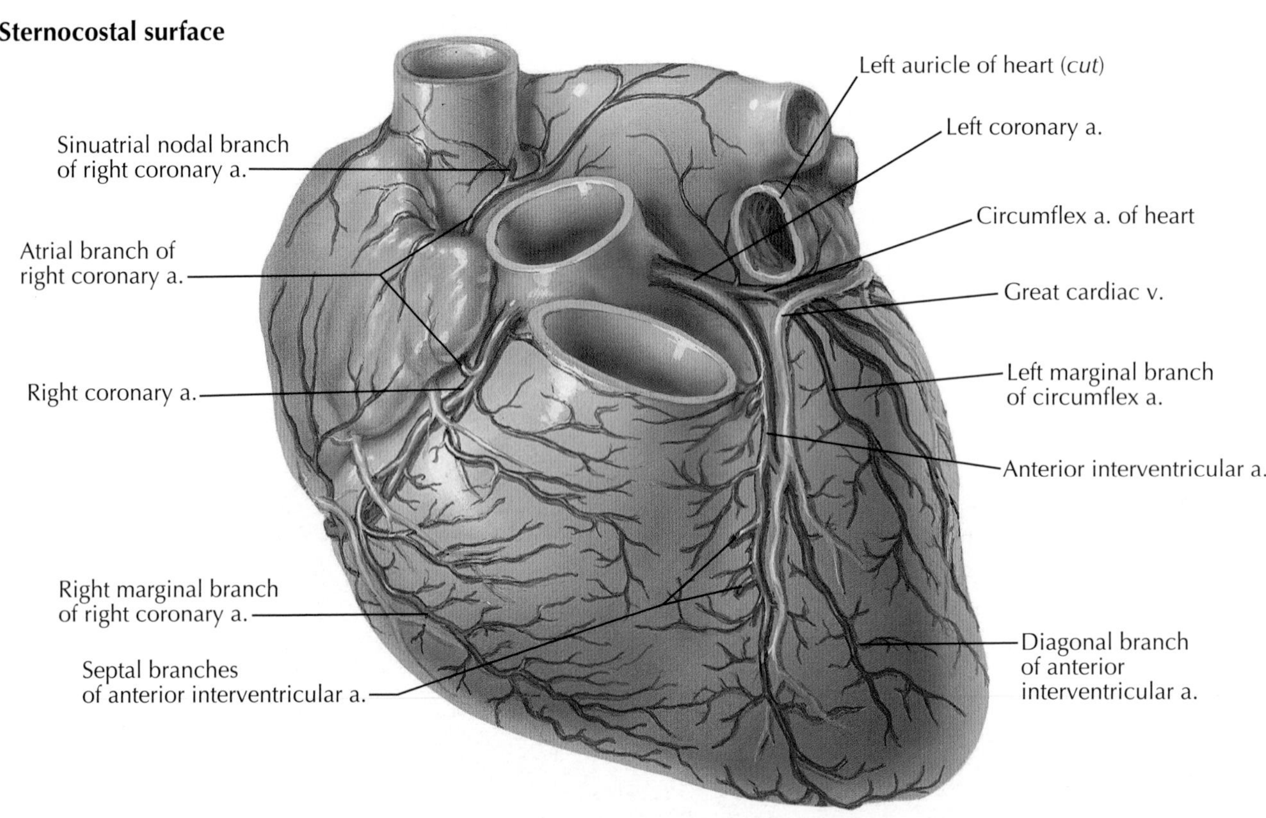
Sternocostal surface
Sinuatrial nodal branch of right coronary a.
Atrial branch of right coronary a.
Right coronary a.
Right marginal branch of right coronary a.
Septal branches of anterior interventricular a.
Left auricle of heart (cut)
Left coronary a.
Circumflex a. of heart
Great cardiac v.
Left marginal branch of circumflex a.
Anterior interventricular a.
Diagonal branch of anterior interventricular a.

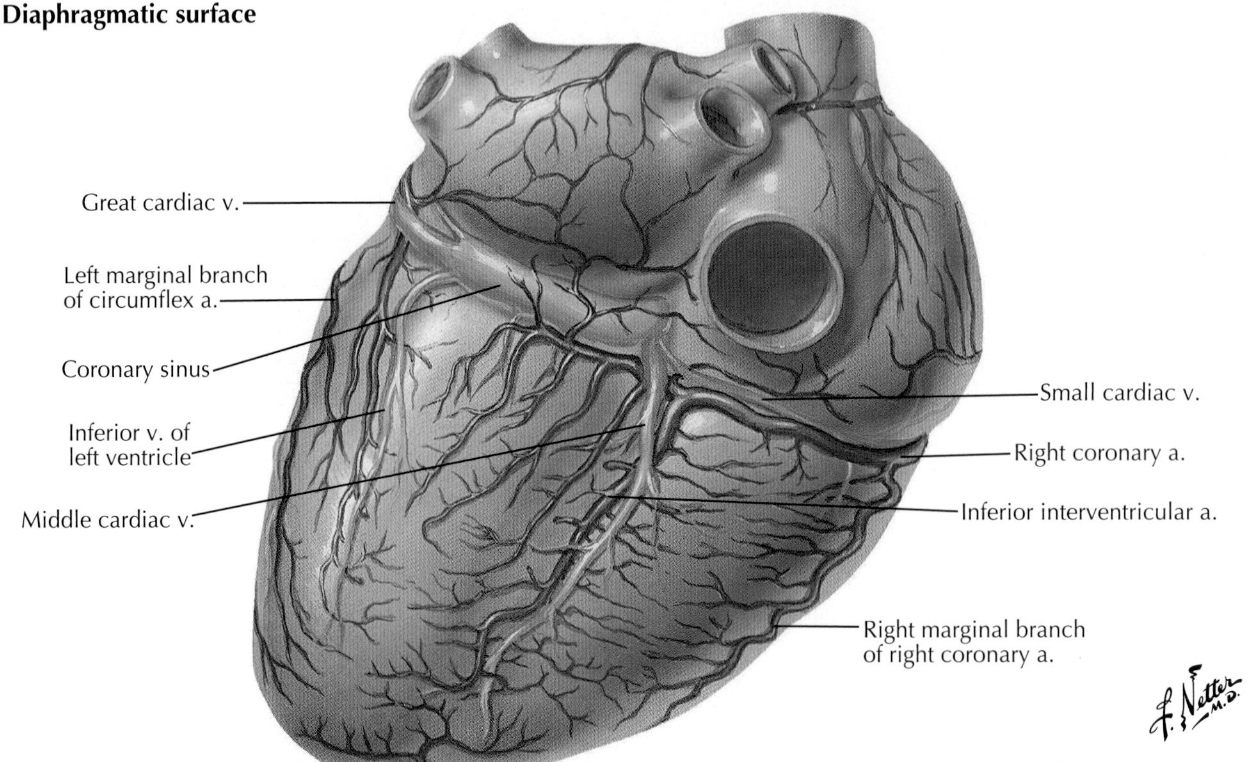
Diaphragmatic surface
Great cardiac v.
Left marginal branch of circumflex a.
Coronary sinus
Inferior v. of left ventricle
Middle cardiac v.
Small cardiac v.
Right coronary a.
Inferior interventricular a.
Right marginal branch of right coronary a.
F. Netter M.D.

Fig. 3.13 Coronary Arteries and Cardiac Veins (Illustration)

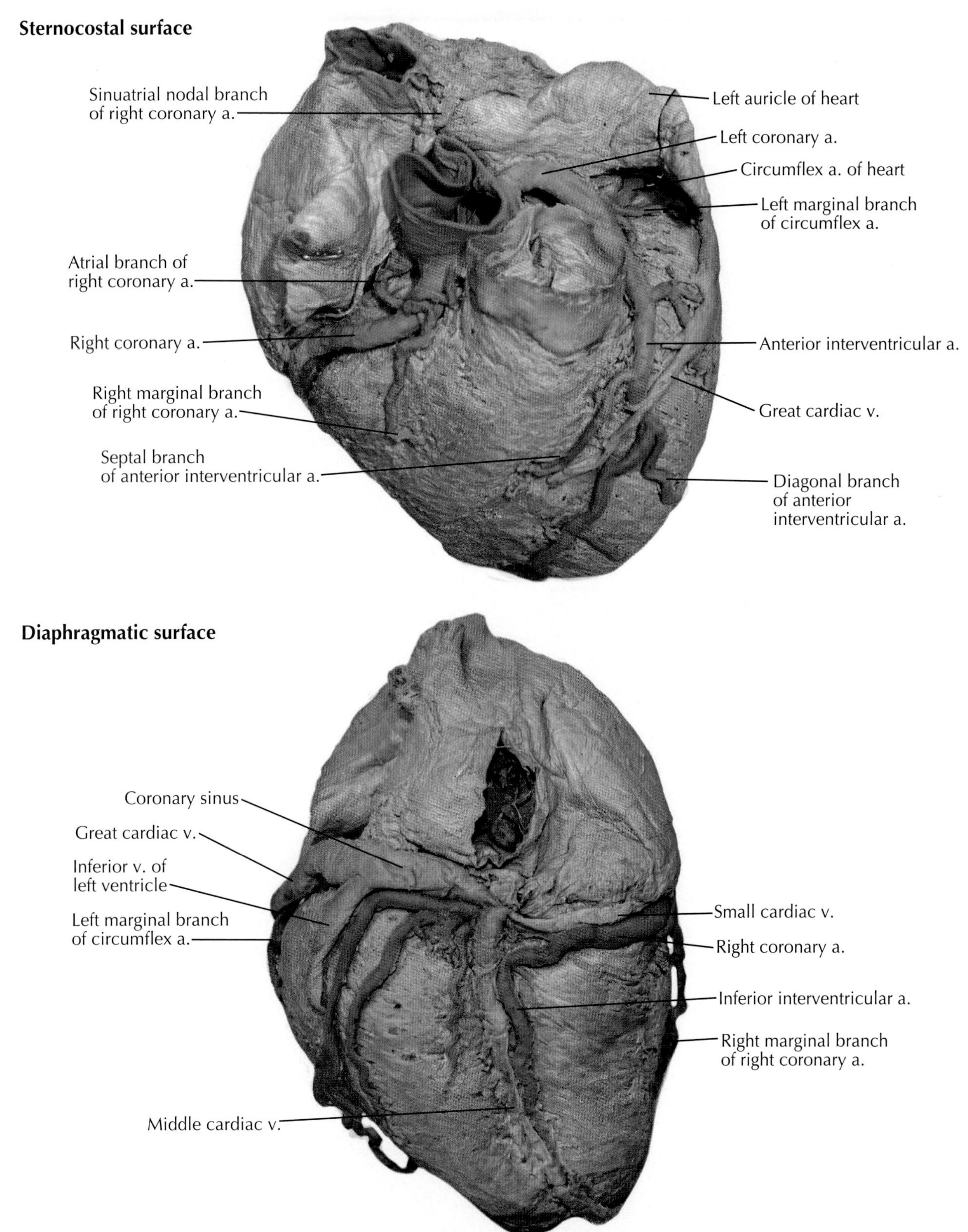
Sternocostal surface
Sinuatrial nodal branch of right coronary a.
Left auricle of heart
Left coronary a.
Circumflex a. of heart
Left marginal branch of circumflex a.
Atrial branch of right coronary a.
Right coronary a.
Anterior interventricular a.
Right marginal branch of right coronary a.
Great cardiac v.
Septal branch of anterior interventricular a.
Diagonal branch of anterior interventricular a.
Diaphragmatic surface
Coronary sinus
Great cardiac v.
Inferior v. of left ventricle
Left marginal branch of circumflex a.
Small cardiac v.
Right coronary a.
Inferior interventricular a.
Right marginal branch of right coronary a.
Middle cardiac v.

Fig. 3.14 Coronary Arteries and Cardiac Veins (Photograph) (see Fig. A.7)

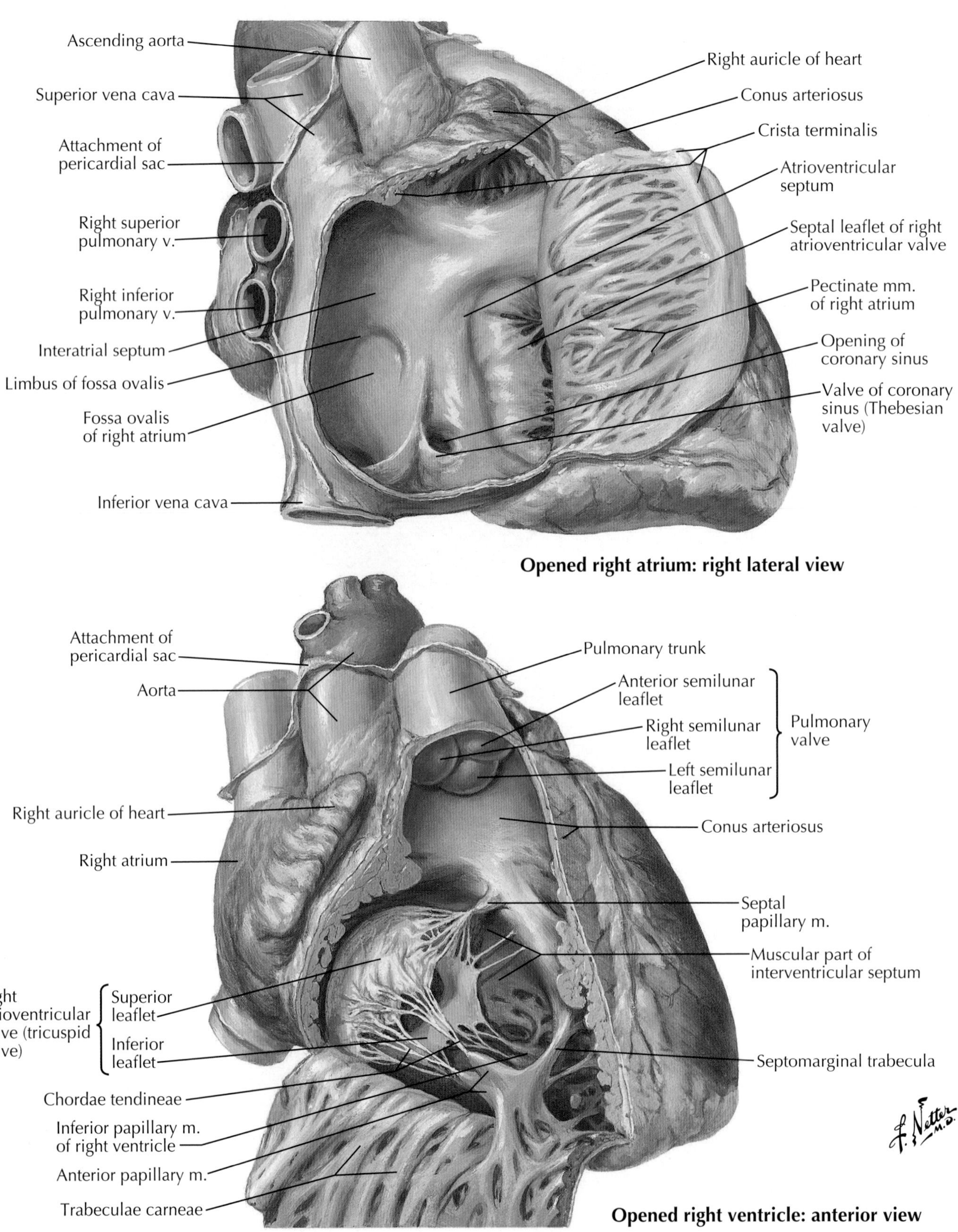
Ascending aorta
Superior vena cava
Attachment of pericardial sac
Right superior pulmonary v.
Right inferior pulmonary v.
Interatrial septum
Limbus of fossa ovalis
Fossa ovalis of right atrium
Inferior vena cava
Right auricle of heart
Conus arteriosus
Crista terminalis
Atrioventricular septum
Septal leaflet of right atrioventricular valve
Pectinate mm. of right atrium
Opening of coronary sinus
Valve of coronary sinus (Thebesian valve)
Opened right atrium: right lateral view
Attachment of pericardial sac
Aorta
Right auricle of heart
Right atrium
Right atrioventricular valve (tricuspid valve)
Superior leaflet
Inferior leaflet
Chordae tendineae
Inferior papillary m. of right ventricle
Anterior papillary m.
Trabeculae carneae
Pulmonary trunk
Anterior semilunar leaflet
Right semilunar leaflet
Left semilunar leaflet
Pulmonary valve
Conus arteriosus
Septal papillary m.
Muscular part of interventricular septum
Septomarginal trabecula
Opened right ventricle: anterior view

Fig. 3.15 Right Atrium and Ventricle (Illustration)

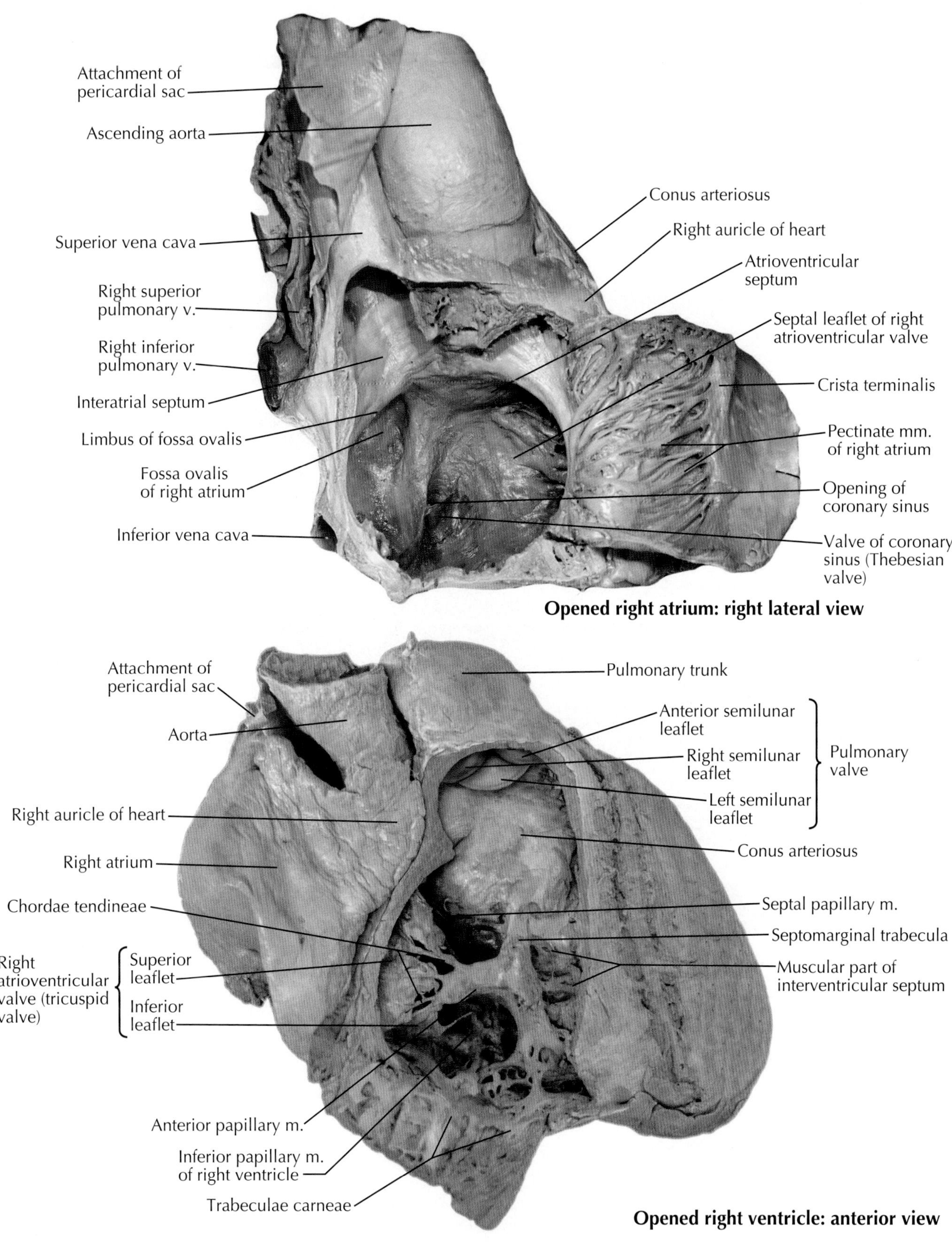
Attachment of pericardial sac
Ascending aorta
Superior vena cava
Right superior pulmonary v.
Right inferior pulmonary v.
Interatrial septum
Limbus of fossa ovalis
Fossa ovalis of right atrium
Inferior vena cava
Conus arteriosus
Right auricle of heart
Atrioventricular septum
Septal leaflet of right atrioventricular valve
Crista terminalis
Pectinate mm. of right atrium
Opening of coronary sinus
Valve of coronary sinus (Thebesian valve)
Opened right atrium: right lateral view
Attachment of pericardial sac
Aorta
Right auricle of heart
Right atrium
Chordae tendineae
Right atrioventricular valve (tricuspid valve)
Superior leaflet
Inferior leaflet
Anterior papillary m.
Inferior papillary m. of right ventricle
Trabeculae carneae
Pulmonary trunk
Anterior semilunar leaflet
Right semilunar leaflet
Left semilunar leaflet
Pulmonary valve
Conus arteriosus
Septal papillary m.
Septomarginal trabecula
Muscular part of interventricular septum
Opened right ventricle: anterior view

Fig. 3.16 Right Atrium and Ventricle (Photograph)

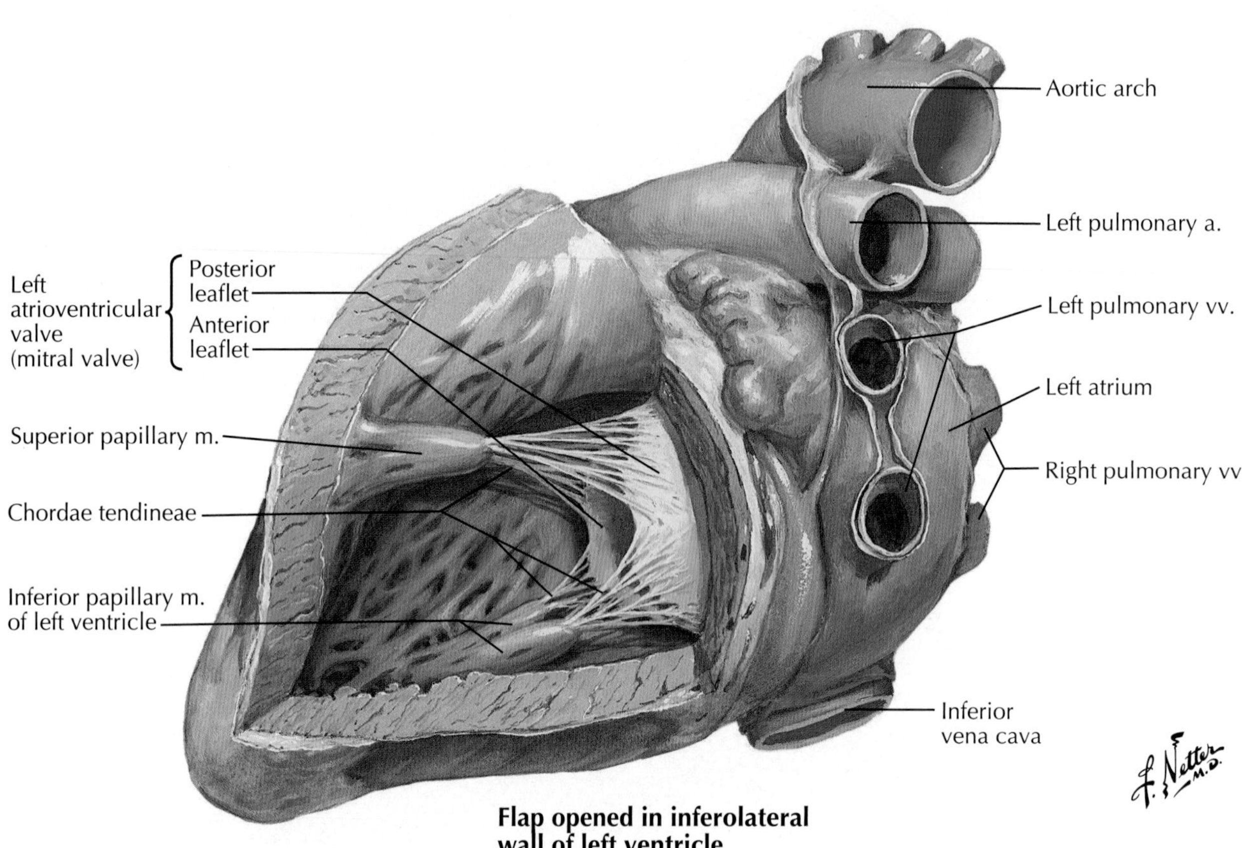
Aortic arch
Left pulmonary a.
Left pulmonary vv.
Left atrium
Right pulmonary vv.
Inferior vena cava
Left atrioventricular valve (mitral valve)
Posterior leaflet
Anterior leaflet
Superior papillary m.
Chordae tendineae
Inferior papillary m. of left ventricle
Flap opened in inferolateral wall of left ventricle

Fig. 3.17 Left Atrium and Ventricle (Illustration)

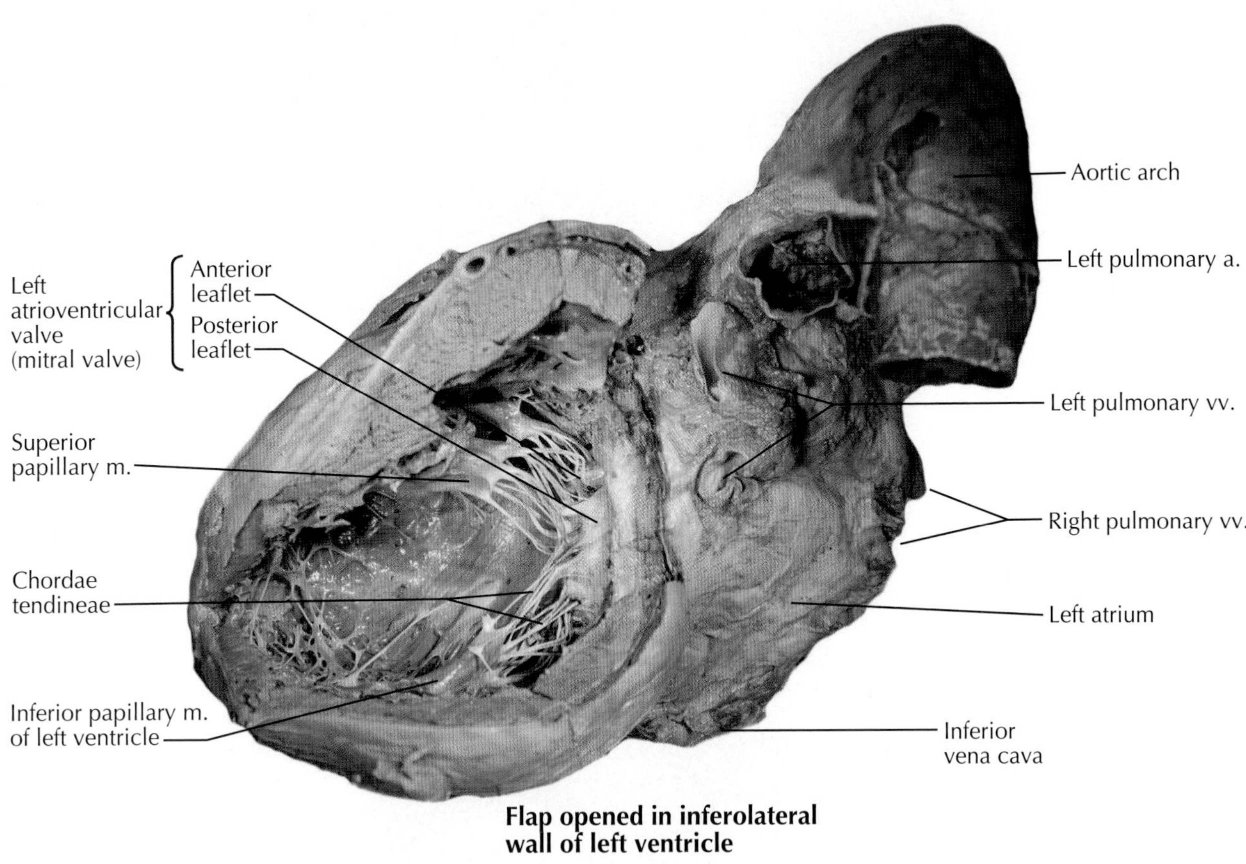
Left atrioventricular valve (mitral valve)
Anterior leaflet
Posterior leaflet
Superior papillary m.
Chordae tendineae
Inferior papillary m. of left ventricle
Aortic arch
Left pulmonary a.
Left pulmonary vv.
Right pulmonary vv.
Left atrium
Inferior vena cava
Flap opened in inferolateral wall of left ventricle

Fig. 3.18 Left Atrium and Ventricle (Photograph)

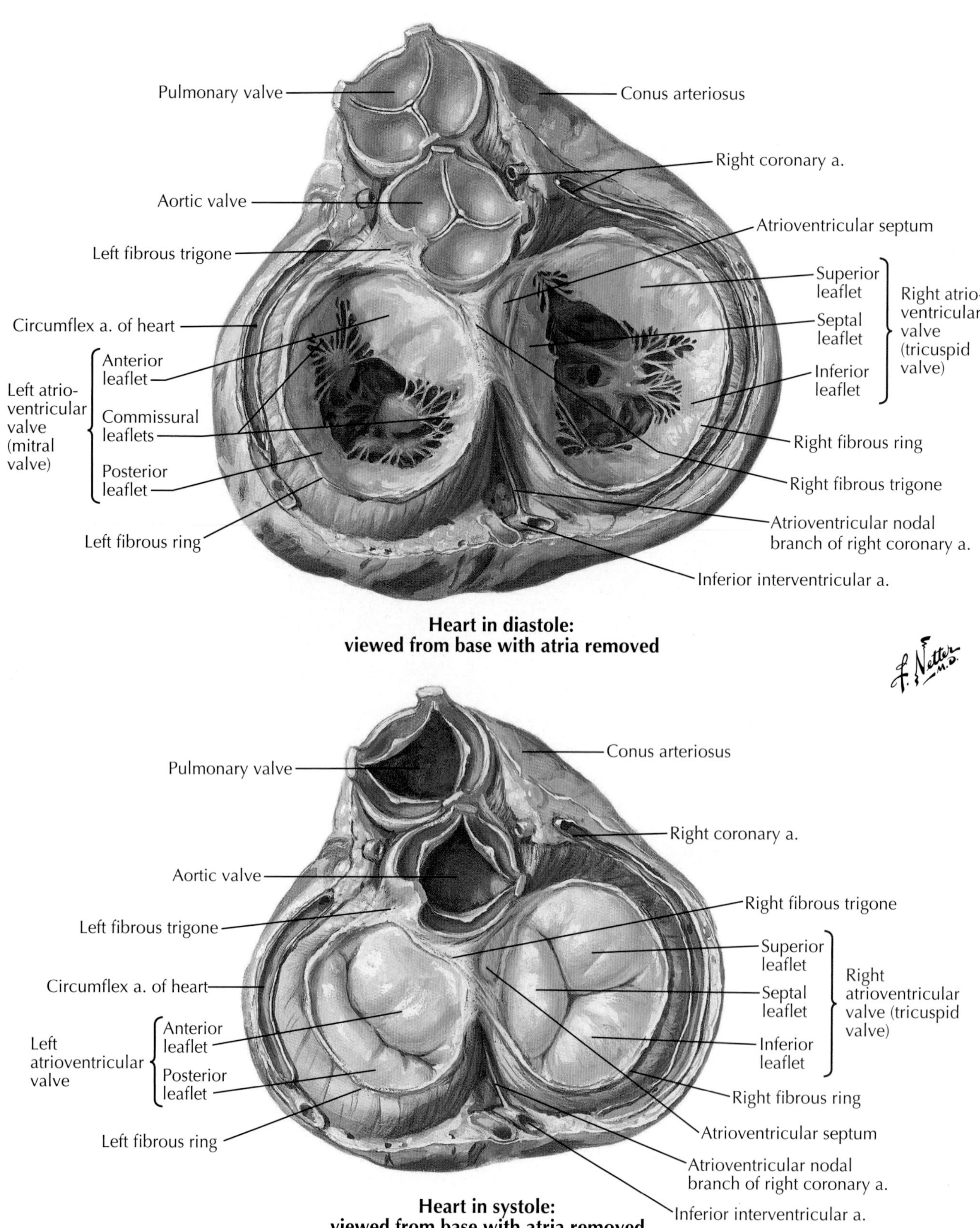
Pulmonary valve
Conus arteriosus
Right coronary a.
Aortic valve
Atrioventricular septum
Left fibrous trigone
Superior leaflet
Right atrio-ventricular valve (tricuspid valve)
Septal leaflet
Circumflex a. of heart
Inferior leaflet
Anterior leaflet
Left atrio-ventricular valve (mitral valve)
Commissural leaflets
Right fibrous ring
Posterior leaflet
Right fibrous trigone
Atrioventricular nodal branch of right coronary a.
Left fibrous ring
Inferior interventricular a.
Heart in diastole: viewed from base with atria removed
F. Netter M.D.
Conus arteriosus
Pulmonary valve
Right coronary a.
Aortic valve
Right fibrous trigone
Left fibrous trigone
Superior leaflet
Right atrioventricular valve (tricuspid valve)
Circumflex a. of heart
Septal leaflet
Anterior leaflet
Left atrioventricular valve
Inferior leaflet
Posterior leaflet
Right fibrous ring
Left fibrous ring
Atrioventricular septum
Atrioventricular nodal branch of right coronary a.
Heart in systole: viewed from base with atria removed
Inferior interventricular a.

Fig. 3.19 Valvular Complex of Heart (Illustration)

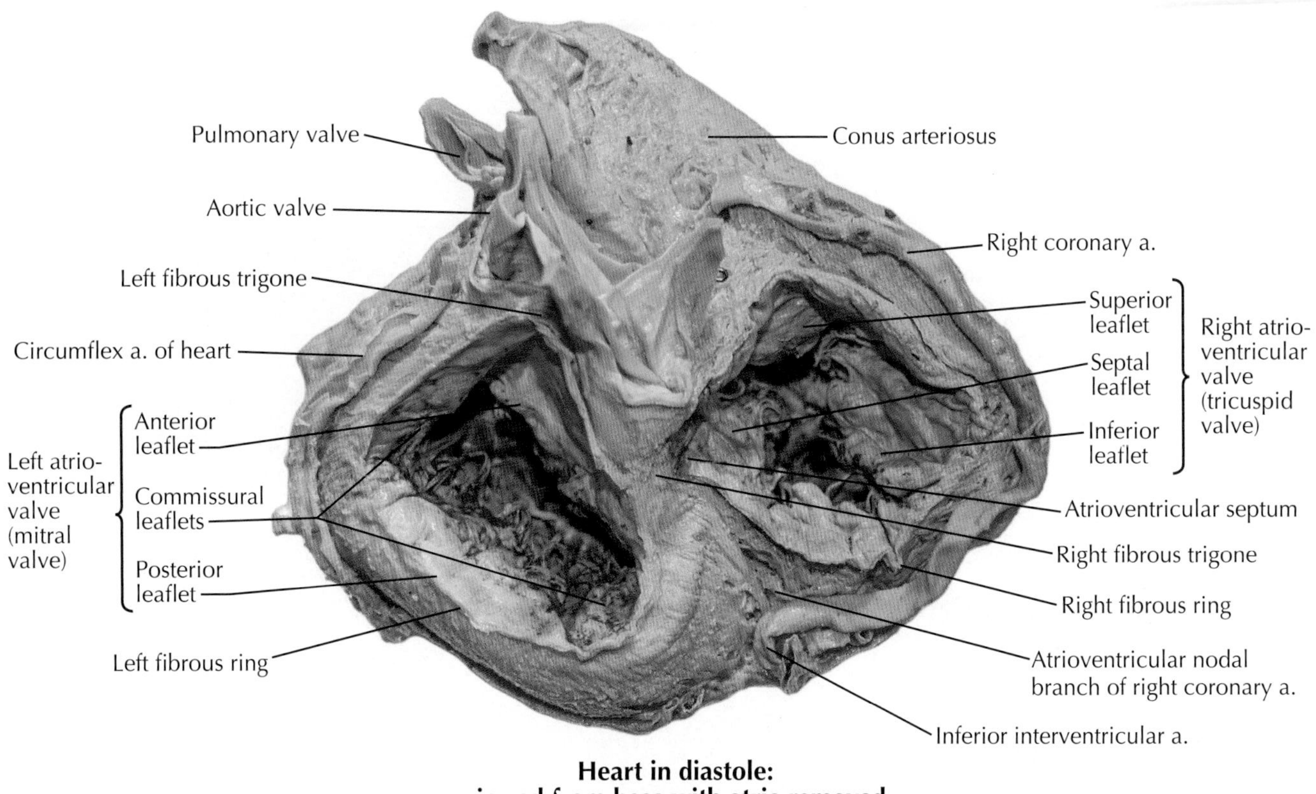
Pulmonary valve
Conus arteriosus
Aortic valve
Right coronary a.
Left fibrous trigone
Superior leaflet
Circumflex a. of heart
Septal leaflet
Right atrioventricular valve (tricuspid valve)
Anterior leaflet
Inferior leaflet
Left atrio-ventricular valve (mitral valve)
Commissural leaflets
Atrioventricular septum
Right fibrous trigone
Posterior leaflet
Right fibrous ring
Left fibrous ring
Atrioventricular nodal branch of right coronary a.
Inferior interventricular a.

Heart in diastole: viewed from base with atria removed

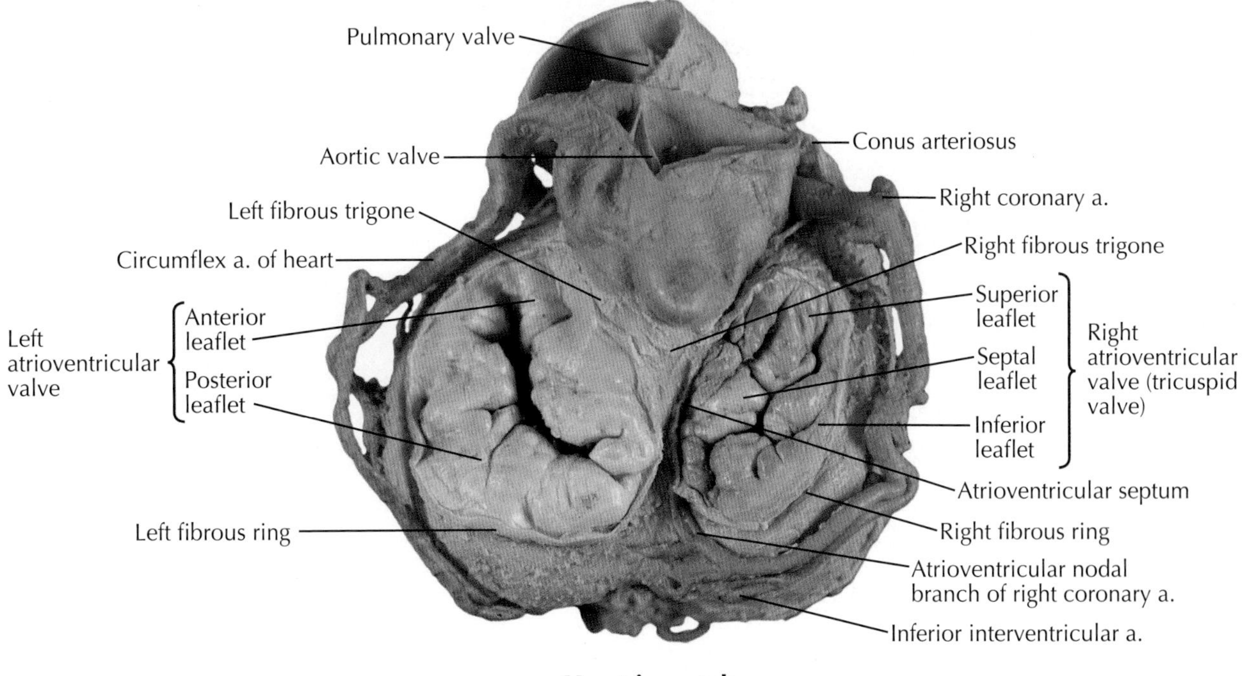
Pulmonary valve
Conus arteriosus
Aortic valve
Right coronary a.
Left fibrous trigone
Right fibrous trigone
Circumflex a. of heart
Superior leaflet
Anterior leaflet
Left atrioventricular valve
Septal leaflet
Right atrioventricular valve (tricuspid valve)
Posterior leaflet
Inferior leaflet
Atrioventricular septum
Left fibrous ring
Right fibrous ring
Atrioventricular nodal branch of right coronary a.
Inferior interventricular a.

Heart in systole: viewed from base with atria removed

Fig. 3.20 Valvular Complex of Heart (Photograph)

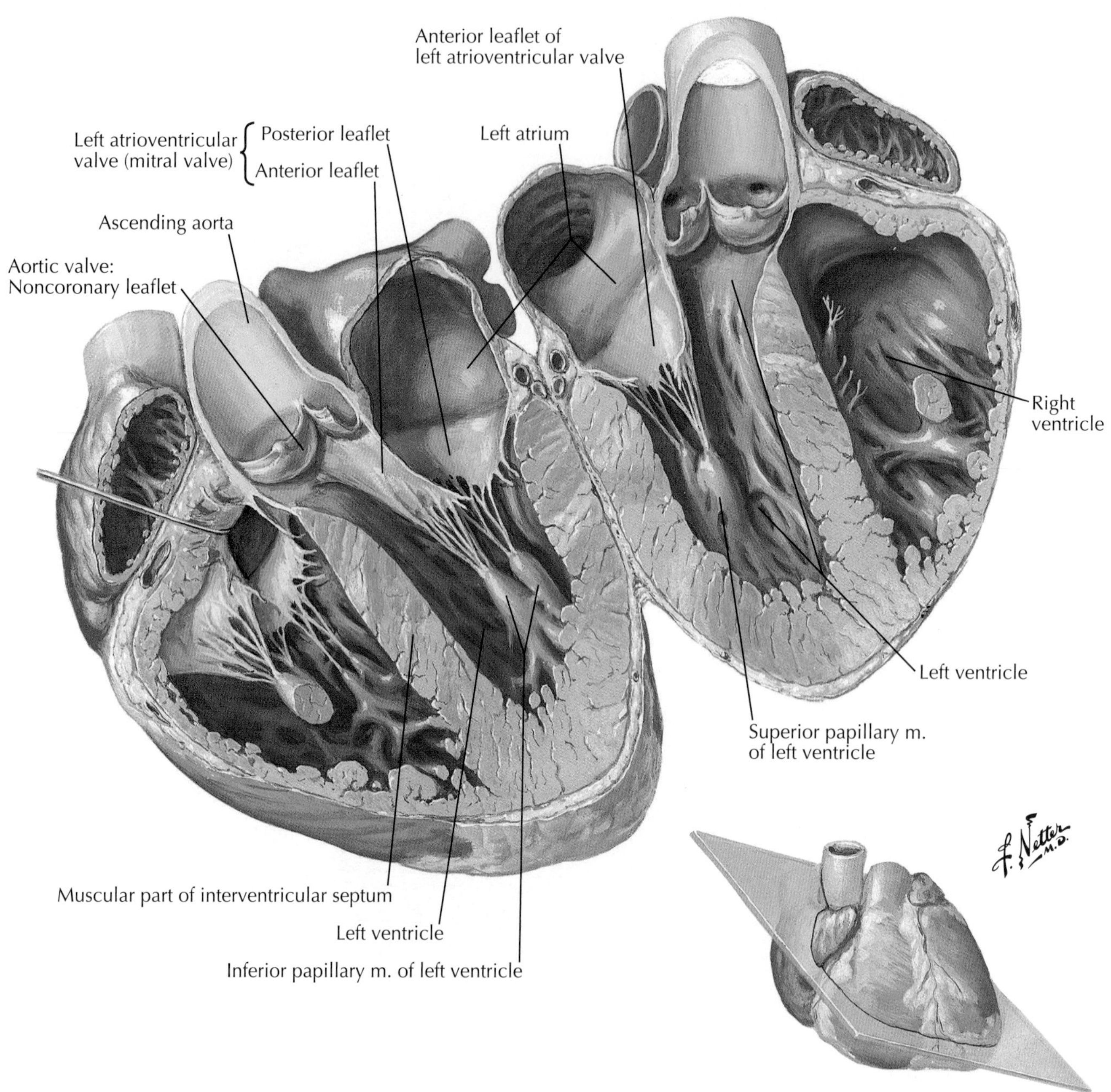
Anterior leaflet of left atrioventricular valve
Left atrioventricular valve (mitral valve)
Posterior leaflet
Anterior leaflet
Left atrium
Ascending aorta
Aortic valve: Noncoronary leaflet
Right ventricle
Left ventricle
Superior papillary m. of left ventricle
Muscular part of interventricular septum
Left ventricle
Inferior papillary m. of left ventricle

Fig. 3.21 Atria, Ventricles, and Interventricular Septum (Illustration)

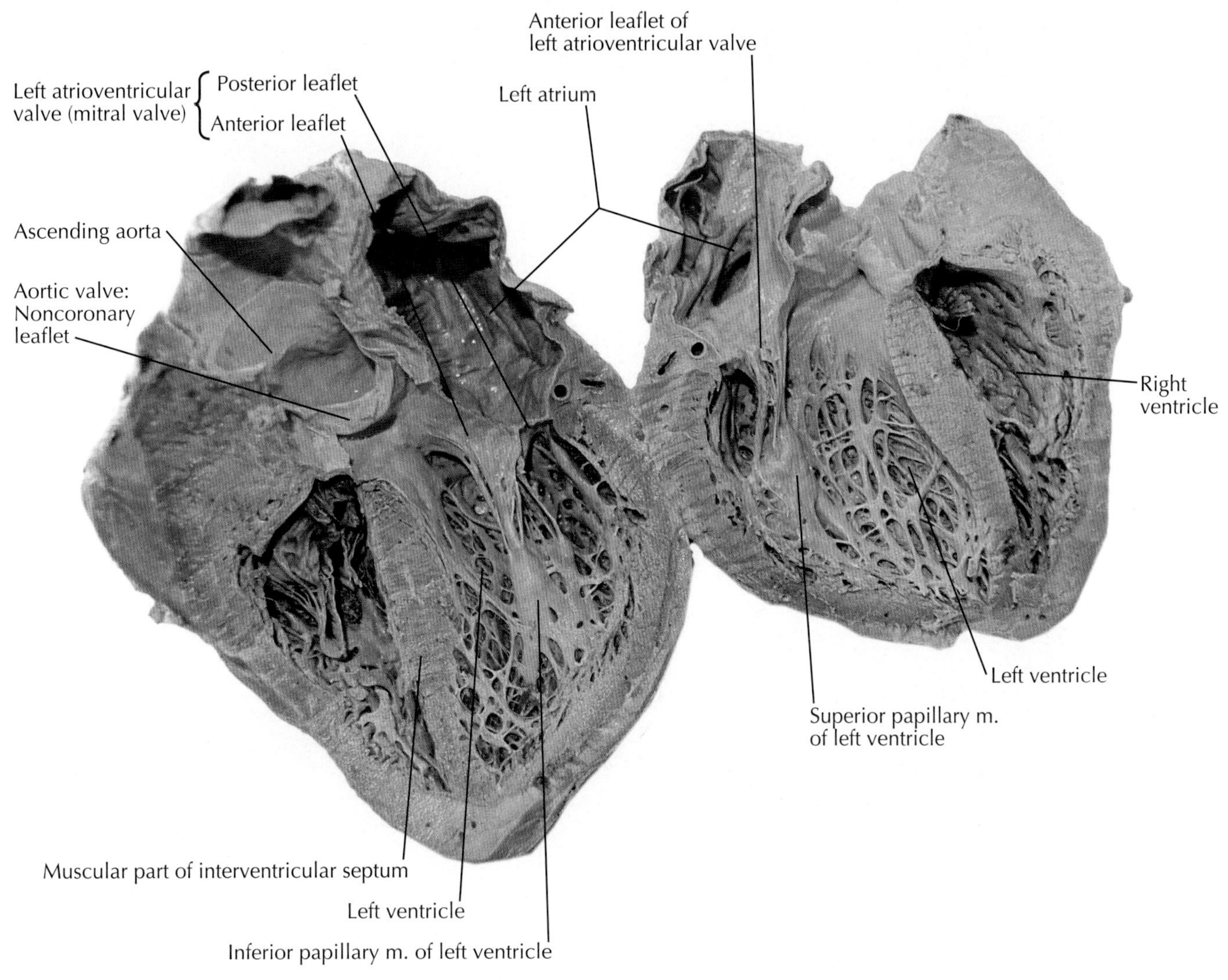
Anterior leaflet of
left atrioventricular valve
Left atrioventricular valve (mitral valve)
Posterior leaflet
Anterior leaflet
Left atrium
Ascending aorta
Aortic valve:
Noncoronary
leaflet
Right
ventricle
Left ventricle
Superior papillary m.
of left ventricle
Muscular part of interventricular septum
Left ventricle
Inferior papillary m. of left ventricle

Fig. 3.22 Atria, Ventricles, and Interventricular Septum (Photograph)

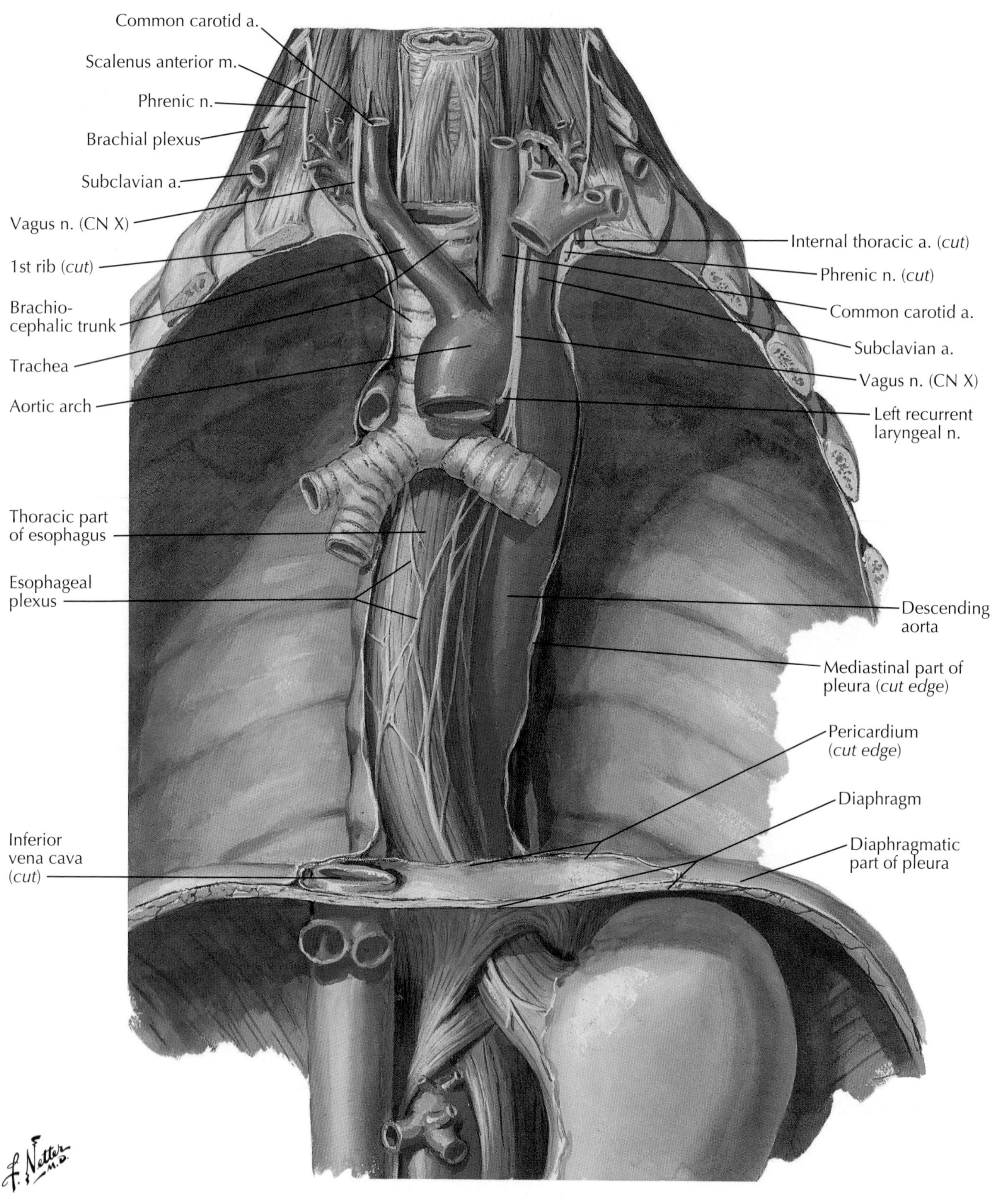
Common carotid a.
Scalenus anterior m.
Phrenic n.
Brachial plexus
Subclavian a.
Vagus n. (CN X)
1st rib (*cut*)
Brachio-cephalic trunk
Trachea
Aortic arch
Thoracic part of esophagus
Esophageal plexus
Inferior vena cava (*cut*)
Internal thoracic a. (*cut*)
Phrenic n. (*cut*)
Common carotid a.
Subclavian a.
Vagus n. (CN X)
Left recurrent laryngeal n.
Descending aorta
Mediastinal part of pleura (*cut edge*)
Pericardium (*cut edge*)
Diaphragm
Diaphragmatic part of pleura

Fig. 3.23 Esophagus In situ (Illustration)

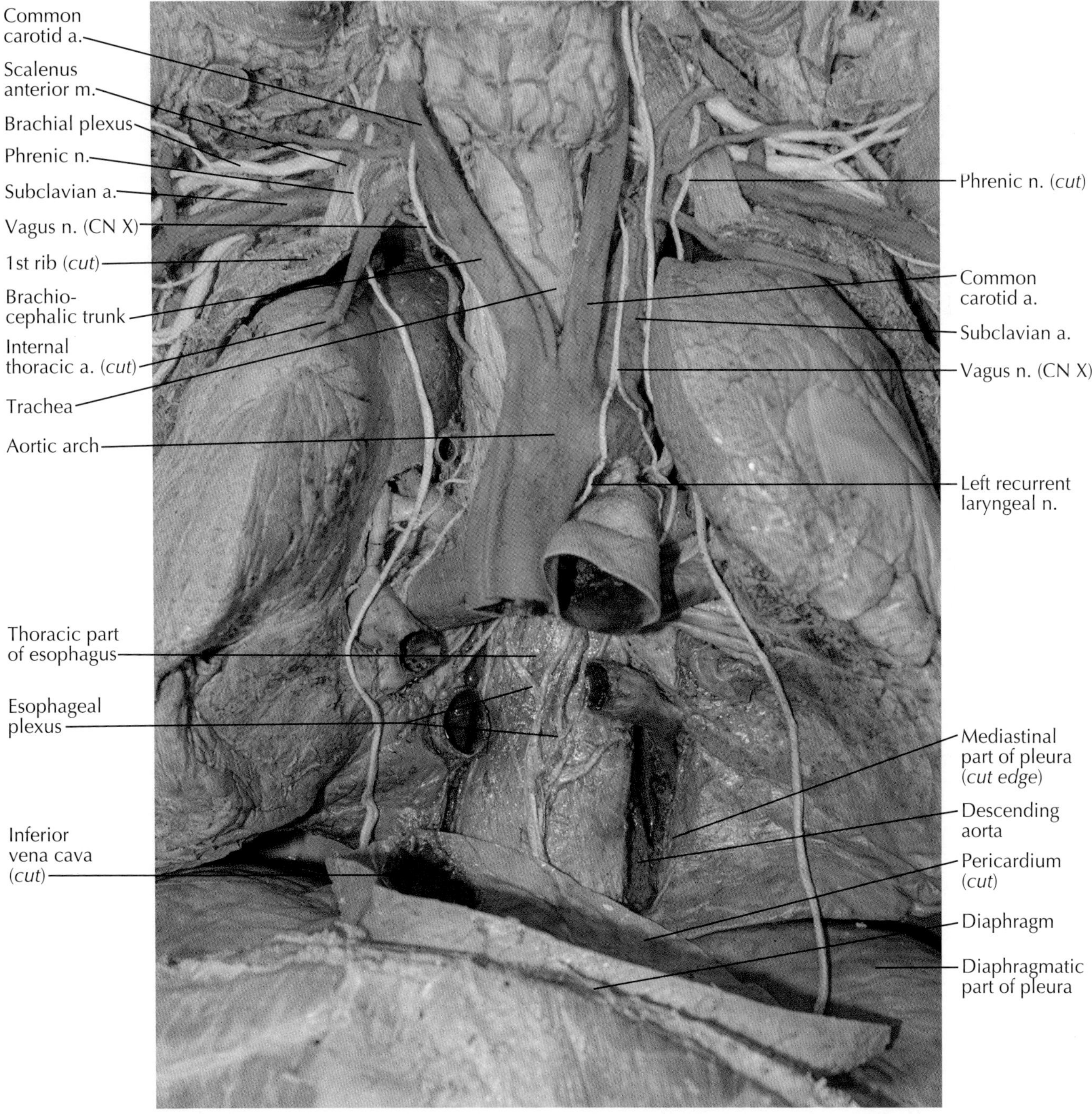
Common carotid a.
Scalenus anterior m.
Brachial plexus
Phrenic n.
Subclavian a.
Vagus n. (CN X)
1st rib (*cut*)
Brachio-cephalic trunk
Internal thoracic a. (*cut*)
Trachea
Aortic arch
Thoracic part of esophagus
Esophageal plexus
Inferior vena cava (*cut*)
Phrenic n. (*cut*)
Common carotid a.
Subclavian a.
Vagus n. (CN X)
Left recurrent laryngeal n.
Mediastinal part of pleura (*cut edge*)
Descending aorta
Pericardium (*cut*)
Diaphragm
Diaphragmatic part of pleura

Fig. 3.24 Esophagus In situ (Photograph) (see Fig. A.8)

CHAPTER

4

ABDOMEN

Alternate Version Available in Appendix

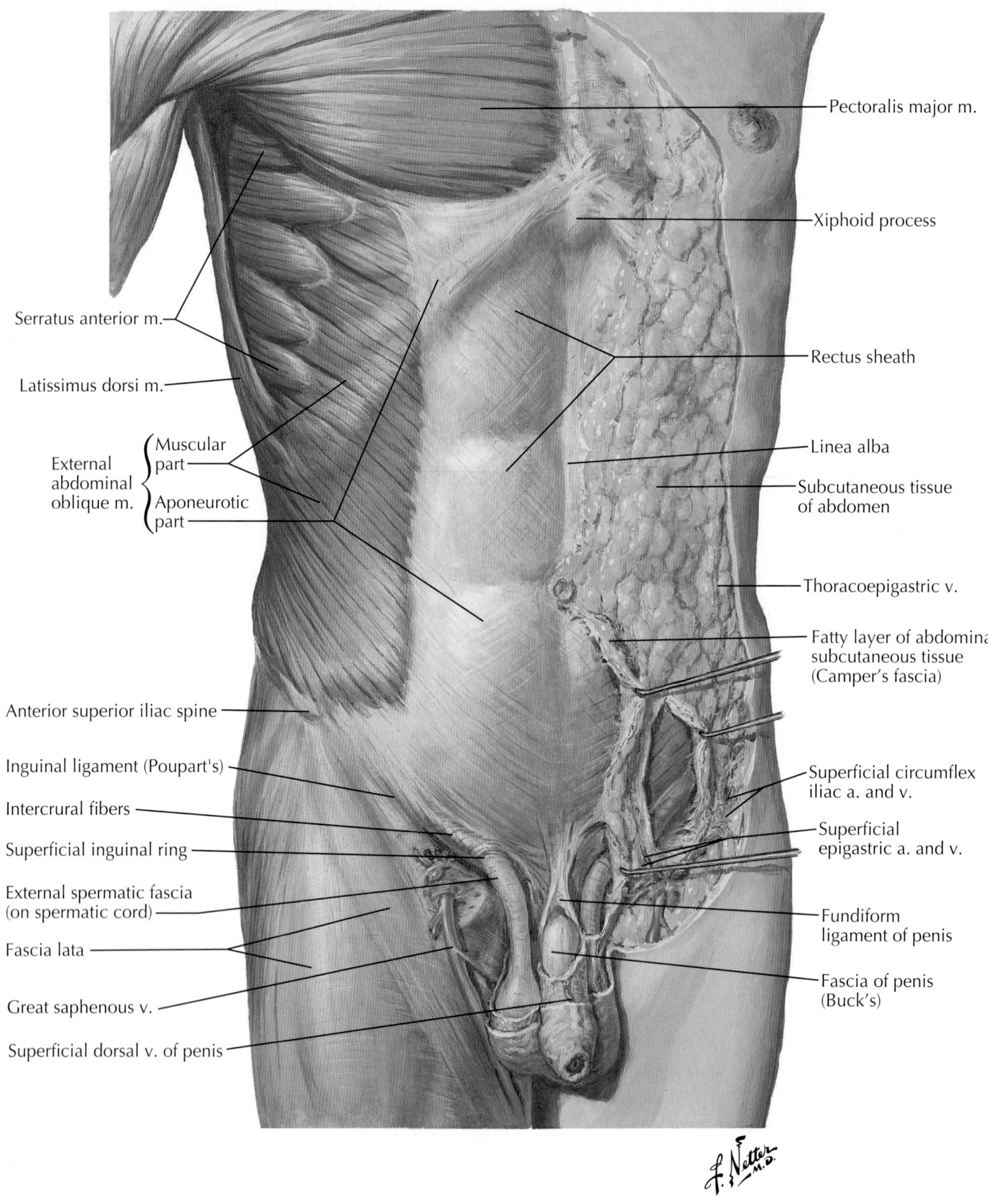
Pectoralis major m.
Xiphoid process
Serratus anterior m.
Rectus sheath
Latissimus dorsi m.
External abdominal oblique m.
Muscular part
Aponeurotic part
Linea alba
Subcutaneous tissue of abdomen
Thoracoepigastric v.
Fatty layer of abdominal subcutaneous tissue (Camper's fascia)
Anterior superior iliac spine
Inguinal ligament (Poupart's)
Superficial circumflex iliac a. and v.
Intercrural fibers
Superficial inguinal ring
Superficial epigastric a. and v.
External spermatic fascia (on spermatic cord)
Fundiform ligament of penis
Fascia lata
Fascia of penis (Buck's)
Great saphenous v.
Superficial dorsal v. of penis
F. Netter M.D.

Fig. 4.1 Anterior Abdominal Wall: Superficial Dissection (Illustration)

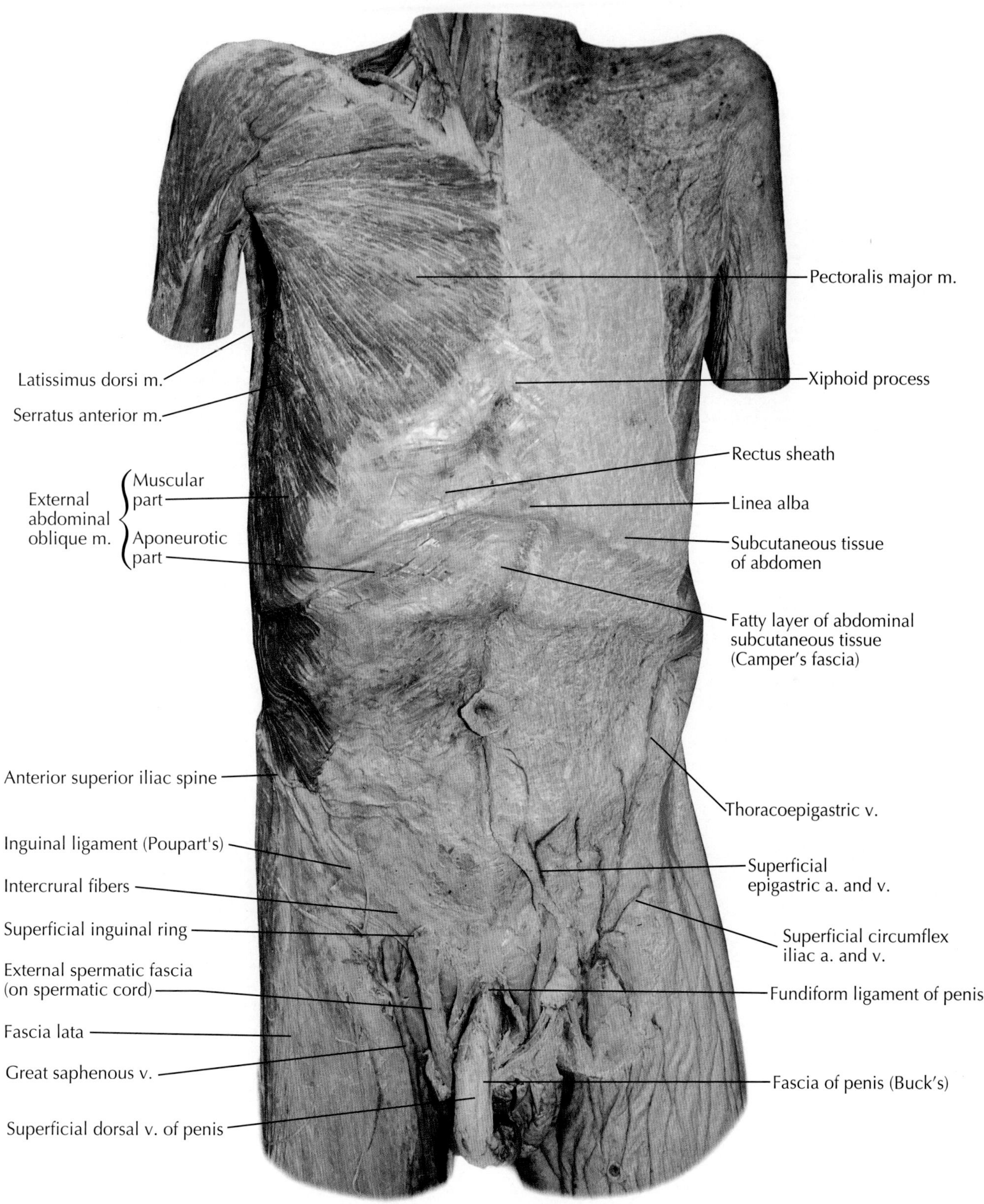
Pectoralis major m.
Latissimus dorsi m.
Xiphoid process
Serratus anterior m.
Rectus sheath
External abdominal oblique m.
Muscular part
Aponeurotic part
Linea alba
Subcutaneous tissue of abdomen
Fatty layer of abdominal subcutaneous tissue (Camper's fascia)
Anterior superior iliac spine
Thoracoepigastric v.
Inguinal ligament (Poupart's)
Superficial epigastric a. and v.
Intercrural fibers
Superficial inguinal ring
Superficial circumflex iliac a. and v.
External spermatic fascia (on spermatic cord)
Fundiform ligament of penis
Fascia lata
Great saphenous v.
Fascia of penis (Buck's)
Superficial dorsal v. of penis

Fig. 4.2 Anterior Abdominal Wall: Superficial Dissection (Photograph)

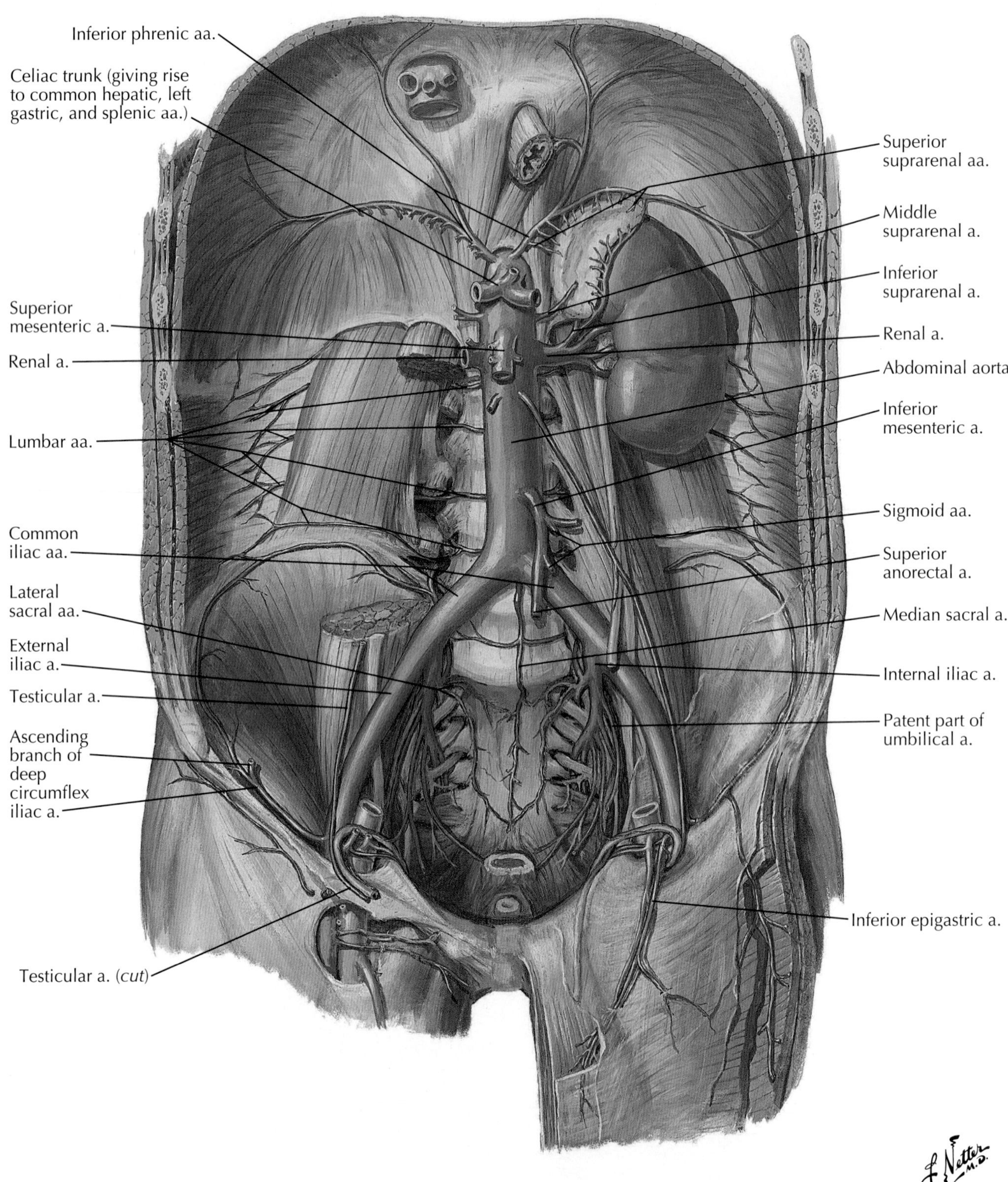
Inferior phrenic aa.
Celiac trunk (giving rise to common hepatic, left gastric, and splenic aa.)
Superior mesenteric a.
Renal a.
Lumbar aa.
Common iliac aa.
Lateral sacral aa.
External iliac a.
Testicular a.
Ascending branch of deep circumflex iliac a.
Testicular a. (cut)
Superior suprarenal aa.
Middle suprarenal a.
Inferior suprarenal a.
Renal a.
Abdominal aorta
Inferior mesenteric a.
Sigmoid aa.
Superior anorectal a.
Median sacral a.
Internal iliac a.
Patent part of umbilical a.
Inferior epigastric a.
F. Netter M.D.

Fig. 4.3 Arteries of Posterior Abdominal Wall (Illustration)

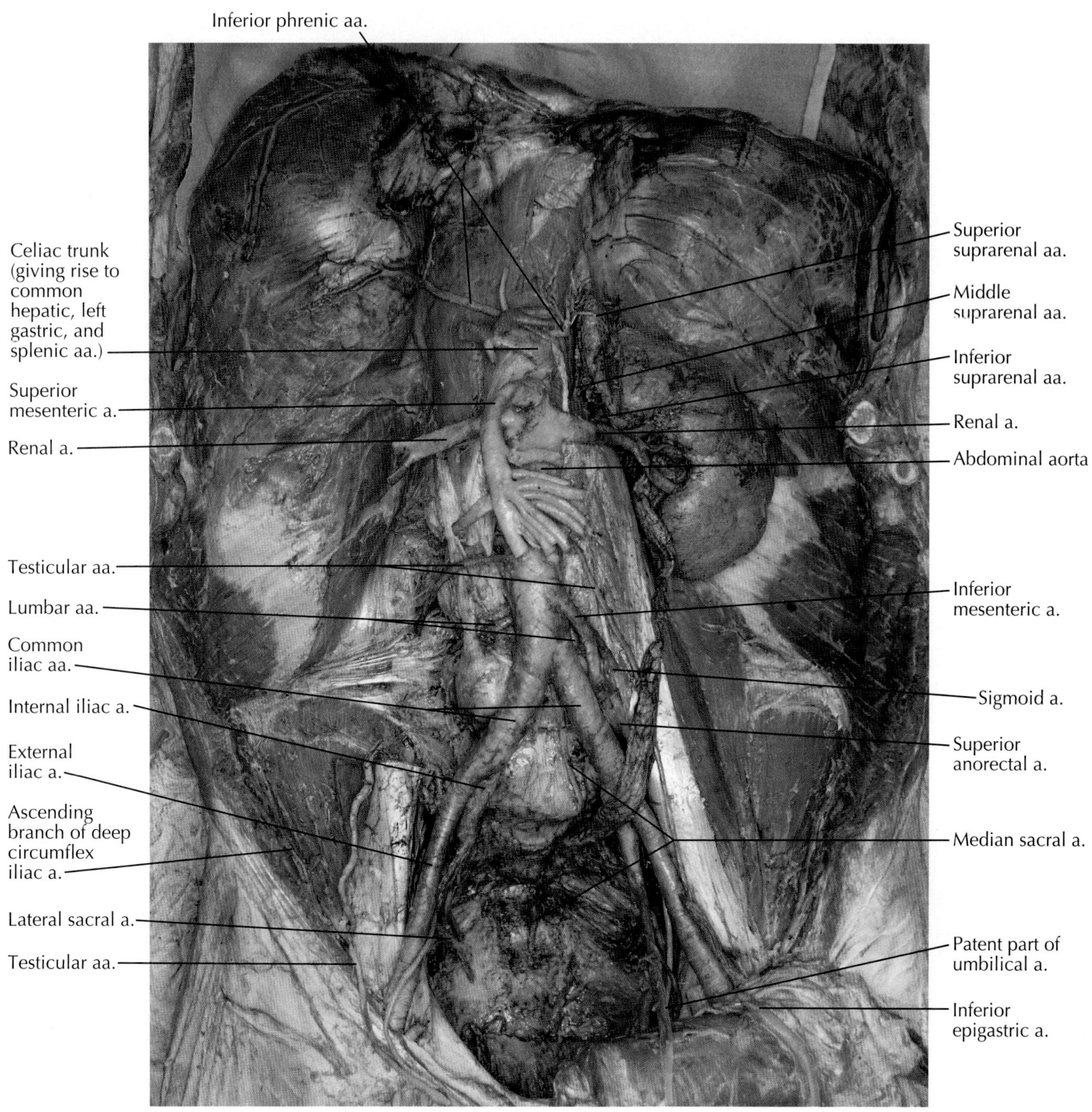
Inferior phrenic aa.
Celiac trunk (giving rise to common hepatic, left gastric, and splenic aa.)
Superior mesenteric a.
Renal a.
Testicular aa.
Lumbar aa.
Common iliac aa.
Internal iliac a.
External iliac a.
Ascending branch of deep circumflex iliac a.
Lateral sacral a.
Testicular aa.
Superior suprarenal aa.
Middle suprarenal aa.
Inferior suprarenal aa.
Renal a.
Abdominal aorta
Inferior mesenteric a.
Sigmoid a.
Superior anorectal a.
Median sacral a.
Patent part of umbilical a.
Inferior epigastric a.

Fig. 4.4 Arteries of Posterior Abdominal Wall (Photograph) (see Fig. A.9)

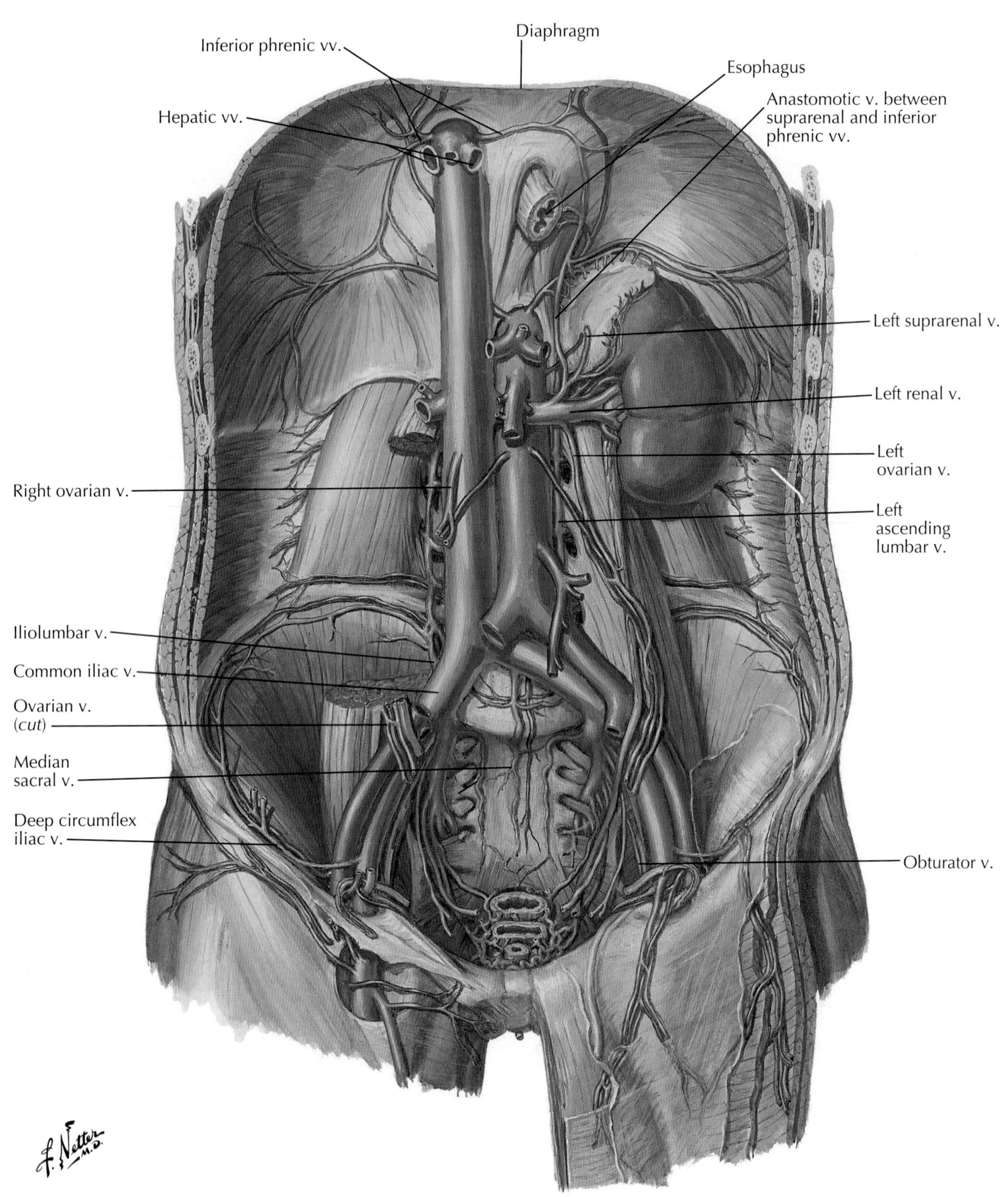
Diaphragm
Inferior phrenic vv.
Esophagus
Anastomotic v. between suprarenal and inferior phrenic vv.
Hepatic vv.
Left suprarenal v.
Left renal v.
Left ovarian v.
Right ovarian v.
Left ascending lumbar v.
Iliolumbar v.
Common iliac v.
Ovarian v. (*cut*)
Median sacral v.
Deep circumflex iliac v.
Obturator v.
F. Netter M.D.

Fig. 4.5 Veins of Posterior Abdominal Wall (Illustration)

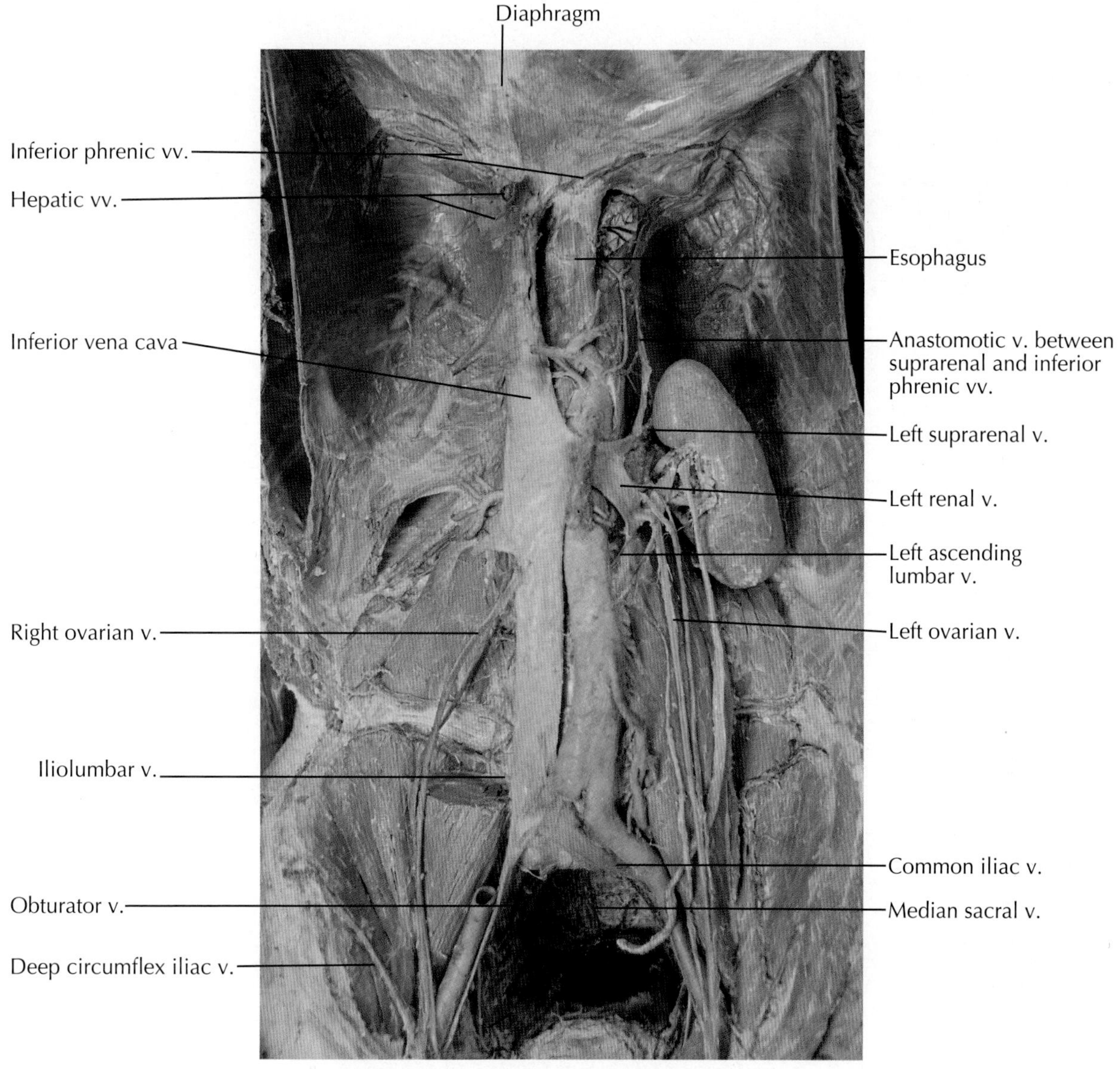
Diaphragm
Inferior phrenic vv.
Hepatic vv.
Esophagus
Inferior vena cava
Anastomotic v. between suprarenal and inferior phrenic vv.
Left suprarenal v.
Left renal v.
Left ascending lumbar v.
Right ovarian v.
Left ovarian v.
Iliolumbar v.
Common iliac v.
Obturator v.
Median sacral v.
Deep circumflex iliac v.

Fig. 4.6 Veins of Posterior Abdominal Wall (Photograph) (see Fig. A.10)

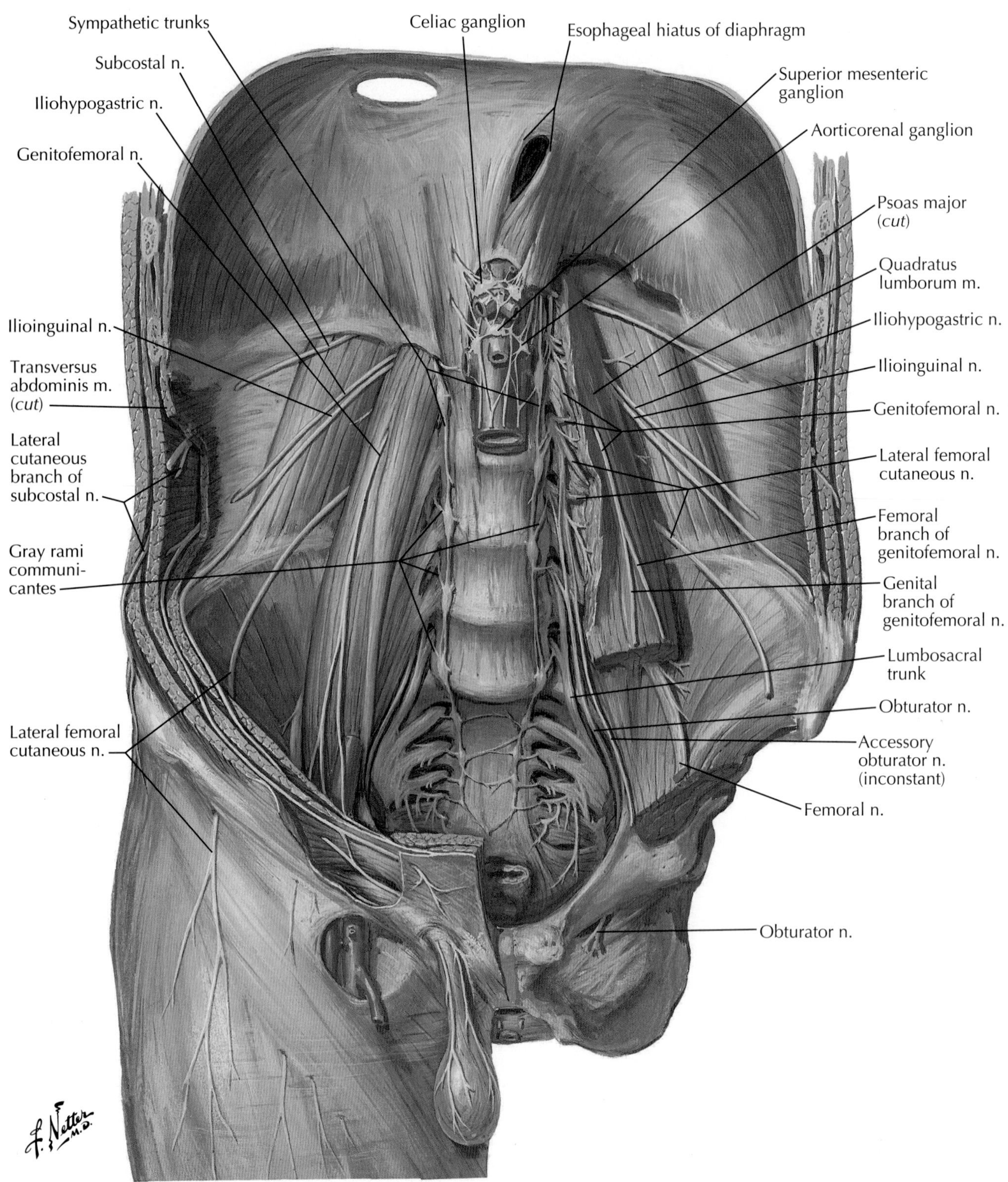
Sympathetic trunks
Celiac ganglion
Esophageal hiatus of diaphragm
Subcostal n.
Superior mesenteric ganglion
Iliohypogastric n.
Aorticorenal ganglion
Genitofemoral n.
Psoas major (cut)
Quadratus lumborum m.
Ilioinguinal n.
Iliohypogastric n.
Ilioinguinal n.
Transversus abdominis m. (cut)
Genitofemoral n.
Lateral cutaneous branch of subcostal n.
Lateral femoral cutaneous n.
Femoral branch of genitofemoral n.
Gray rami communi- cantes
Genital branch of genitofemoral n.
Lumbosacral trunk
Obturator n.
Lateral femoral cutaneous n.
Accessory obturator n. (inconstant)
Femoral n.
Obturator n.
F. Netter M.D.

Fig. 4.7 Nerves of Posterior Abdominal Wall (Illustration)

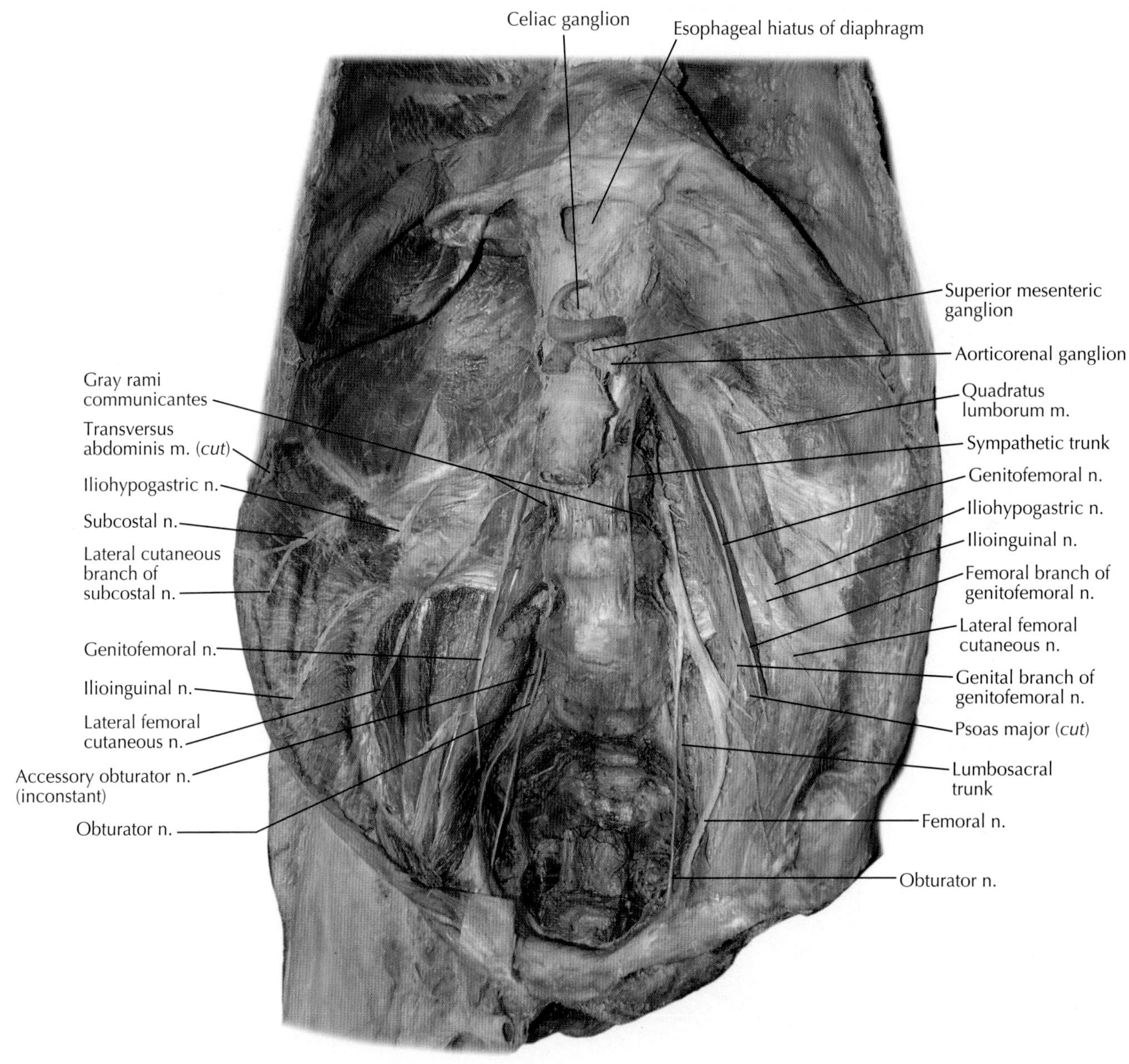

Celiac ganglion
Esophageal hiatus of diaphragm
Superior mesenteric ganglion
Aorticorenal ganglion
Quadratus lumborum m.
Sympathetic trunk
Genitofemoral n.
Iliohypogastric n.
Ilioinguinal n.
Femoral branch of genitofemoral n.
Lateral femoral cutaneous n.
Genital branch of genitofemoral n.
Psoas major (cut)
Lumbosacral trunk
Femoral n.
Obturator n.
Gray rami communicantes
Transversus abdominis m. (cut)
Iliohypogastric n.
Subcostal n.
Lateral cutaneous branch of subcostal n.
Genitofemoral n.
Ilioinguinal n.
Lateral femoral cutaneous n.
Accessory obturator n. (inconstant)
Obturator n.

Fig. 4.8 Nerves of Posterior Abdominal Wall (Photograph)

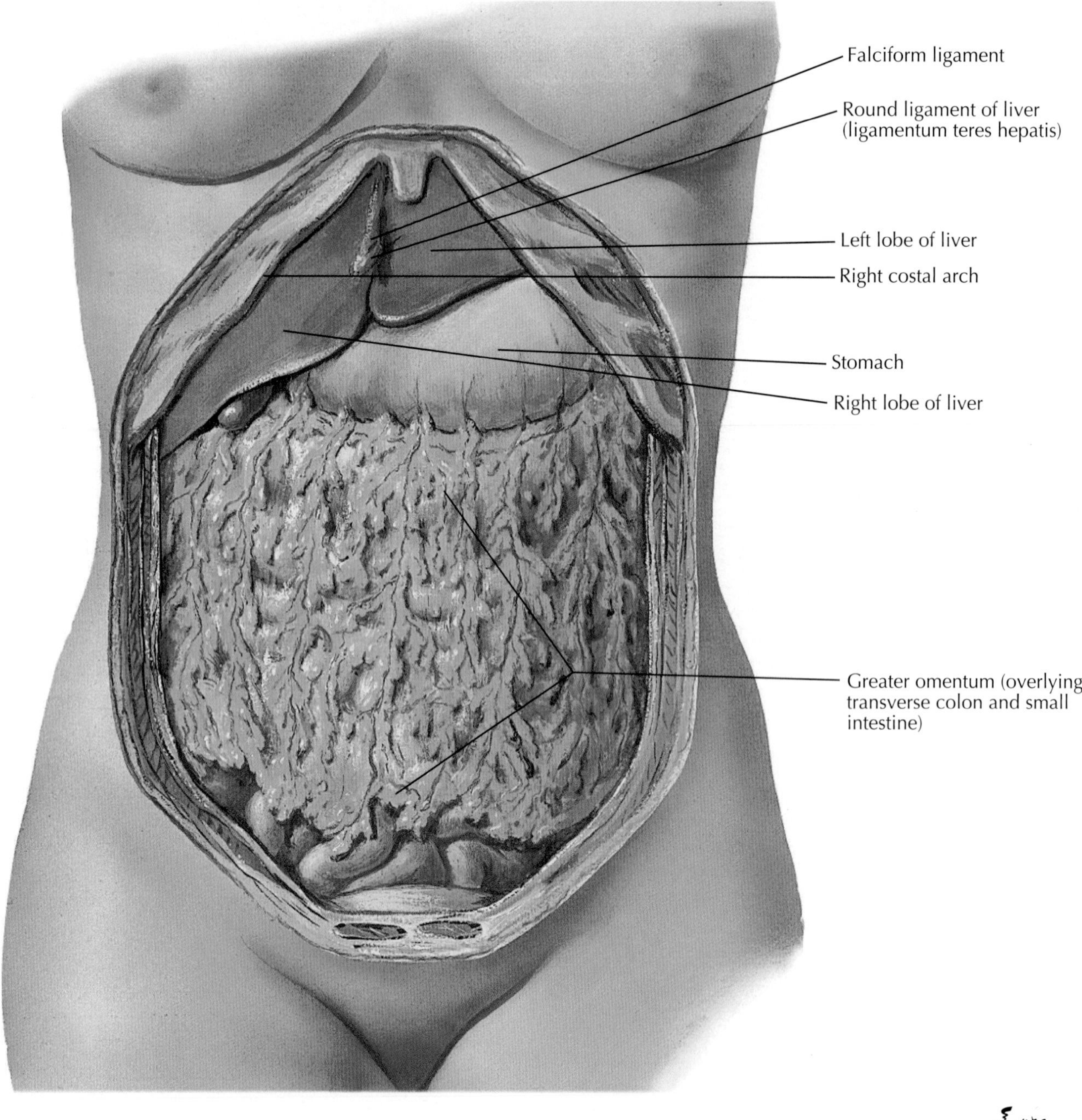
Falciform ligament
Round ligament of liver (ligamentum teres hepatis)
Left lobe of liver
Right costal arch
Stomach
Right lobe of liver
Greater omentum (overlying transverse colon and small intestine)
F. Netter M.D.

Fig. 4.9 Greater Omentum and Abdominal Viscera (Illustration)

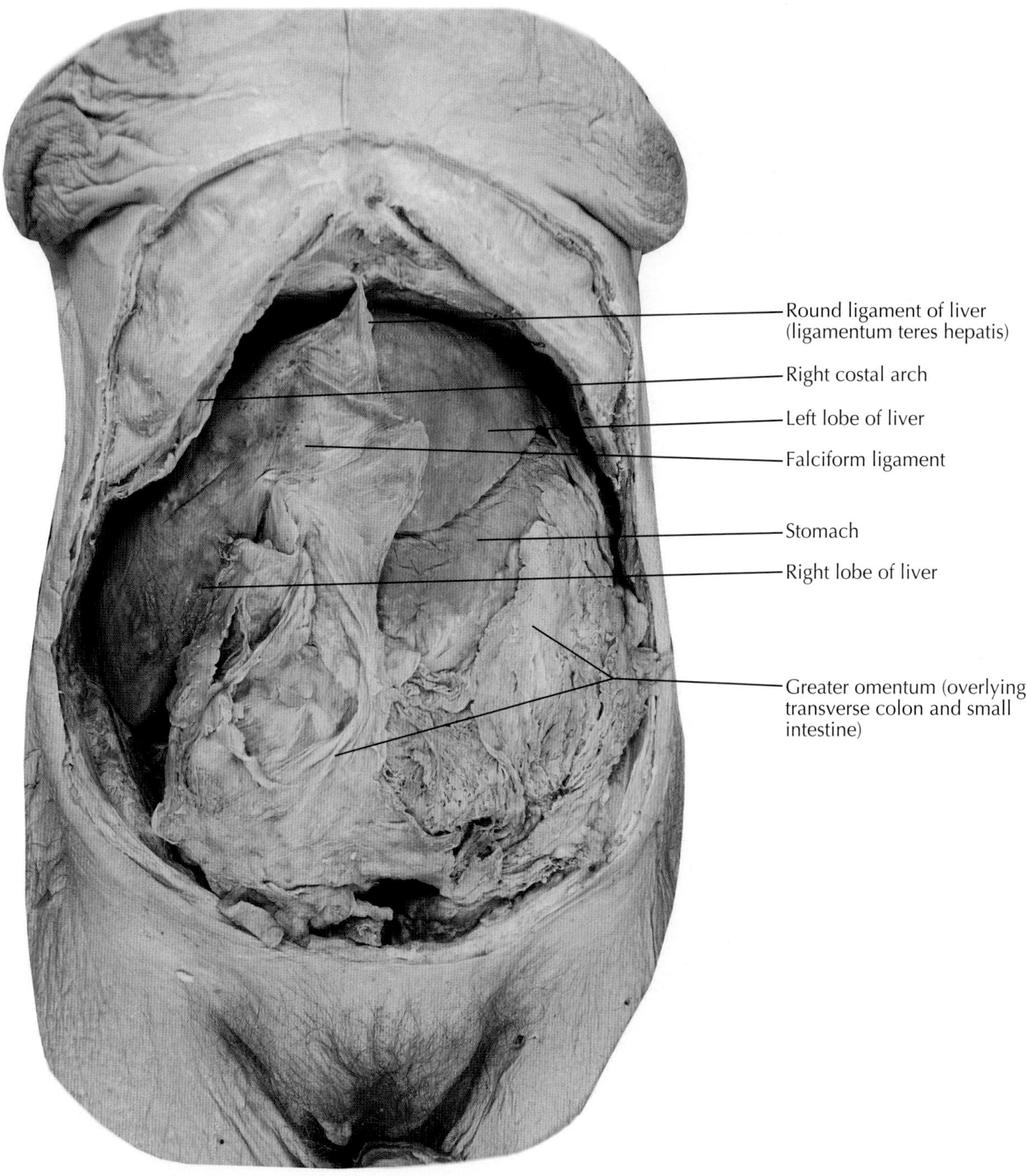
Round ligament of liver (ligamentum teres hepatis)
Right costal arch
Left lobe of liver
Falciform ligament
Stomach
Right lobe of liver
Greater omentum (overlying transverse colon and small intestine)

Fig. 4.10 Greater Omentum and Abdominal Viscera (Photograph)

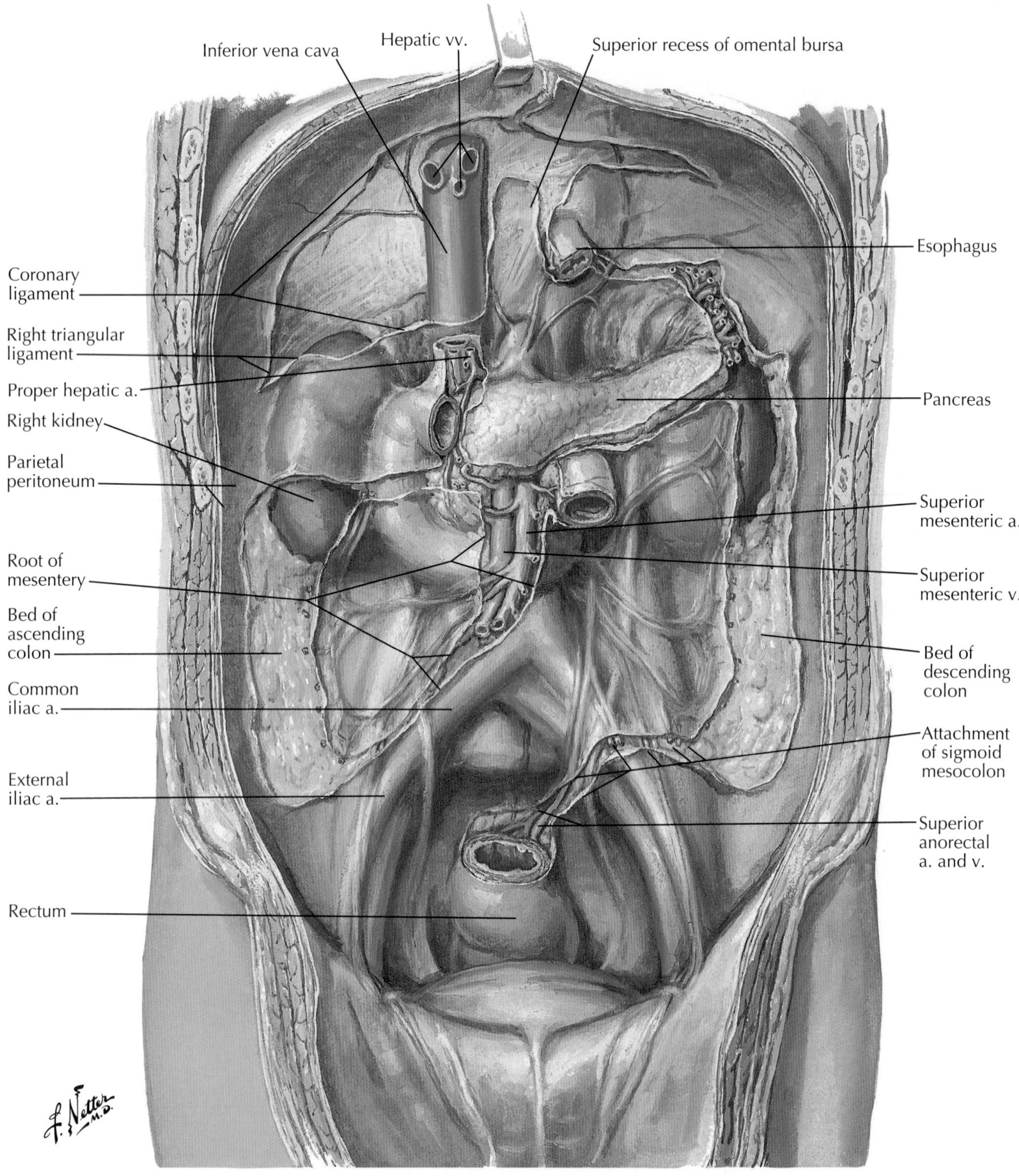
Inferior vena cava
Hepatic vv.
Superior recess of omental bursa
Esophagus
Coronary ligament
Right triangular ligament
Proper hepatic a.
Pancreas
Right kidney
Parietal peritoneum
Superior mesenteric a.
Root of mesentery
Superior mesenteric v.
Bed of ascending colon
Bed of descending colon
Common iliac a.
Attachment of sigmoid mesocolon
External iliac a.
Superior anorectal a. and v.
Rectum

Fig. 4.11 Peritoneum of Posterior Abdominal Wall (Illustration)

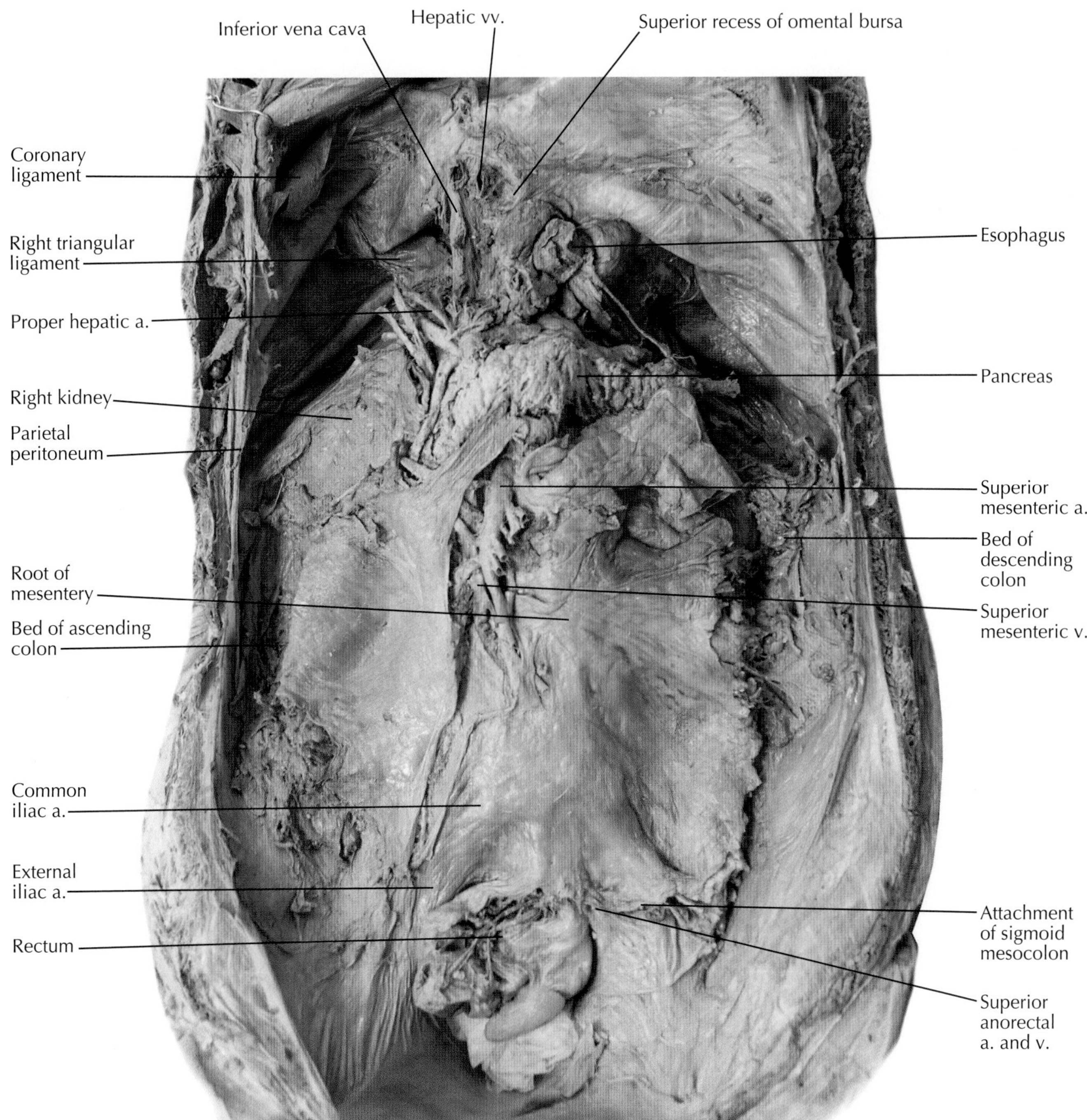
Inferior vena cava
Hepatic vv.
Superior recess of omental bursa
Coronary ligament
Right triangular ligament
Proper hepatic a.
Right kidney
Parietal peritoneum
Root of mesentery
Bed of ascending colon
Common iliac a.
External iliac a.
Rectum
Esophagus
Pancreas
Superior mesenteric a.
Bed of descending colon
Superior mesenteric v.
Attachment of sigmoid mesocolon
Superior anorectal a. and v.

Fig. 4.12 Peritoneum of Posterior Abdominal Wall (Photograph)

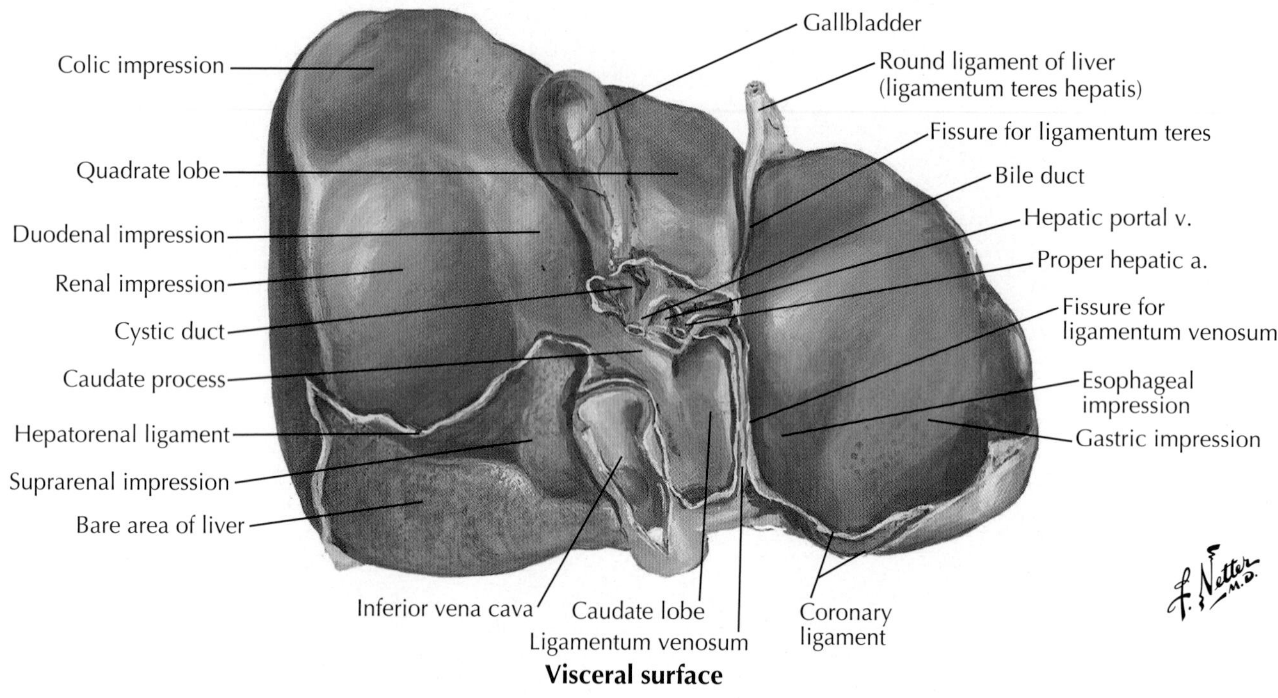
Gallbladder
Round ligament of liver
(ligamentum teres hepatis)
Fissure for ligamentum teres
Bile duct
Hepatic portal v.
Proper hepatic a.
Fissure for
ligamentum venosum
Esophageal
impression
Gastric impression
Colic impression
Quadrate lobe
Duodenal impression
Renal impression
Cystic duct
Caudate process
Hepatorenal ligament
Suprarenal impression
Bare area of liver
Inferior vena cava
Caudate lobe
Ligamentum venosum
Coronary
ligament
Visceral surface

Fig. 4.13 Surfaces and Bed of Liver (Illustration)

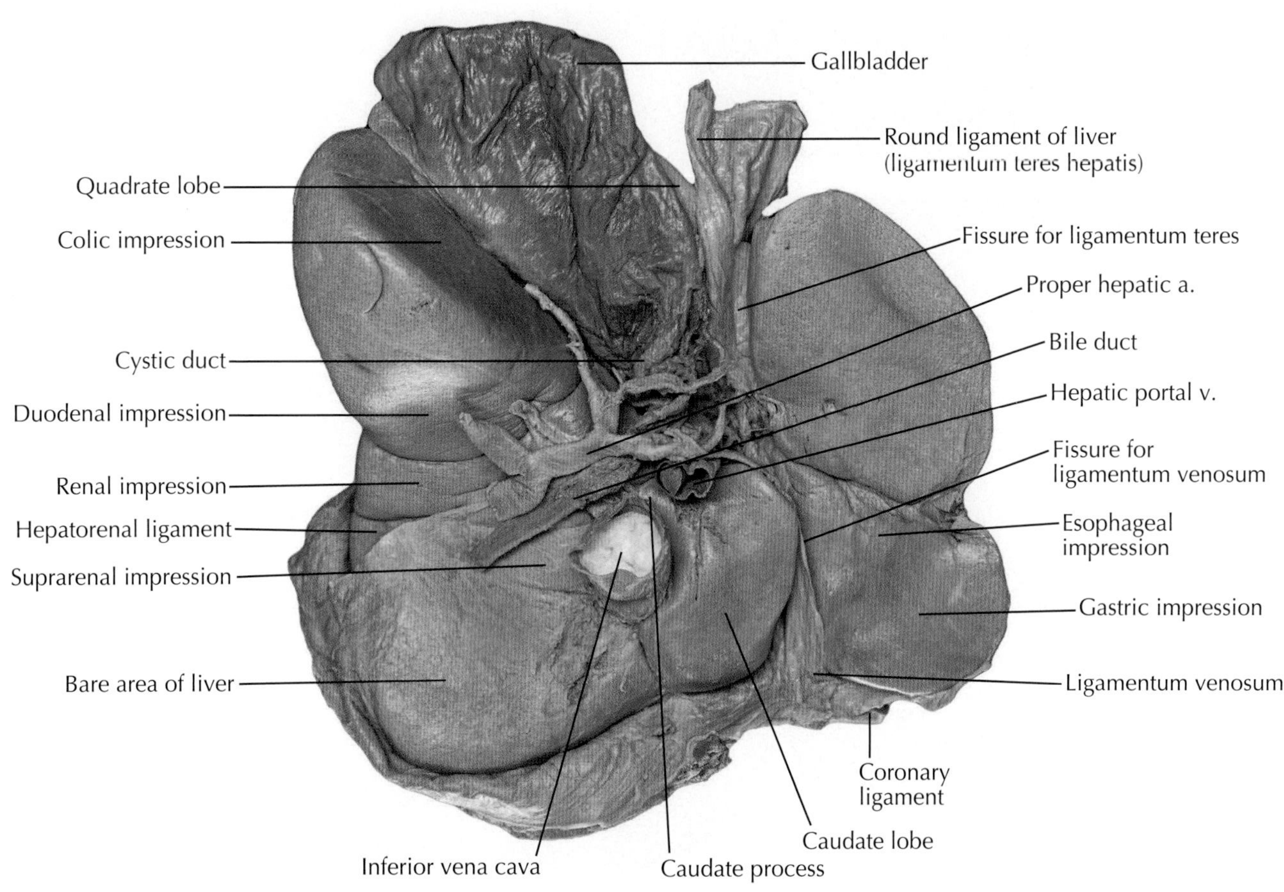
Gallbladder
Round ligament of liver (ligamentum teres hepatis)
Quadrate lobe
Colic impression
Fissure for ligamentum teres
Proper hepatic a.
Cystic duct
Bile duct
Hepatic portal v.
Duodenal impression
Fissure for ligamentum venosum
Renal impression
Hepatorenal ligament
Esophageal impression
Suprarenal impression
Gastric impression
Bare area of liver
Ligamentum venosum
Coronary ligament
Caudate lobe
Inferior vena cava
Caudate process

Visceral surface

Fig. 4.14 Surfaces and Bed of Liver (Photograph)

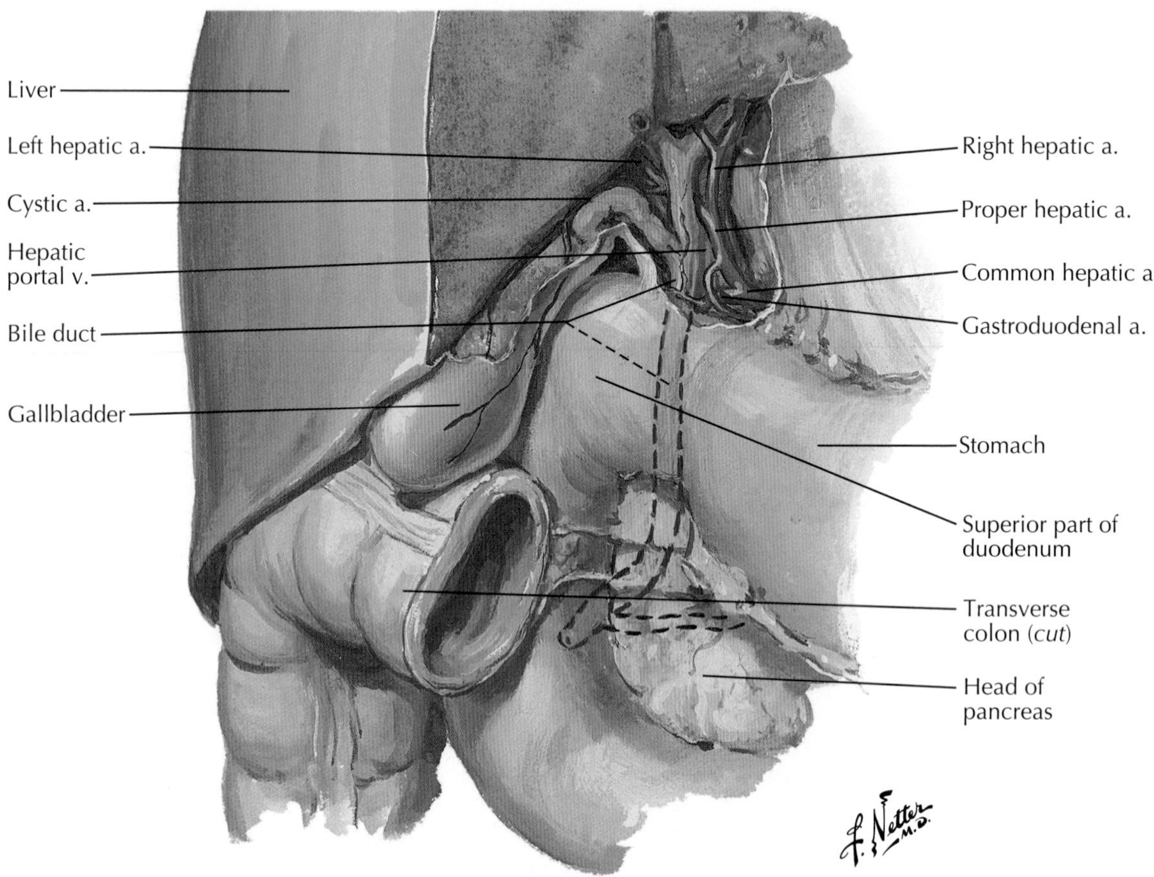
Liver
Left hepatic a.
Cystic a.
Hepatic portal v.
Bile duct
Gallbladder
Right hepatic a.
Proper hepatic a.
Common hepatic a.
Gastroduodenal a.
Stomach
Superior part of duodenum
Transverse colon (*cut*)
Head of pancreas

Fig. 4.15 Gallbladder, Extrahepatic Bile Ducts, and Pancreatic Duct (Illustration)

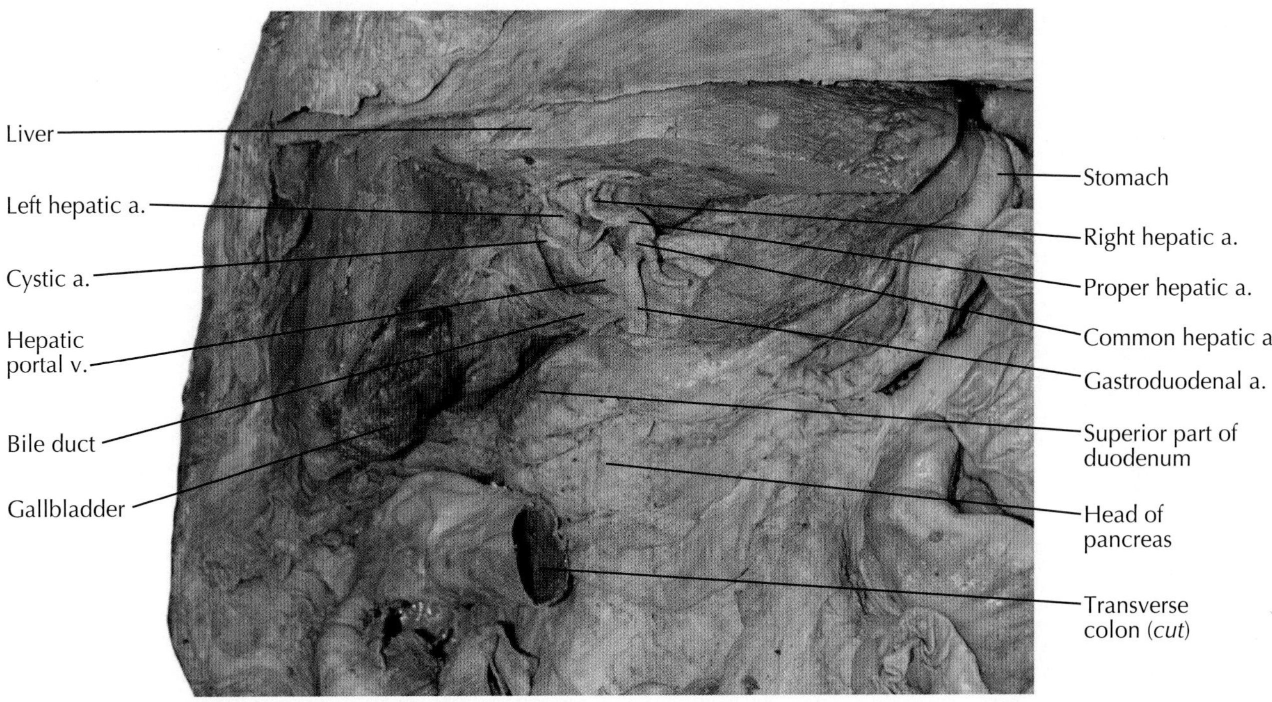
Liver
Left hepatic a.
Cystic a.
Hepatic portal v.
Bile duct
Gallbladder
Stomach
Right hepatic a.
Proper hepatic a.
Common hepatic a.
Gastroduodenal a.
Superior part of duodenum
Head of pancreas
Transverse colon (*cut*)

Fig. 4.16 Gallbladder, Extrahepatic Bile Ducts, and Pancreatic Duct (Photograph)

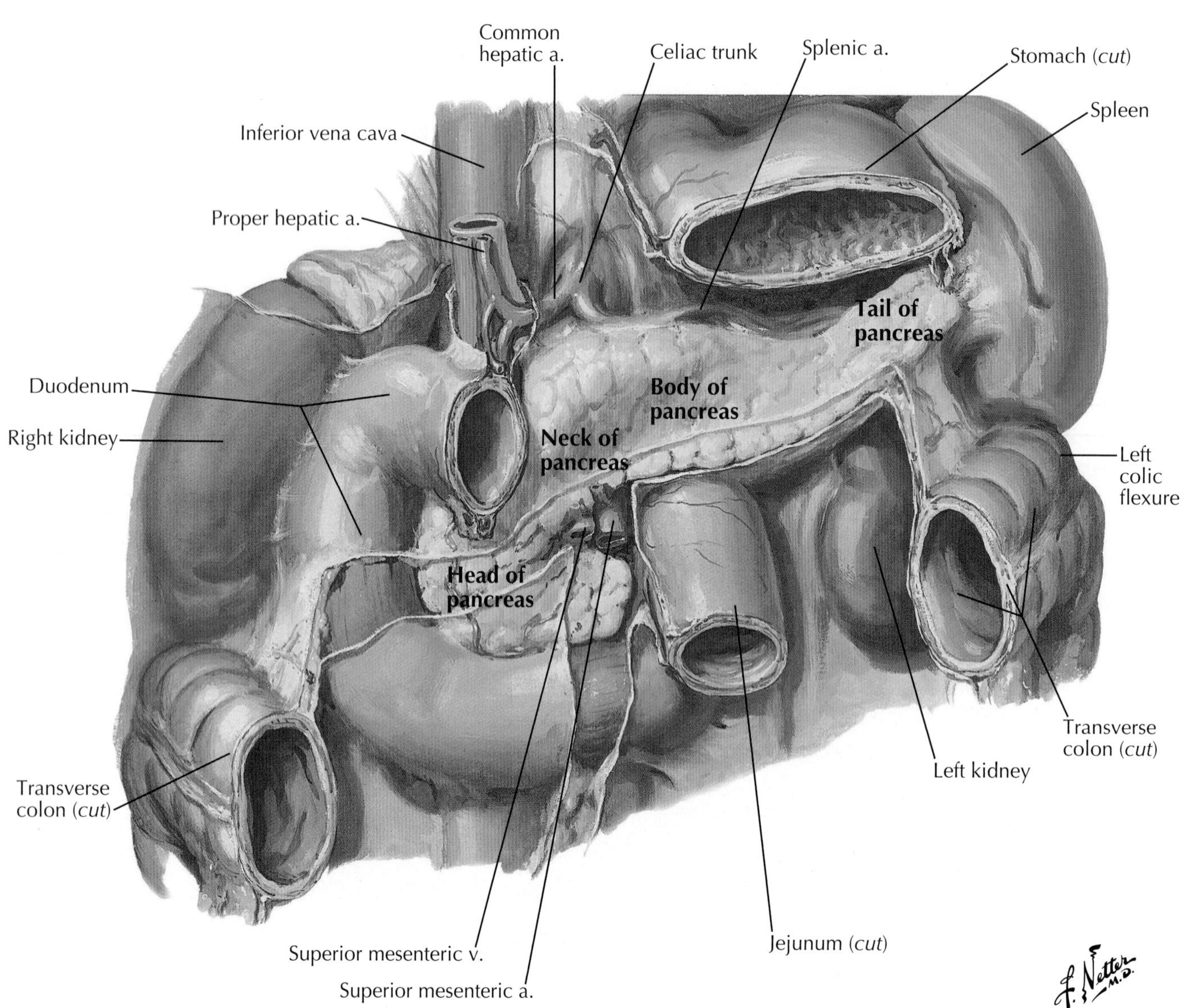
Common hepatic a.
Celiac trunk
Splenic a.
Stomach (cut)
Spleen
Inferior vena cava
Proper hepatic a.
Tail of pancreas
Body of pancreas
Neck of pancreas
Duodenum
Right kidney
Left colic flexure
Head of pancreas
Transverse colon (cut)
Left kidney
Transverse colon (cut)
Superior mesenteric v.
Superior mesenteric a.
Jejunum (cut)
F. Netter M.D.

Fig. 4.17 Pancreas In situ (Illustration)

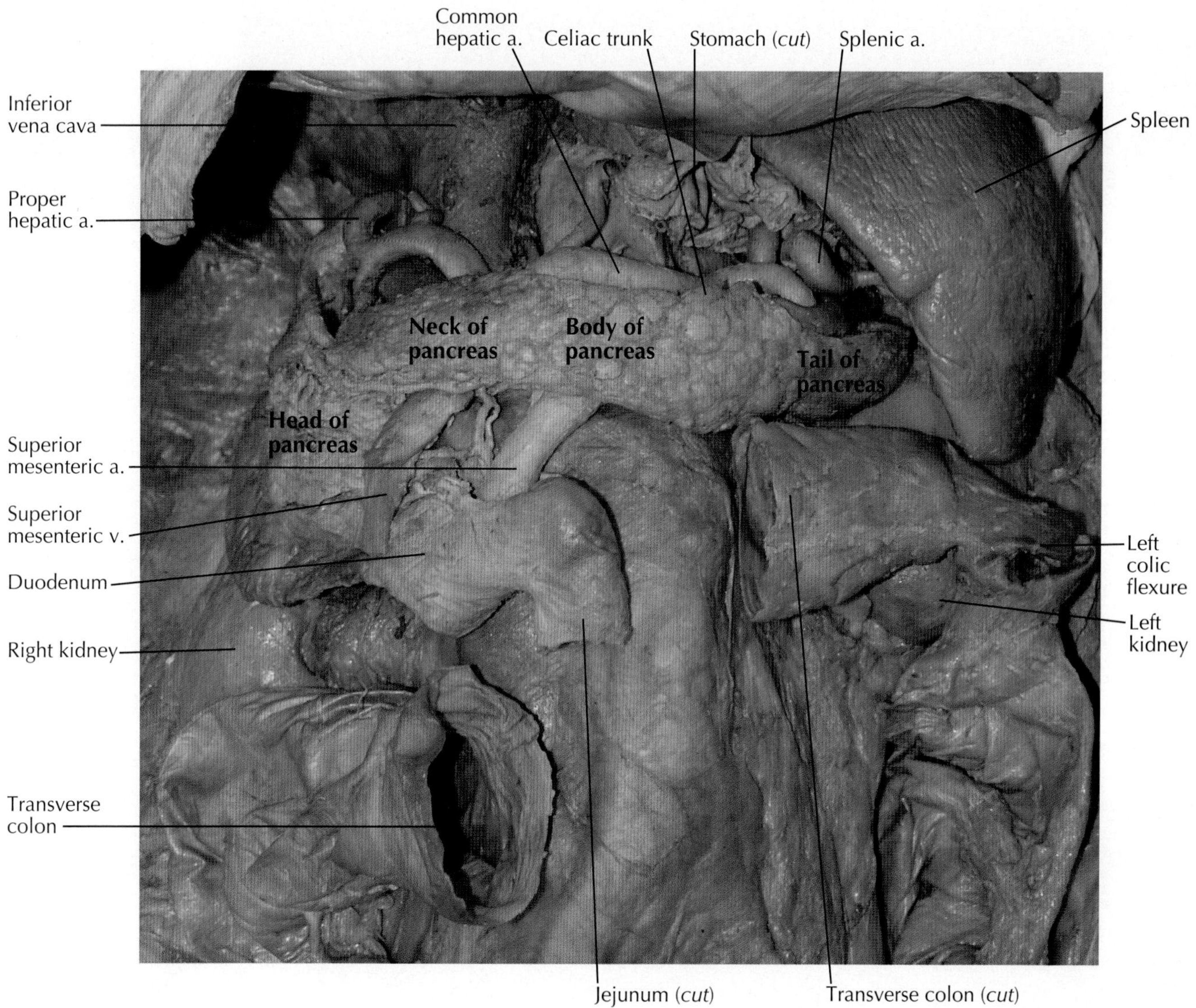
Common hepatic a.
Celiac trunk
Stomach (*cut*)
Splenic a.
Inferior vena cava
Spleen
Proper hepatic a.
Neck of pancreas
Body of pancreas
Tail of pancreas
Head of pancreas
Superior mesenteric a.
Superior mesenteric v.
Duodenum
Left colic flexure
Left kidney
Right kidney
Transverse colon
Jejunum (*cut*)
Transverse colon (*cut*)

Fig. 4.18 Pancreas In situ (Photograph)

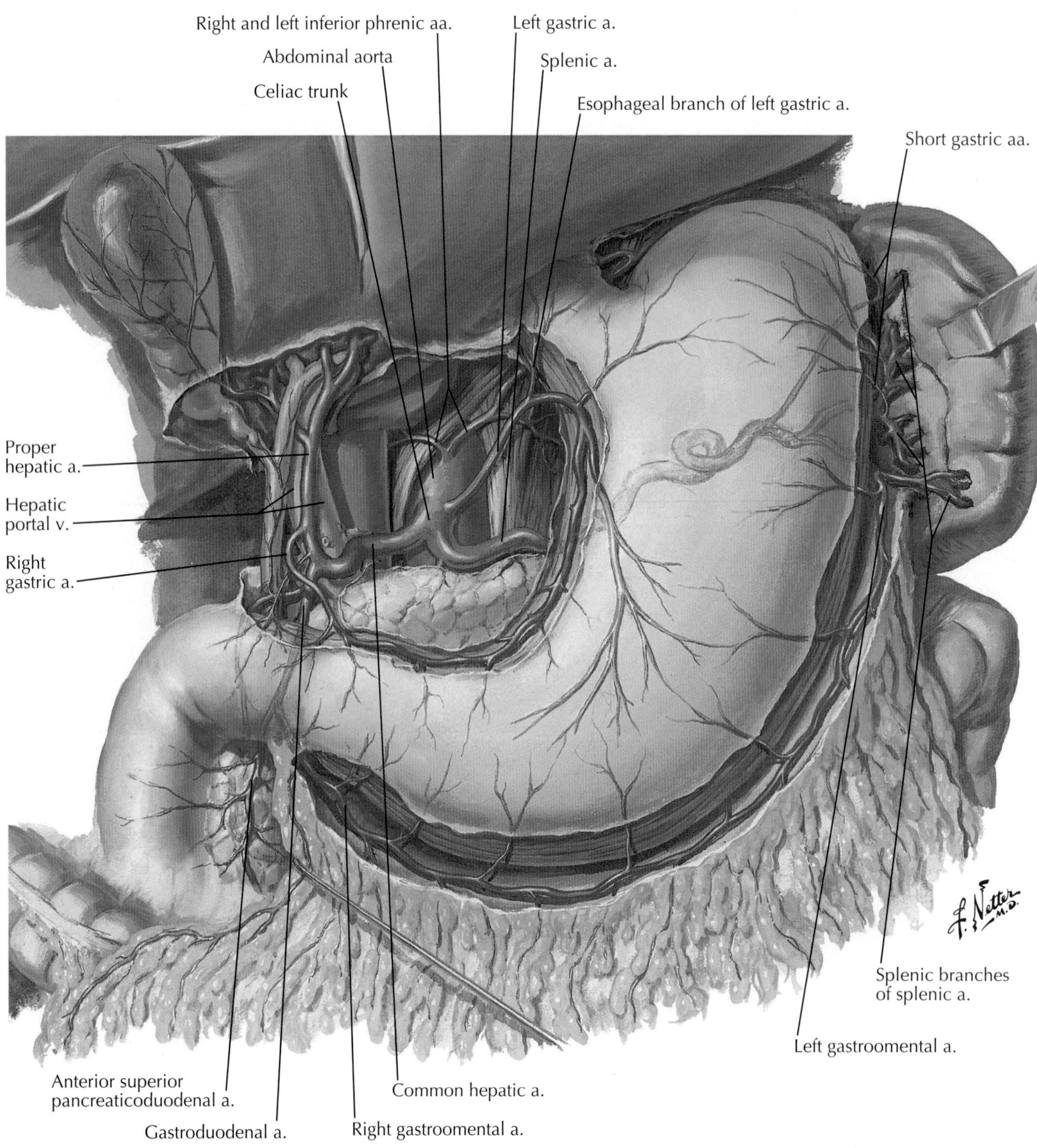
Right and left inferior phrenic aa.
Abdominal aorta
Celiac trunk
Left gastric a.
Splenic a.
Esophageal branch of left gastric a.
Short gastric aa.
Proper hepatic a.
Hepatic portal v.
Right gastric a.
Splenic branches of splenic a.
Left gastroomental a.
Anterior superior pancreaticoduodenal a.
Common hepatic a.
Gastroduodenal a.
Right gastroomental a.

Fig. 4.19 Arteries of Stomach, Liver, and Spleen (Illustration)

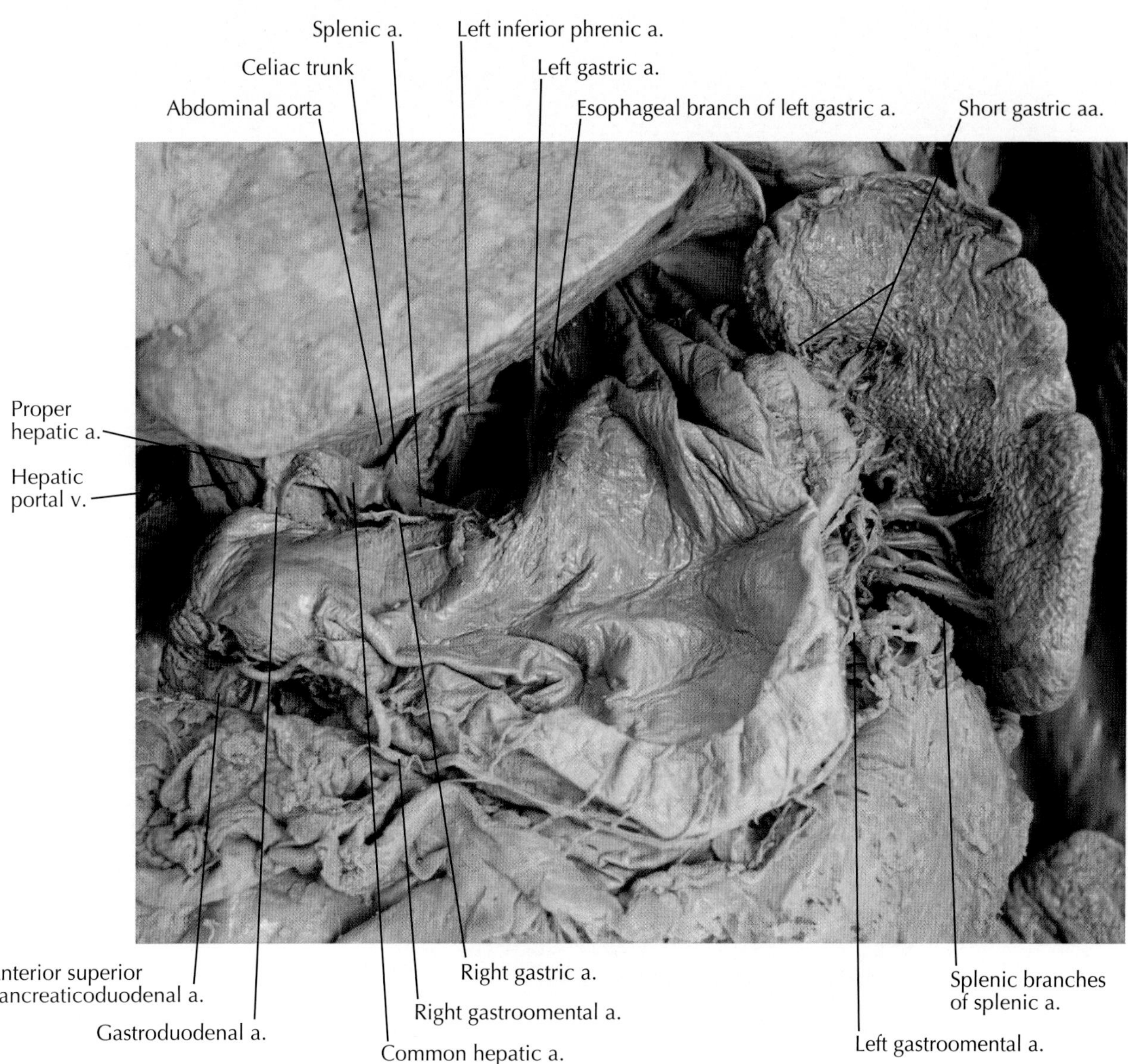
Splenic a.
Left inferior phrenic a.
Celiac trunk
Left gastric a.
Abdominal aorta
Esophageal branch of left gastric a.
Short gastric aa.
Proper hepatic a.
Hepatic portal v.
Anterior superior pancreaticoduodenal a.
Gastroduodenal a.
Right gastric a.
Right gastroomental a.
Common hepatic a.
Splenic branches of splenic a.
Left gastroomental a.

Fig. 4.20 Arteries of Stomach, Liver, and Spleen (Photograph)

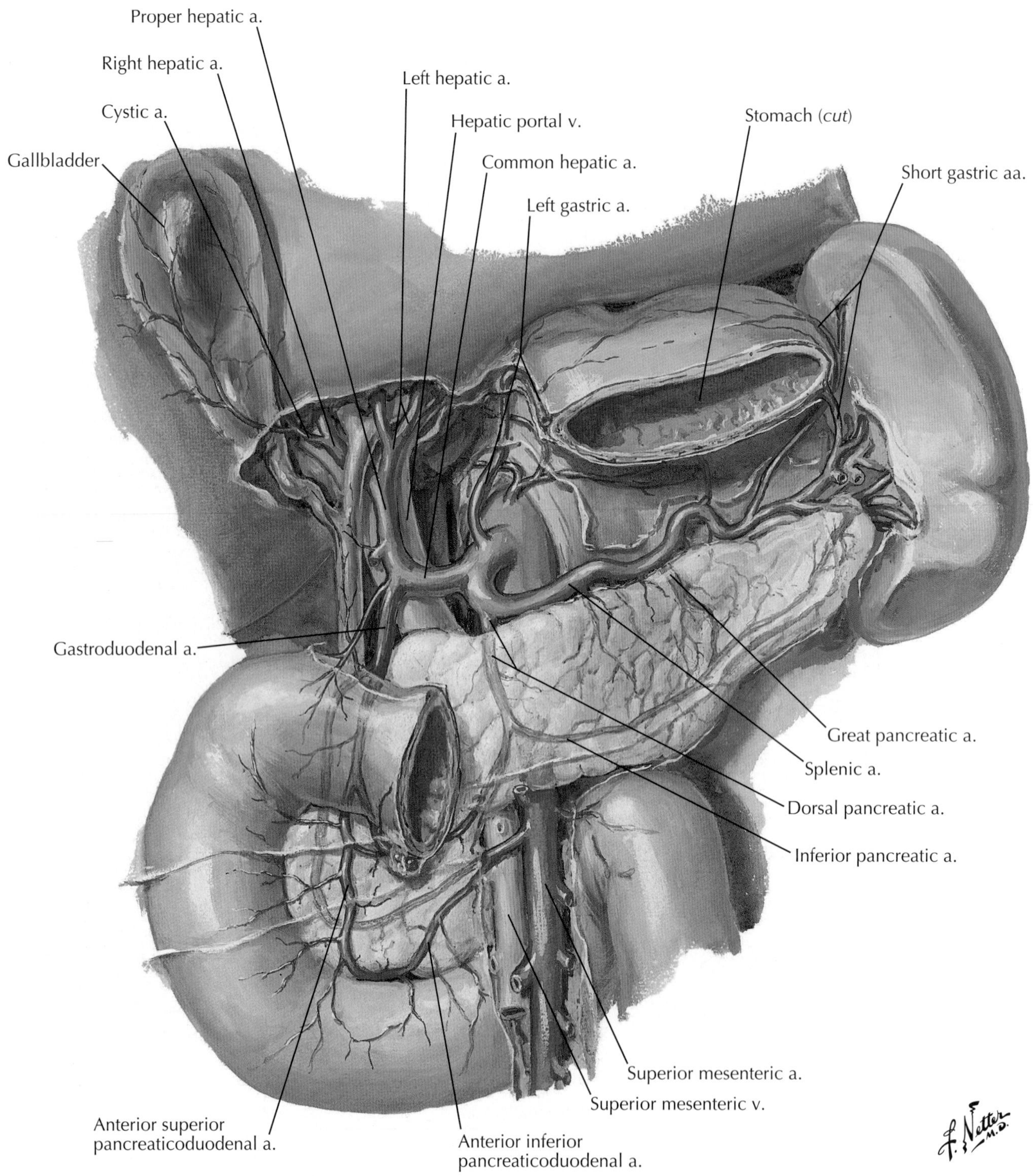
Proper hepatic a.
Right hepatic a.
Left hepatic a.
Cystic a.
Hepatic portal v.
Stomach (*cut*)
Gallbladder
Common hepatic a.
Short gastric aa.
Left gastric a.
Gastroduodenal a.
Great pancreatic a.
Splenic a.
Dorsal pancreatic a.
Inferior pancreatic a.
Superior mesenteric a.
Superior mesenteric v.
Anterior superior pancreaticoduodenal a.
Anterior inferior pancreaticoduodenal a.

Fig. 4.21 Arteries of Liver, Pancreas, Duodenum, and Spleen (Illustration)

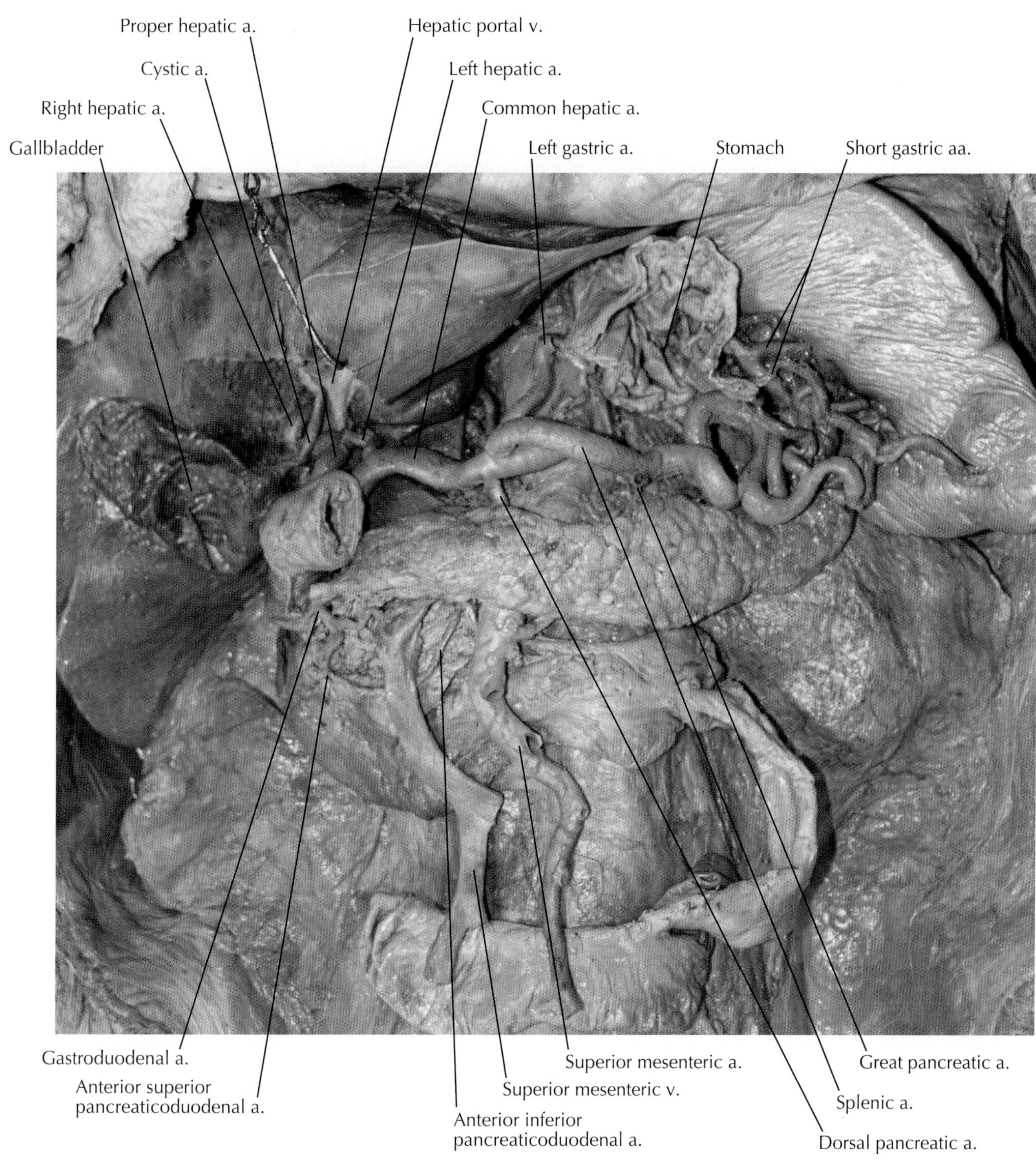
Proper hepatic a.
Hepatic portal v.
Cystic a.
Left hepatic a.
Right hepatic a.
Common hepatic a.
Gallbladder
Left gastric a.
Stomach
Short gastric aa.
Gastroduodenal a.
Anterior superior pancreaticoduodenal a.
Superior mesenteric a.
Superior mesenteric v.
Anterior inferior pancreaticoduodenal a.
Great pancreatic a.
Splenic a.
Dorsal pancreatic a.

Fig. 4.22 Arteries of Liver, Pancreas, Duodenum, and Spleen (Photograph) (see Fig. A.11)

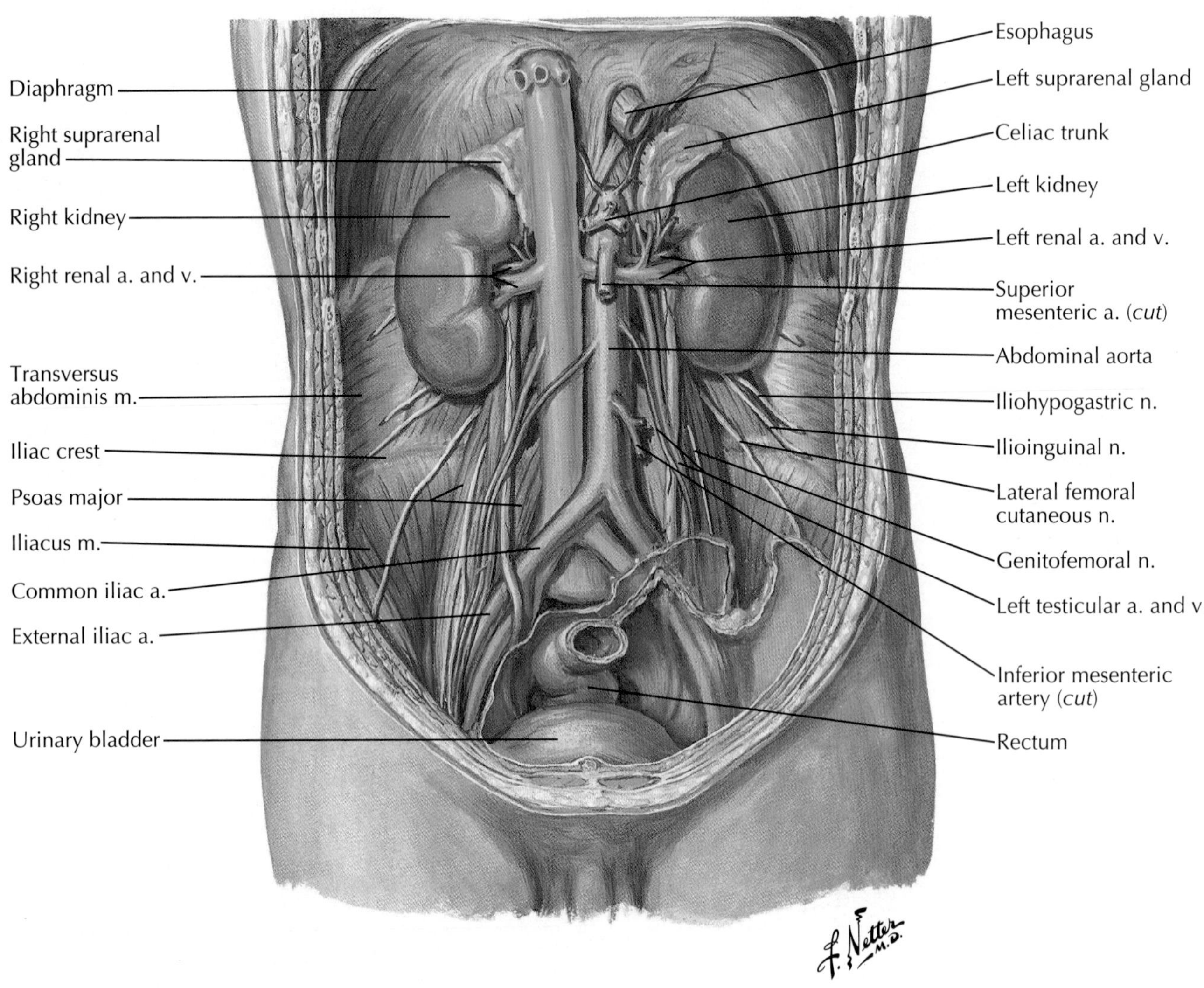
Diaphragm
Right suprarenal gland
Right kidney
Right renal a. and v.
Transversus abdominis m.
Iliac crest
Psoas major
Iliacus m.
Common iliac a.
External iliac a.
Urinary bladder
Esophagus
Left suprarenal gland
Celiac trunk
Left kidney
Left renal a. and v.
Superior mesenteric a. (*cut*)
Abdominal aorta
Iliohypogastric n.
Ilioinguinal n.
Lateral femoral cutaneous n.
Genitofemoral n.
Left testicular a. and v.
Inferior mesenteric artery (*cut*)
Rectum
F. Netter M.D.

Fig. 4.23 Kidneys In situ: Anterior Views (Illustration)

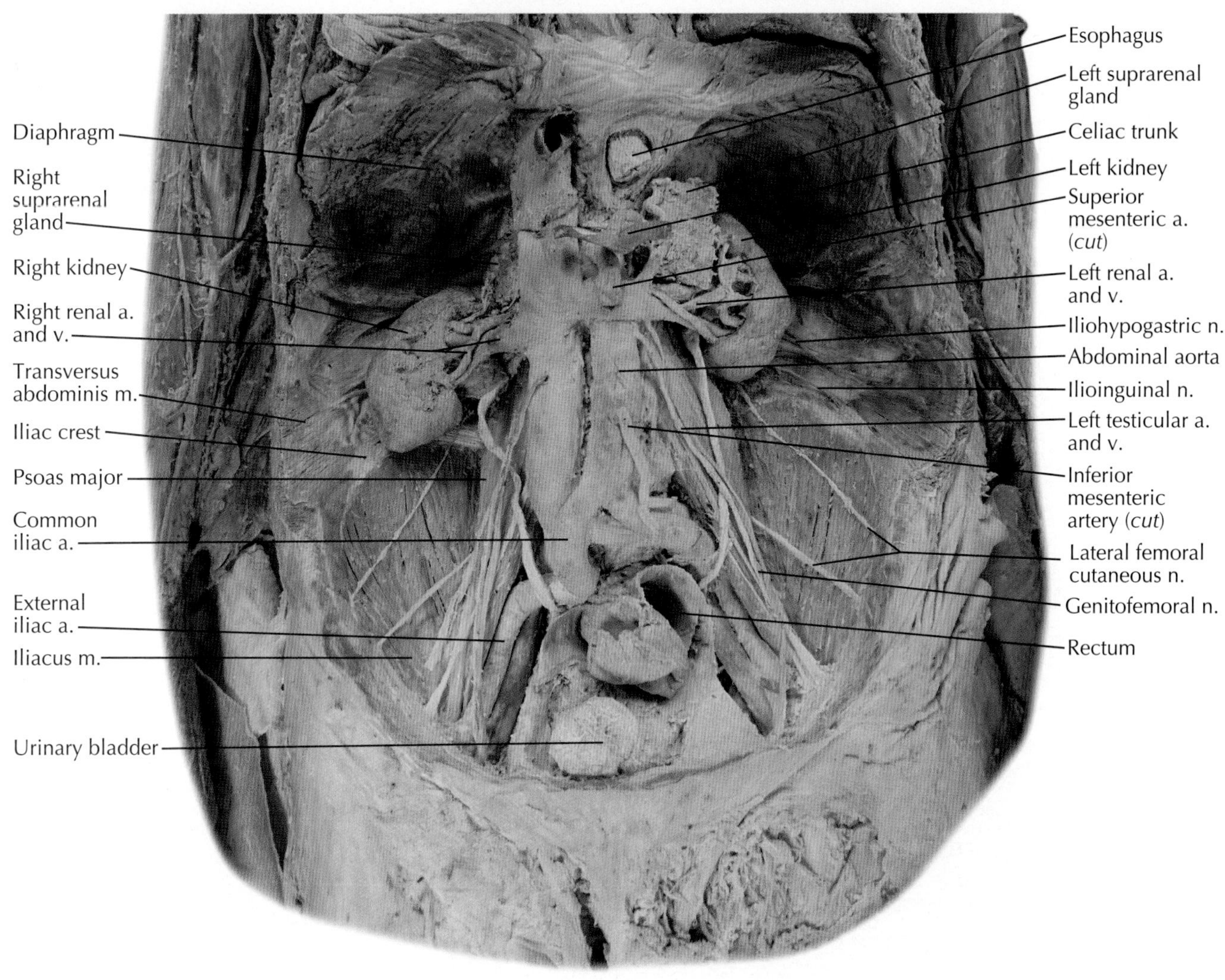
Esophagus
Left suprarenal gland
Celiac trunk
Left kidney
Superior mesenteric a. (*cut*)
Left renal a. and v.
Iliohypogastric n.
Abdominal aorta
Ilioinguinal n.
Left testicular a. and v.
Inferior mesenteric artery (*cut*)
Lateral femoral cutaneous n.
Genitofemoral n.
Rectum
Diaphragm
Right suprarenal gland
Right kidney
Right renal a. and v.
Transversus abdominis m.
Iliac crest
Psoas major
Common iliac a.
External iliac a.
Iliacus m.
Urinary bladder

Fig. 4.24 Kidneys In situ: Anterior Views (Photograph)

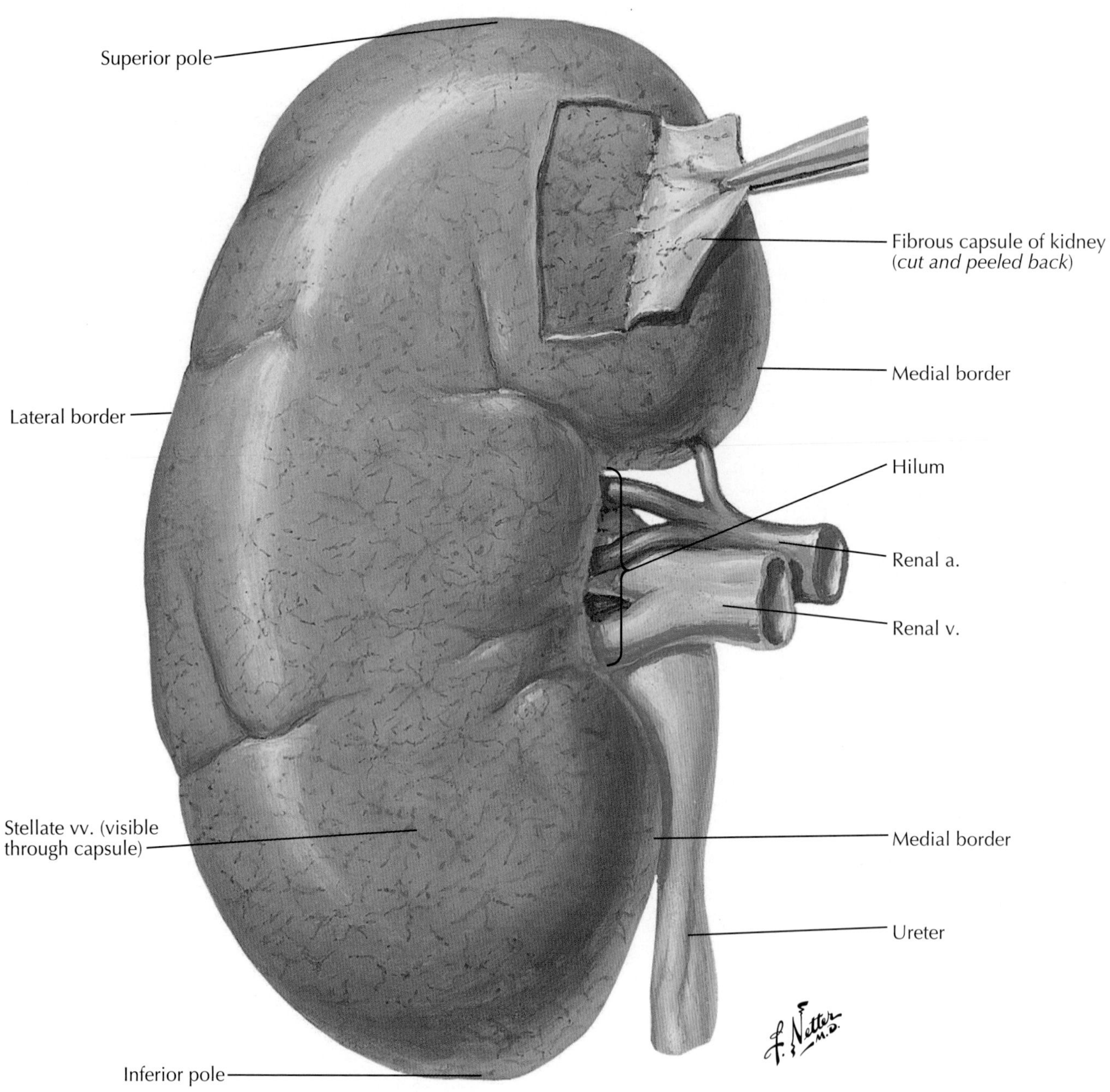
Superior pole
Fibrous capsule of kidney
(cut and peeled back)
Medial border
Lateral border
Hilum
Renal a.
Renal v.
Stellate vv. (visible
through capsule)
Medial border
Ureter
F. Netter M.D.
Inferior pole

Fig. 4.25 Gross Structure of Kidney (Illustration)

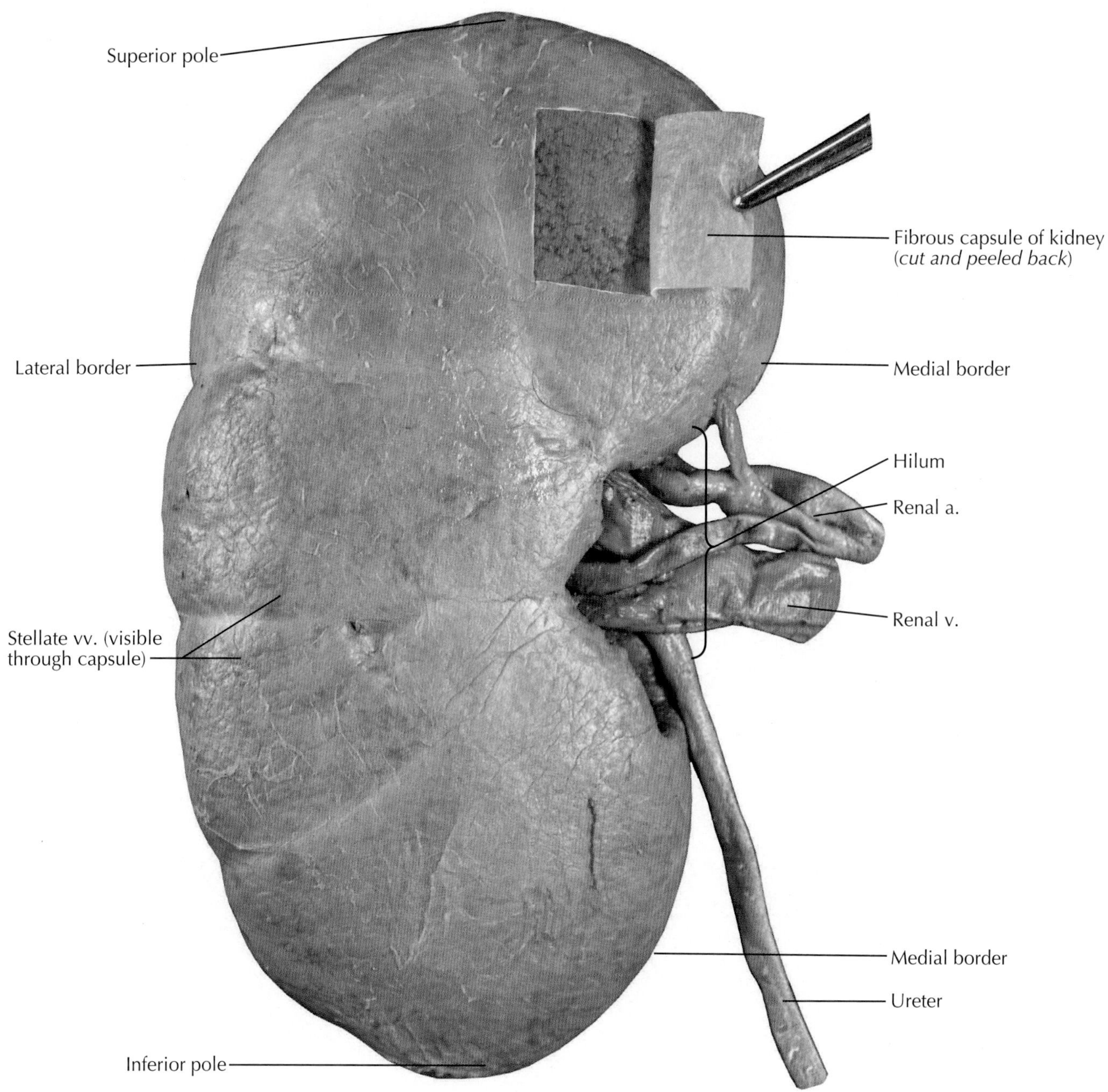
Superior pole
Fibrous capsule of kidney (*cut and peeled back*)
Lateral border
Medial border
Hilum
Renal a.
Renal v.
Stellate vv. (visible through capsule)
Medial border
Ureter
Inferior pole

Fig. 4.26 Gross Structure of Kidney (Photograph) (see Fig. A.12)

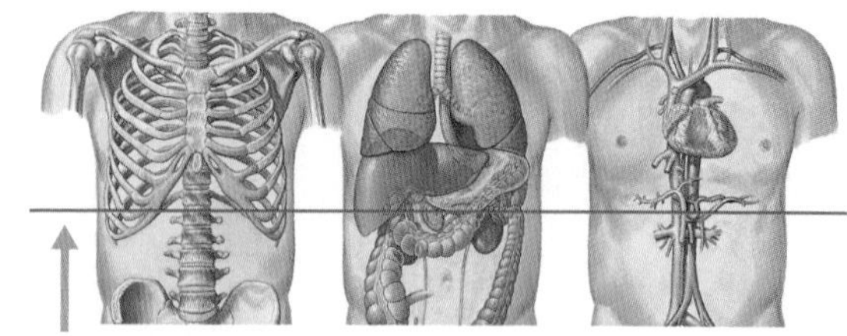

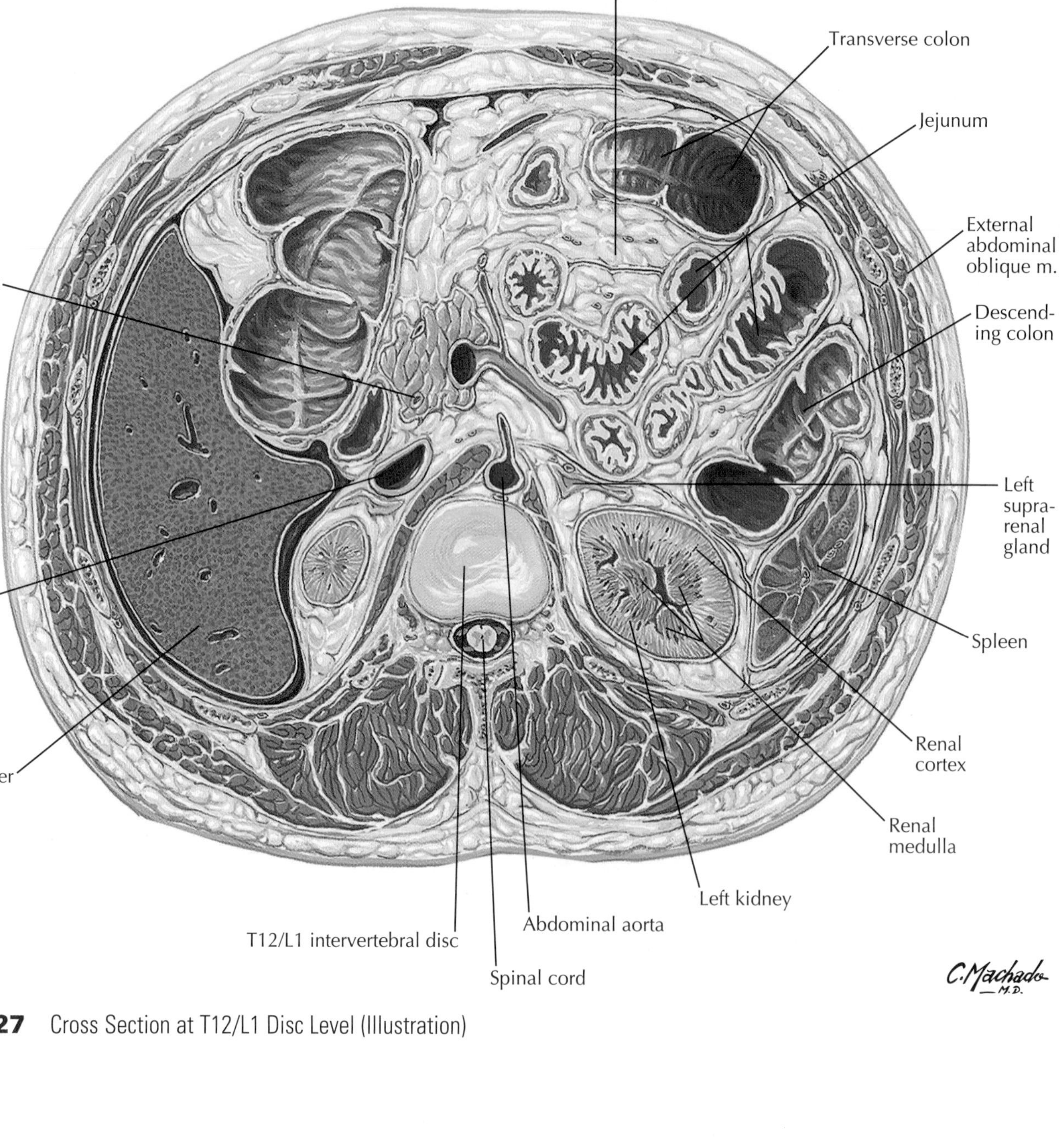

Messentery
Transverse colon
Jejunum
External abdominal oblique m.
Descending colon
Left suprarenal gland
Spleen
Renal cortex
Renal medulla
Left kidney
Abdominal aorta
Spinal cord
T12/L1 intervertebral disc
Liver
Inferior vena cava
Bile duct

Fig. 4.27 Cross Section at T12/L1 Disc Level (Illustration)

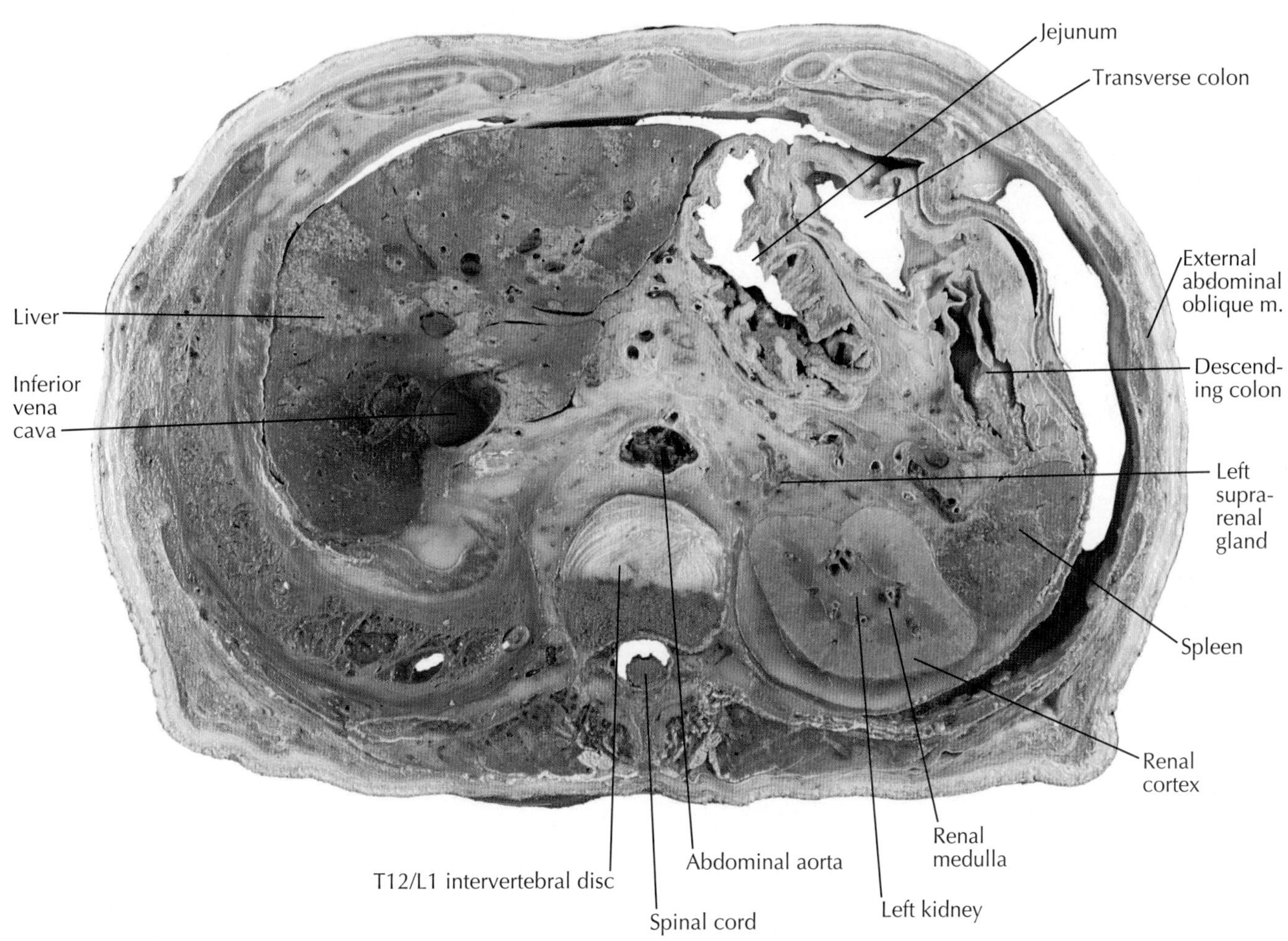
Jejunum
Transverse colon
External abdominal oblique m.
Liver
Inferior vena cava
Descend-ing colon
Left supra-renal gland
Spleen
Renal cortex
Renal medulla
Abdominal aorta
T12/L1 intervertebral disc
Left kidney
Spinal cord

Fig. 4.28 Cross Section at T12/L1 Disc Level (Photograph)

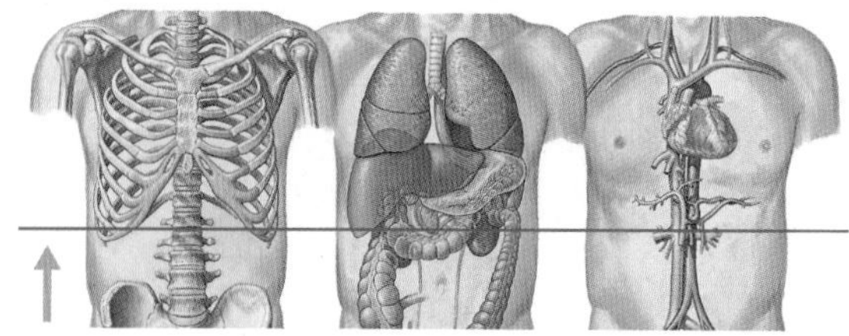

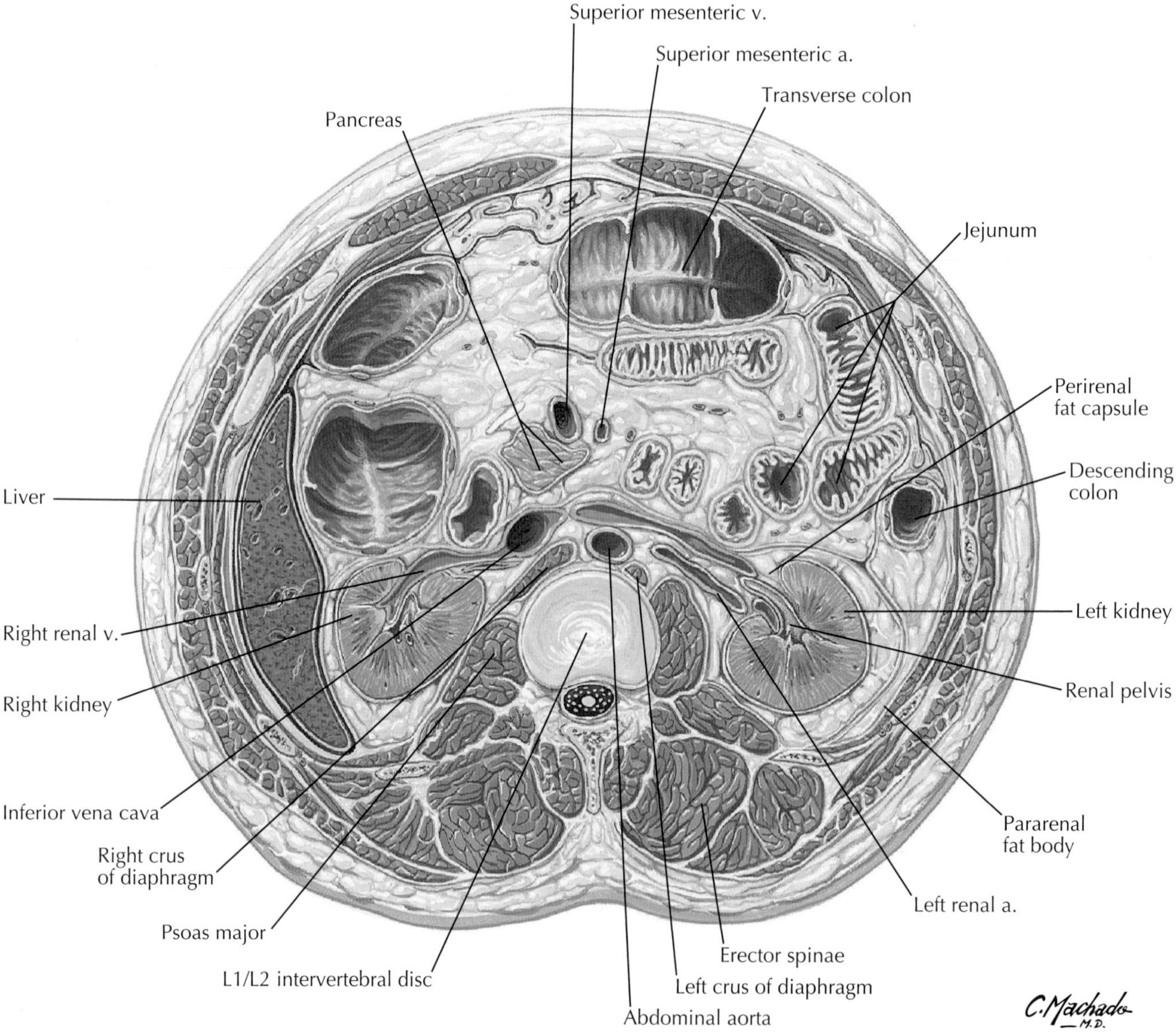

Superior mesenteric v.
Superior mesenteric a.
Transverse colon
Pancreas
Jejunum
Perirenal fat capsule
Descending colon
Liver
Left kidney
Right renal v.
Renal pelvis
Right kidney
Inferior vena cava
Pararenal fat body
Right crus of diaphragm
Left renal a.
Psoas major
Erector spinae
L1/L2 intervertebral disc
Left crus of diaphragm
Abdominal aorta
C. Machado — M.D.

Fig. 4.29 Cross Section at L1/L2 Disc Level (Illustration)

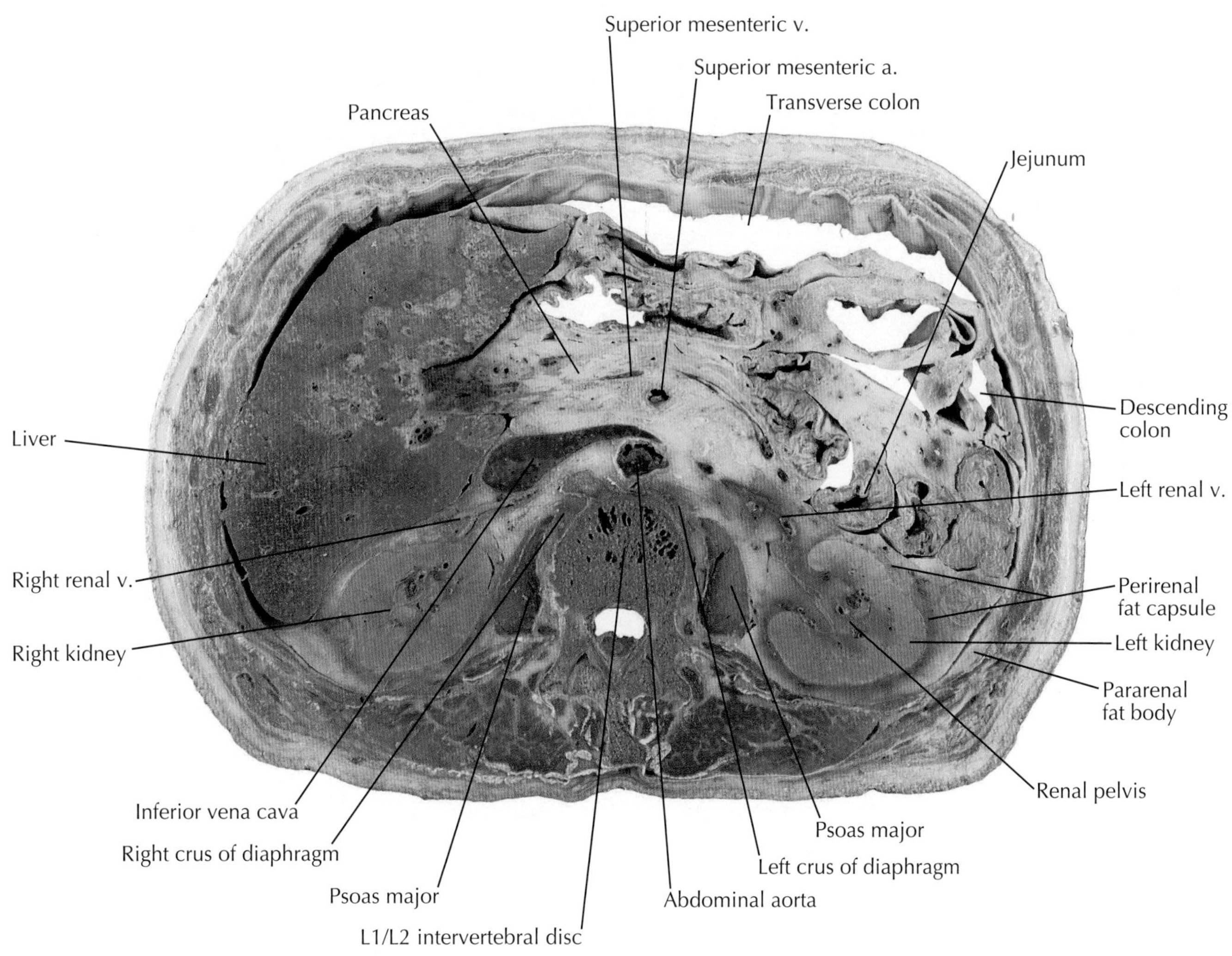
Superior mesenteric v.
Superior mesenteric a.
Transverse colon
Pancreas
Jejunum
Descending colon
Liver
Left renal v.
Right renal v.
Perirenal fat capsule
Left kidney
Right kidney
Pararenal fat body
Renal pelvis
Inferior vena cava
Psoas major
Right crus of diaphragm
Left crus of diaphragm
Psoas major
Abdominal aorta
L1/L2 intervertebral disc

Fig. 4.30 Cross Section at L1/L2 Disc Level (Photograph)

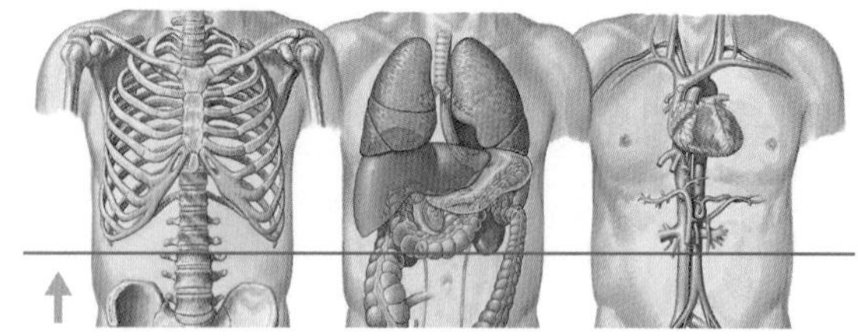

Round ligament of liver
Transverse colon
Linea alba
Rectus abdominis m.
Rectus sheath
Greater omentum
Parietal peritoneum
Aponeurosis of internal and external abdominal oblique mm.
Transversalis fascia
Transversus abdominis m.
Internal abdominal oblique m.
External abdominal oblique m.
Descending colon
Quadratus lumborum m.
Testicular a. and v.
Psoas major
Inferior vena cava
Sympathetic trunk
Abdominal aorta
Erector spinae
L3/L4 intervertebral disc

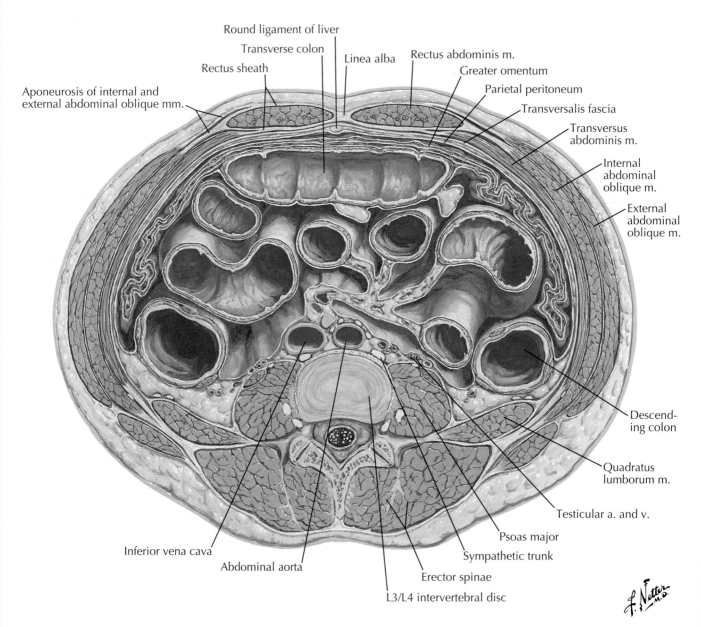

Fig. 4.31 Cross Section at L3/L4 Disc Level (Illustration)

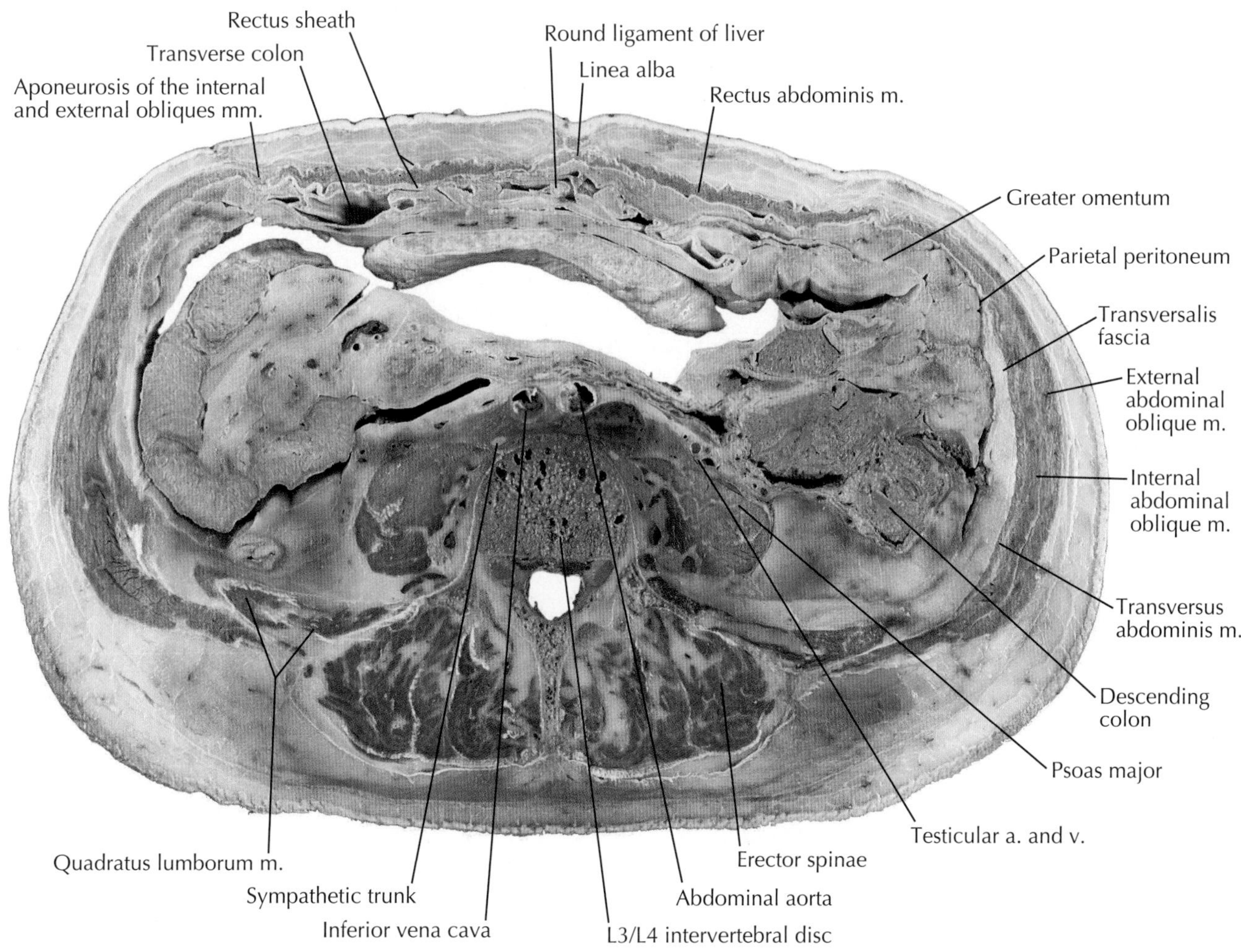
Rectus sheath
Transverse colon
Aponeurosis of the internal and external obliques mm.
Round ligament of liver
Linea alba
Rectus abdominis m.
Greater omentum
Parietal peritoneum
Transversalis fascia
External abdominal oblique m.
Internal abdominal oblique m.
Transversus abdominis m.
Descending colon
Psoas major
Testicular a. and v.
Erector spinae
Abdominal aorta
L3/L4 intervertebral disc
Inferior vena cava
Sympathetic trunk
Quadratus lumborum m.

Fig. 4.32 Cross Section at L3/L4 Disc Level (Photograph)

PELVIS

CHAPTER 5

Paramedian (sagittal) dissection

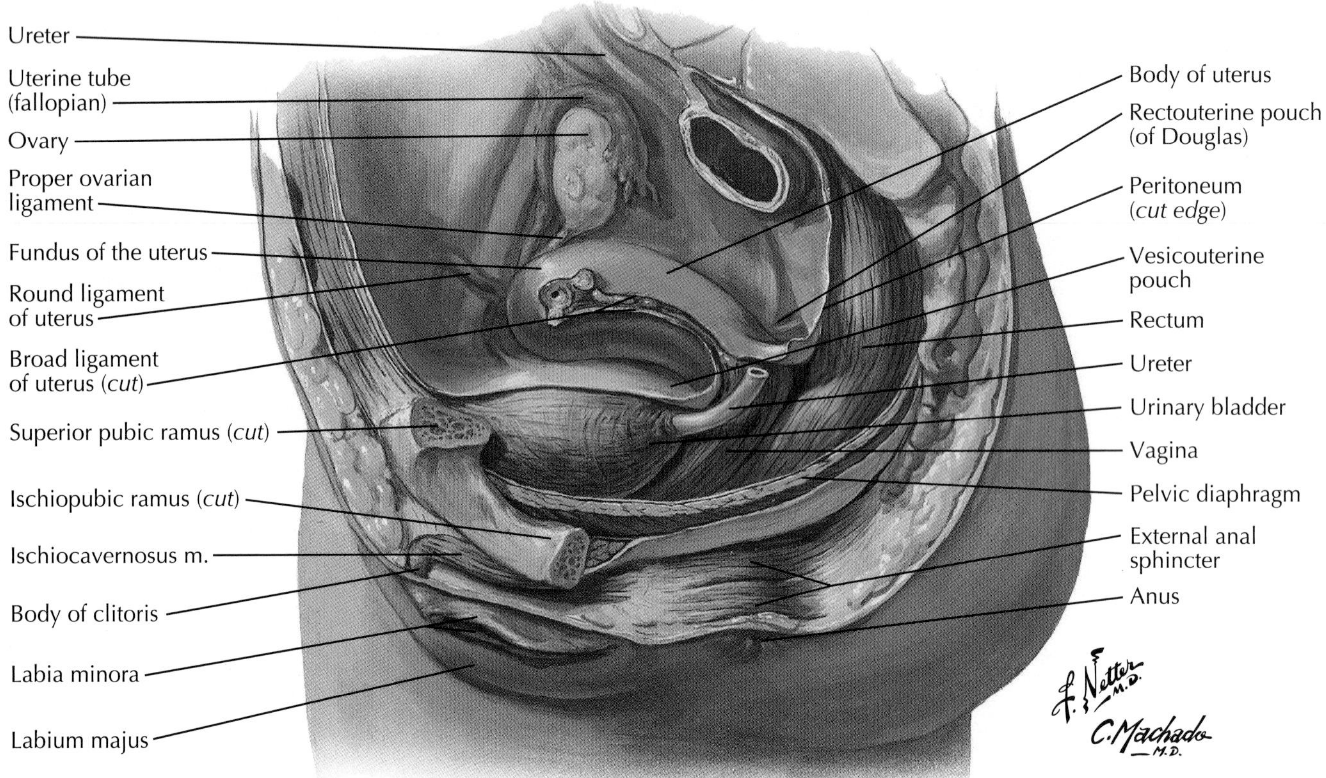
Ureter
Uterine tube (fallopian)
Ovary
Proper ovarian ligament
Fundus of the uterus
Round ligament of uterus
Broad ligament of uterus (*cut*)
Superior pubic ramus (*cut*)
Ischiopubic ramus (*cut*)
Ischiocavernosus m.
Body of clitoris
Labia minora
Labium majus
Body of uterus
Rectouterine pouch (of Douglas)
Peritoneum (*cut edge*)
Vesicouterine pouch
Rectum
Ureter
Urinary bladder
Vagina
Pelvic diaphragm
External anal sphincter
Anus

Fig. 5.1 Pelvic Viscera and Perineum: Female (Illustration)

Paramedian (sagittal) dissection

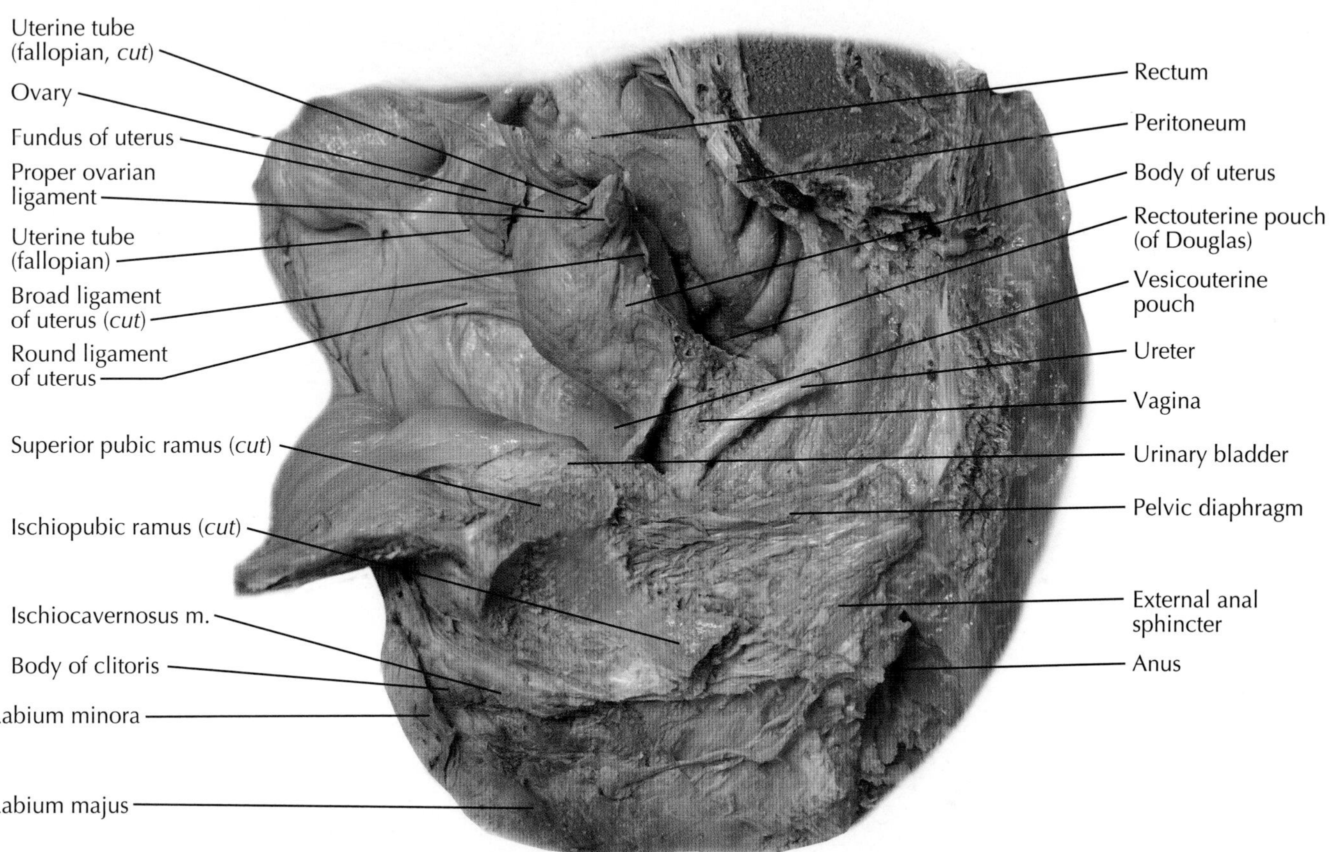
Uterine tube (fallopian, *cut*)
Ovary
Fundus of uterus
Proper ovarian ligament
Uterine tube (fallopian)
Broad ligament of uterus (*cut*)
Round ligament of uterus
Superior pubic ramus (*cut*)
Ischiopubic ramus (*cut*)
Ischiocavernosus m.
Body of clitoris
Labium minora
Labium majus
Rectum
Peritoneum
Body of uterus
Rectouterine pouch (of Douglas)
Vesicouterine pouch
Ureter
Vagina
Urinary bladder
Pelvic diaphragm
External anal sphincter
Anus

Fig. 5.2 Pelvic Viscera and Perineum: Female (Photograph)

Superior view with peritoneum intact

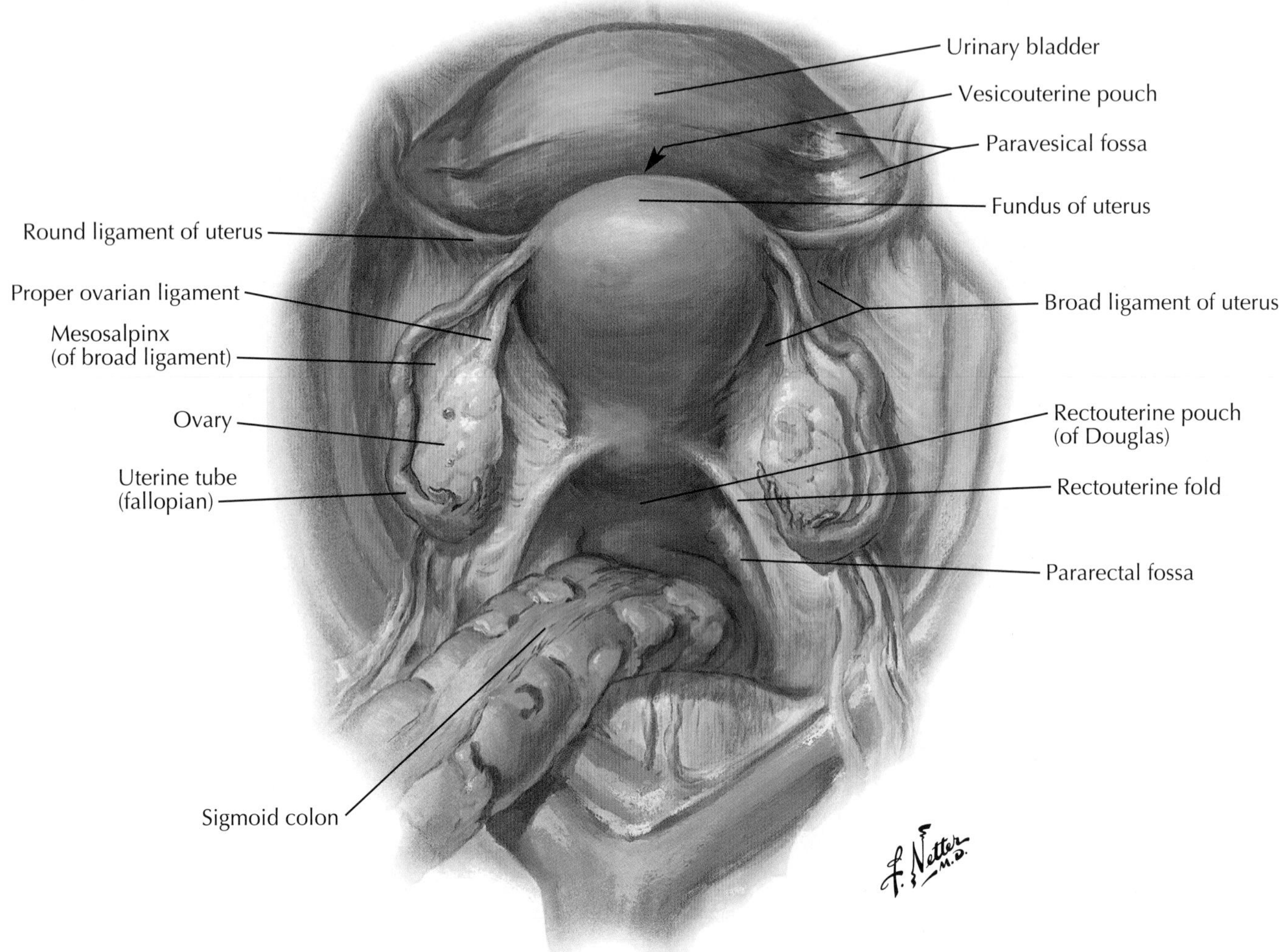
Urinary bladder
Vesicouterine pouch
Paravesical fossa
Fundus of uterus
Round ligament of uterus
Proper ovarian ligament
Broad ligament of uterus
Mesosalpinx
(of broad ligament)
Rectouterine pouch
(of Douglas)
Ovary
Uterine tube
(fallopian)
Rectouterine fold
Pararectal fossa
Sigmoid colon

Fig. 5.3 Female Internal Genital Organs (Illustration)

Superior view with peritoneum intact

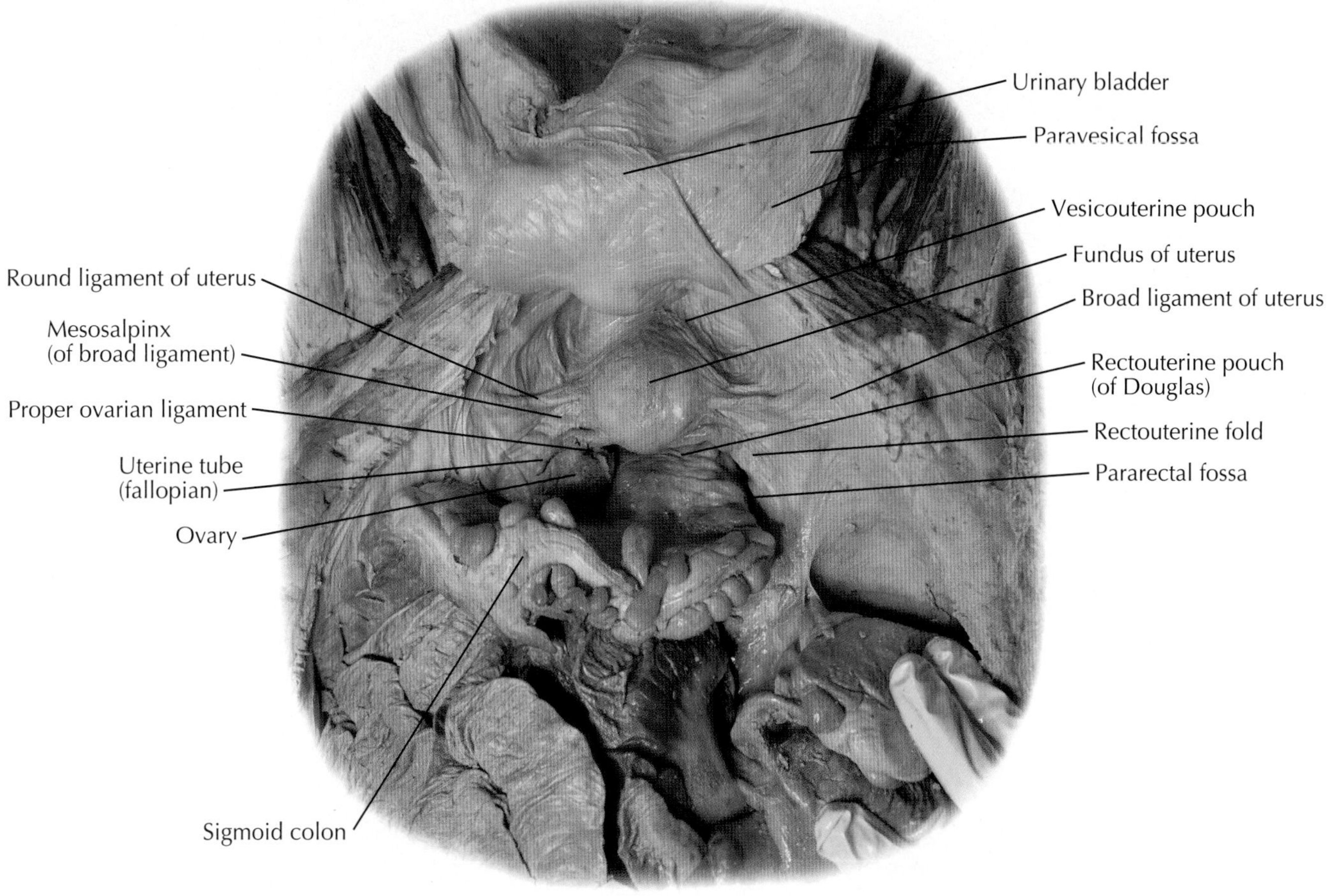
Urinary bladder
Paravesical fossa
Vesicouterine pouch
Fundus of uterus
Broad ligament of uterus
Rectouterine pouch
(of Douglas)
Rectouterine fold
Pararectal fossa
Round ligament of uterus
Mesosalpinx
(of broad ligament)
Proper ovarian ligament
Uterine tube
(fallopian)
Ovary
Sigmoid colon

Fig. 5.4 Female Internal Genital Organs (Photograph)

Superior view

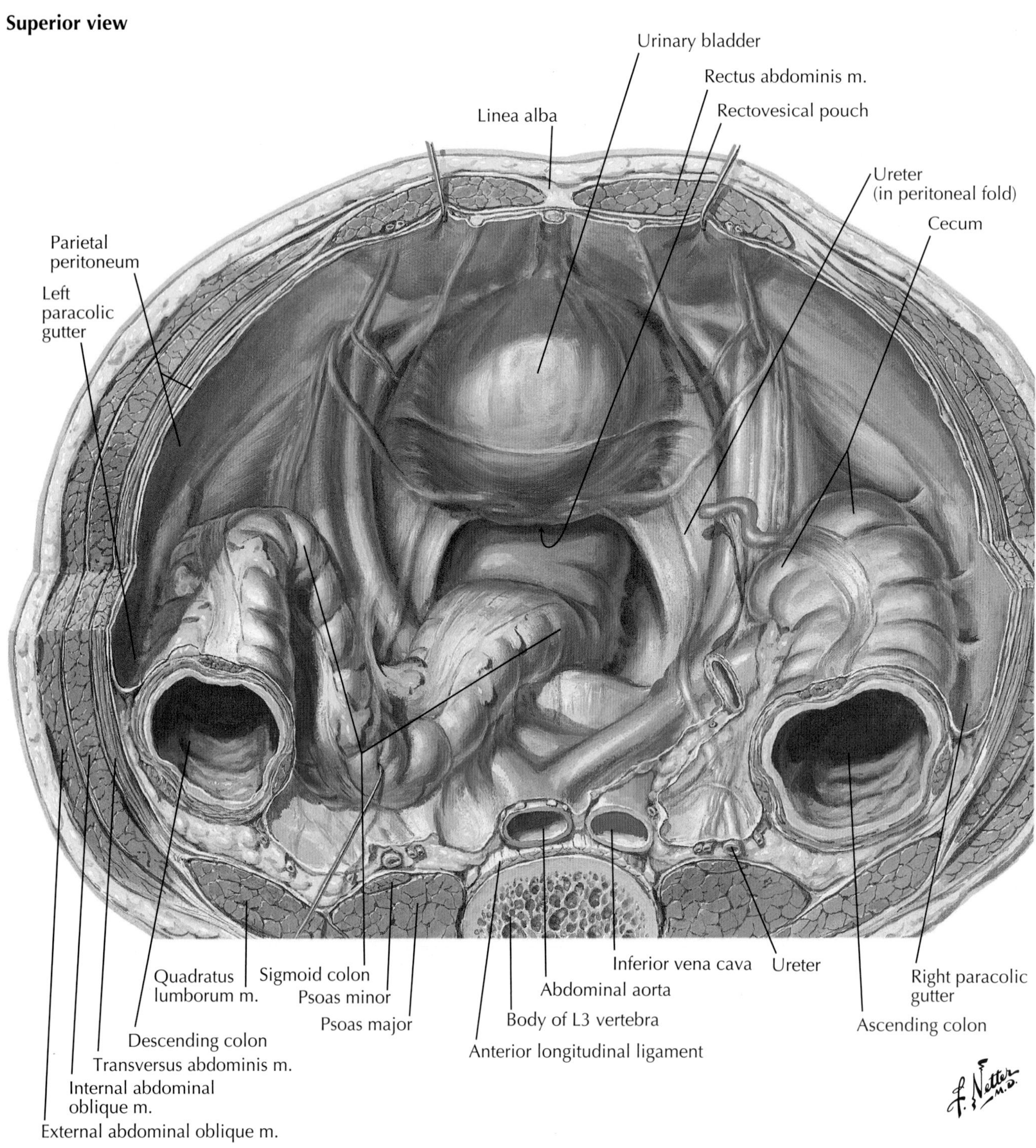
Urinary bladder
Rectus abdominis m.
Linea alba
Rectovesical pouch
Ureter
(in peritoneal fold)
Cecum
Parietal
peritoneum
Left
paracolic
gutter
Quadratus
lumborum m.
Sigmoid colon
Psoas minor
Psoas major
Inferior vena cava
Ureter
Abdominal aorta
Body of L3 vertebra
Anterior longitudinal ligament
Right paracolic
gutter
Ascending colon
Descending colon
Transversus abdominis m.
Internal abdominal
oblique m.
External abdominal oblique m.

Fig. 5.5 Pelvic Cavity: Male (Illustration)

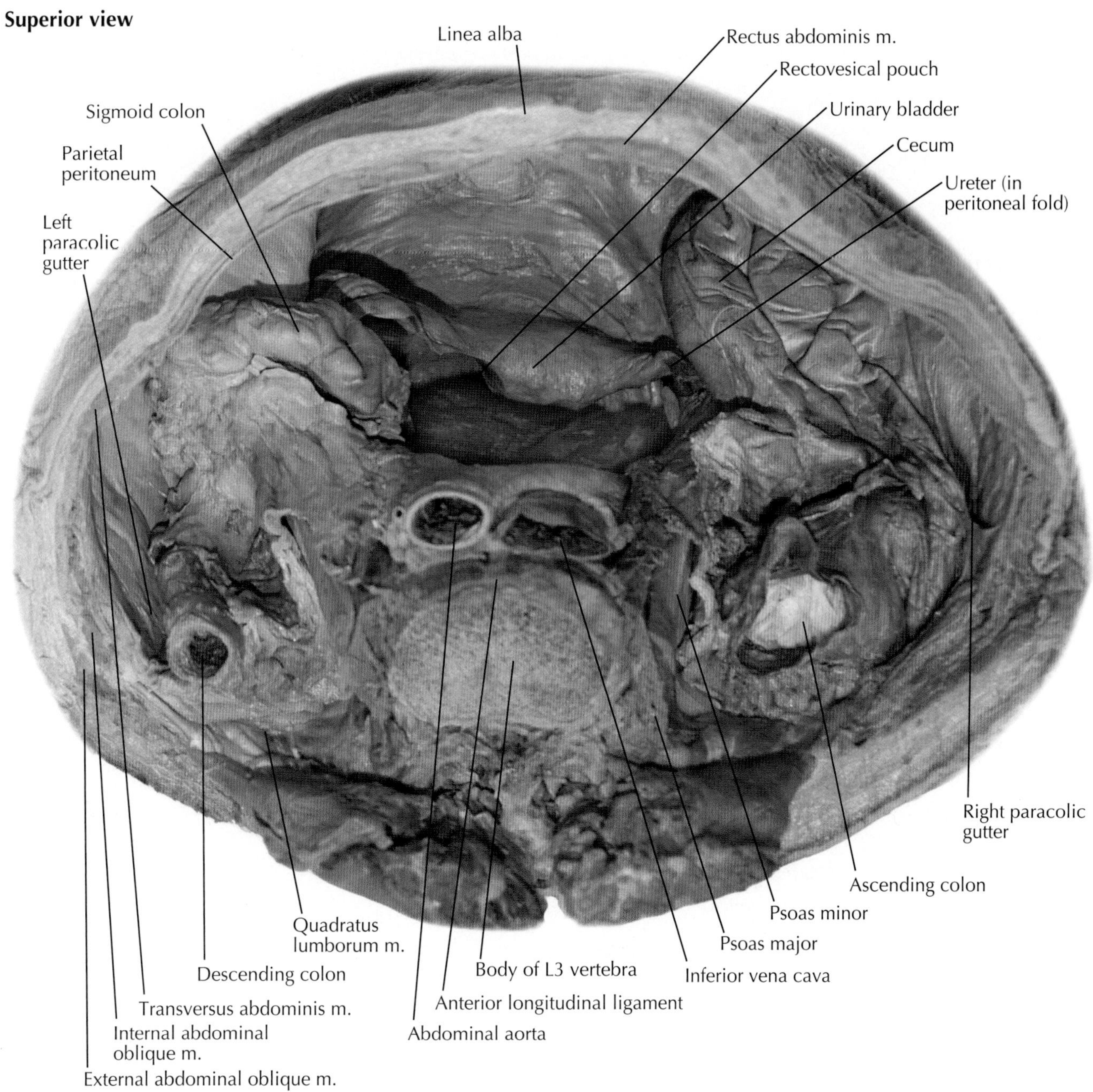
Superior view
Linea alba
Rectus abdominis m.
Rectovesical pouch
Urinary bladder
Cecum
Ureter (in peritoneal fold)
Sigmoid colon
Parietal peritoneum
Left paracolic gutter
Right paracolic gutter
Ascending colon
Psoas minor
Psoas major
Inferior vena cava
Body of L3 vertebra
Anterior longitudinal ligament
Abdominal aorta
Quadratus lumborum m.
Descending colon
Transversus abdominis m.
Internal abdominal oblique m.
External abdominal oblique m.

Fig. 5.6 Pelvic Cavity: Male (Photograph)

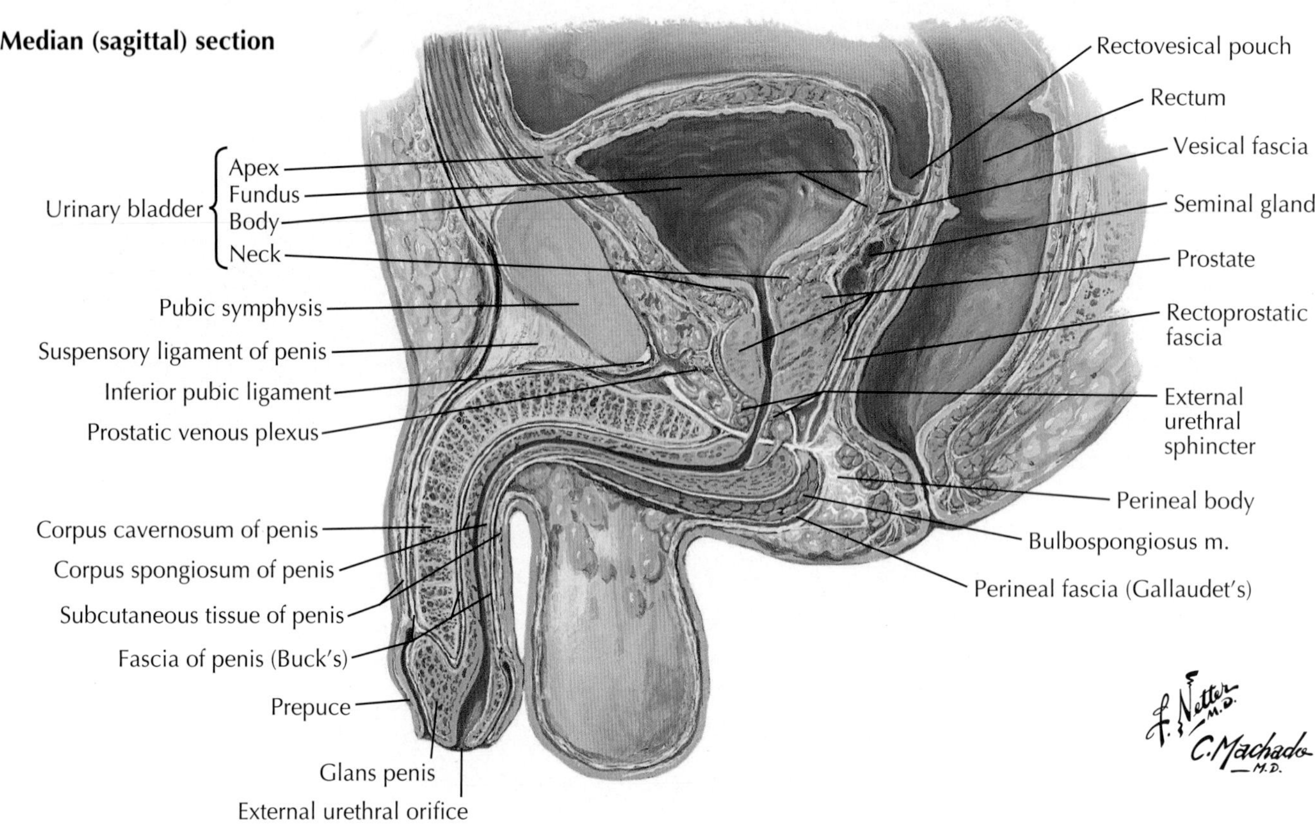
Median (sagittal) section
Urinary bladder
Apex
Fundus
Body
Neck
Pubic symphysis
Suspensory ligament of penis
Inferior pubic ligament
Prostatic venous plexus
Corpus cavernosum of penis
Corpus spongiosum of penis
Subcutaneous tissue of penis
Fascia of penis (Buck's)
Prepuce
Glans penis
External urethral orifice
Rectovesical pouch
Rectum
Vesical fascia
Seminal gland
Prostate
Rectoprostatic fascia
External urethral sphincter
Perineal body
Bulbospongiosus m.
Perineal fascia (Gallaudet's)
F. Netter M.D.
C. Machado M.D.

Fig. 5.7 Pelvic Viscera and Perineum: Male (Illustration)

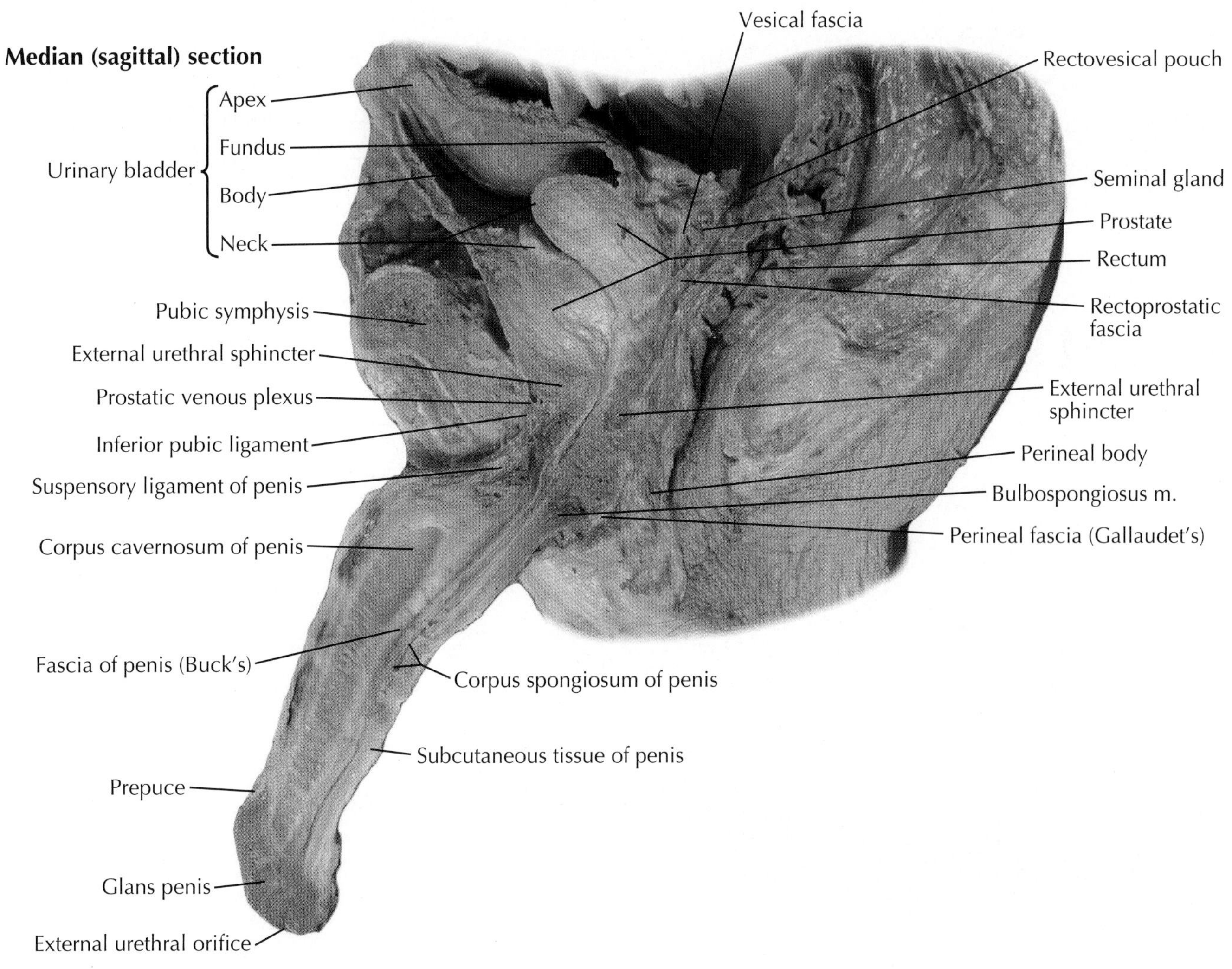
Median (sagittal) section
Urinary bladder
Apex
Fundus
Body
Neck
Pubic symphysis
External urethral sphincter
Prostatic venous plexus
Inferior pubic ligament
Suspensory ligament of penis
Corpus cavernosum of penis
Fascia of penis (Buck's)
Prepuce
Glans penis
External urethral orifice
Vesical fascia
Rectovesical pouch
Seminal gland
Prostate
Rectum
Rectoprostatic fascia
External urethral sphincter
Perineal body
Bulbospongiosus m.
Perineal fascia (Gallaudet's)
Corpus spongiosum of penis
Subcutaneous tissue of penis

Fig. 5.8 Pelvic Viscera and Perineum: Male (Photograph)

Female: median section

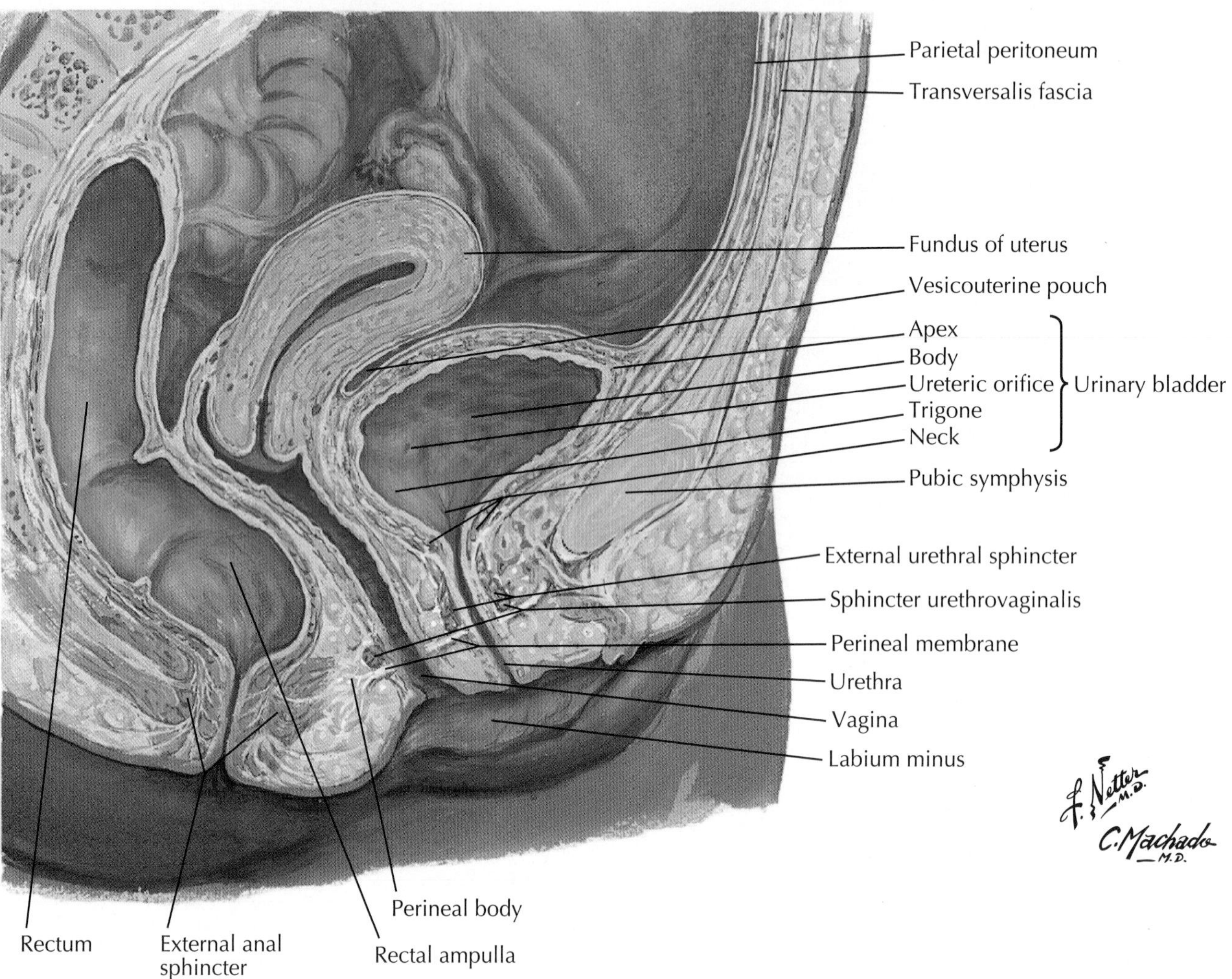
Parietal peritoneum
Transversalis fascia
Fundus of uterus
Vesicouterine pouch
Apex
Body
Ureteric orifice
Trigone
Neck
Urinary bladder
Pubic symphysis
External urethral sphincter
Sphincter urethrovaginalis
Perineal membrane
Urethra
Vagina
Labium minus
Perineal body
Rectum
External anal sphincter
Rectal ampulla

Fig. 5.9 Urinary Bladder: Orientation and Supports (Illustration)

Female: median section

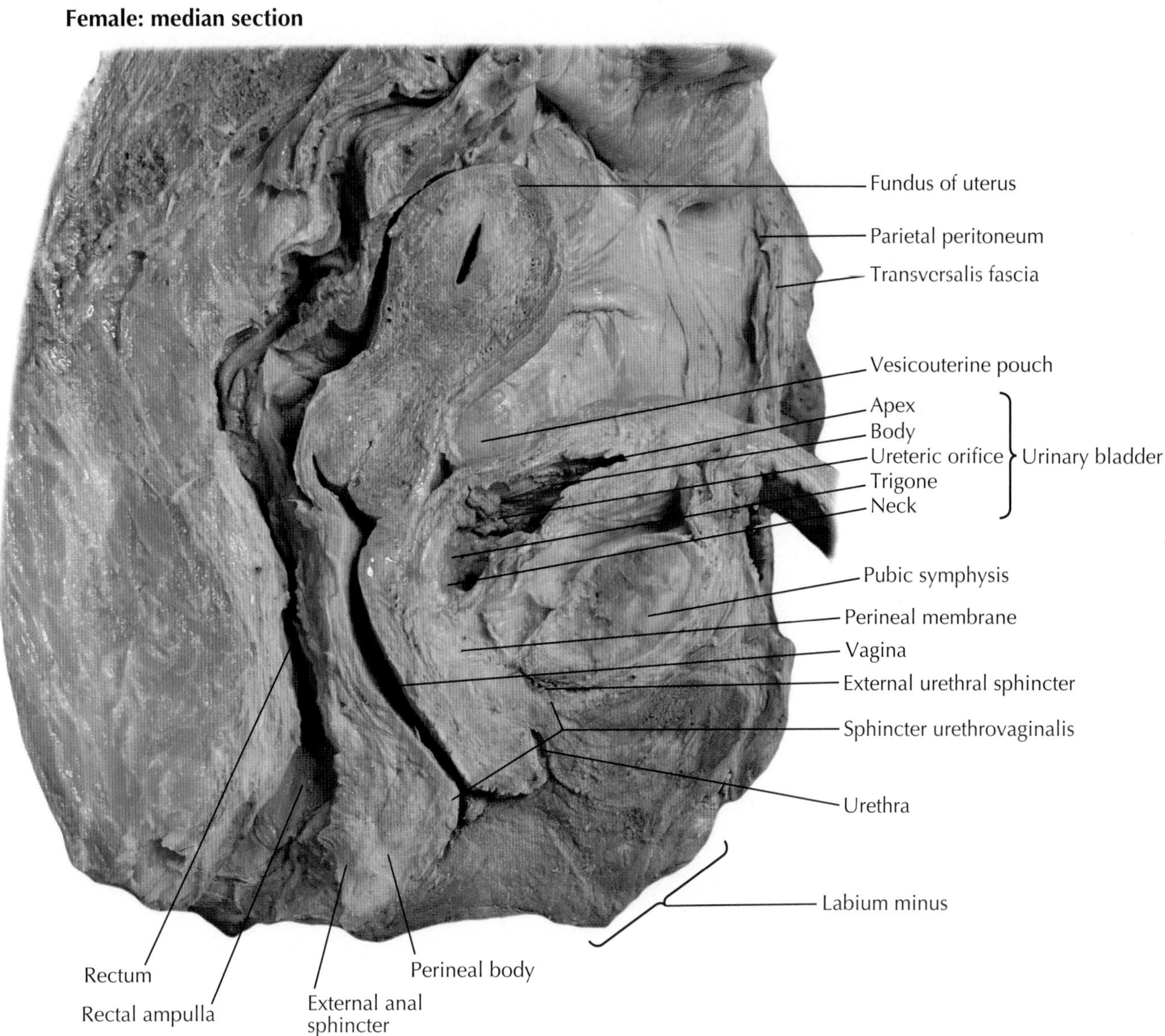

Fundus of uterus
Parietal peritoneum
Transversalis fascia
Vesicouterine pouch
Apex
Body
Ureteric orifice
Trigone
Neck
Urinary bladder
Pubic symphysis
Perineal membrane
Vagina
External urethral sphincter
Sphincter urethrovaginalis
Urethra
Labium minus
Rectum
Rectal ampulla
External anal sphincter
Perineal body

Fig. 5.10 Urinary Bladder: Orientation and Supports (Photograph)

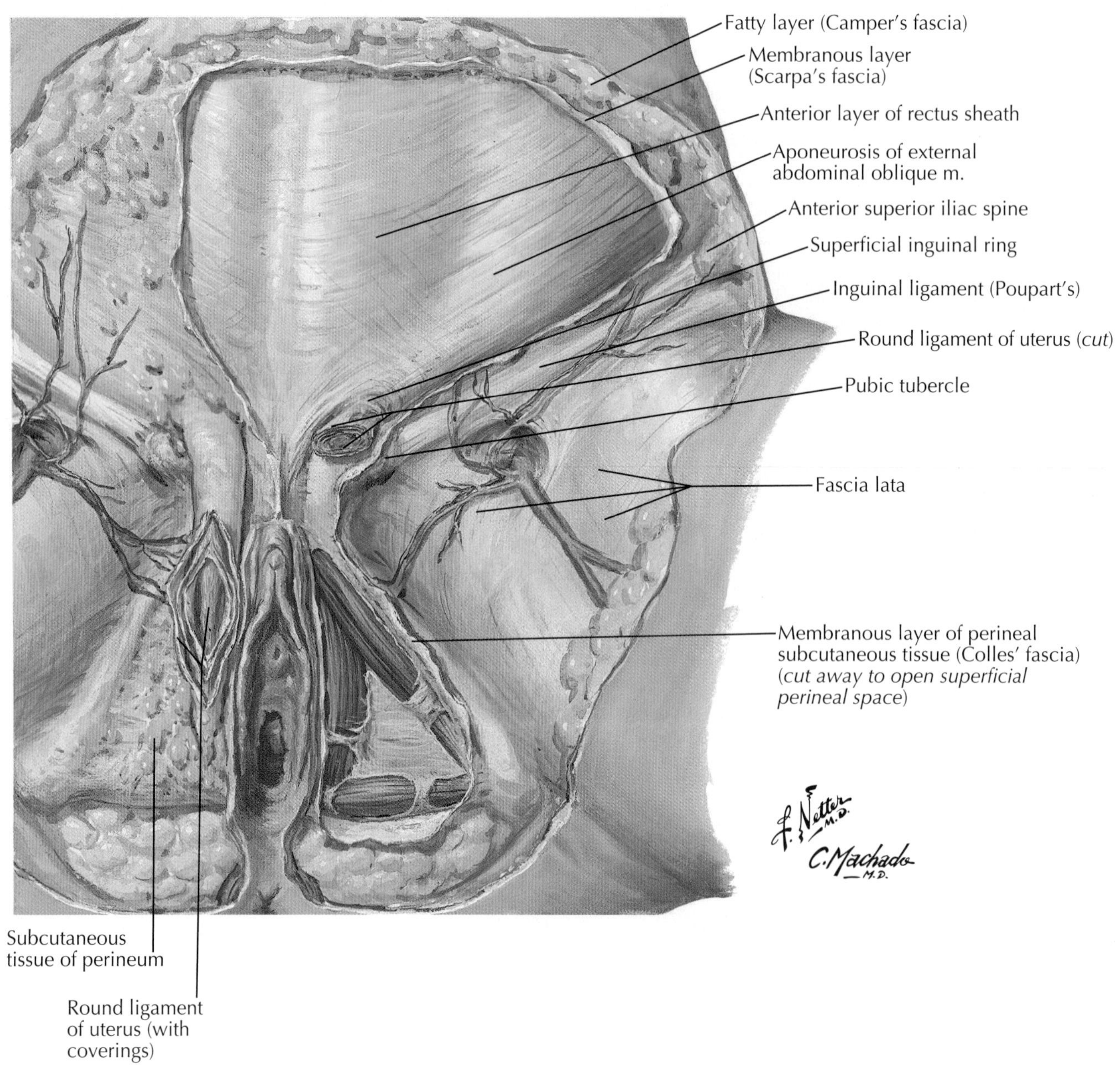
Fatty layer (Camper's fascia)
Membranous layer (Scarpa's fascia)
Anterior layer of rectus sheath
Aponeurosis of external abdominal oblique m.
Anterior superior iliac spine
Superficial inguinal ring
Inguinal ligament (Poupart's)
Round ligament of uterus (*cut*)
Pubic tubercle
Fascia lata
Membranous layer of perineal subcutaneous tissue (Colles' fascia) (*cut away to open superficial perineal space*)
Subcutaneous tissue of perineum
Round ligament of uterus (with coverings)
F. Netter M.D.
C. Machado M.D.

Fig. 5.11 Female Perineum (Superficial Dissection) (Illustration)

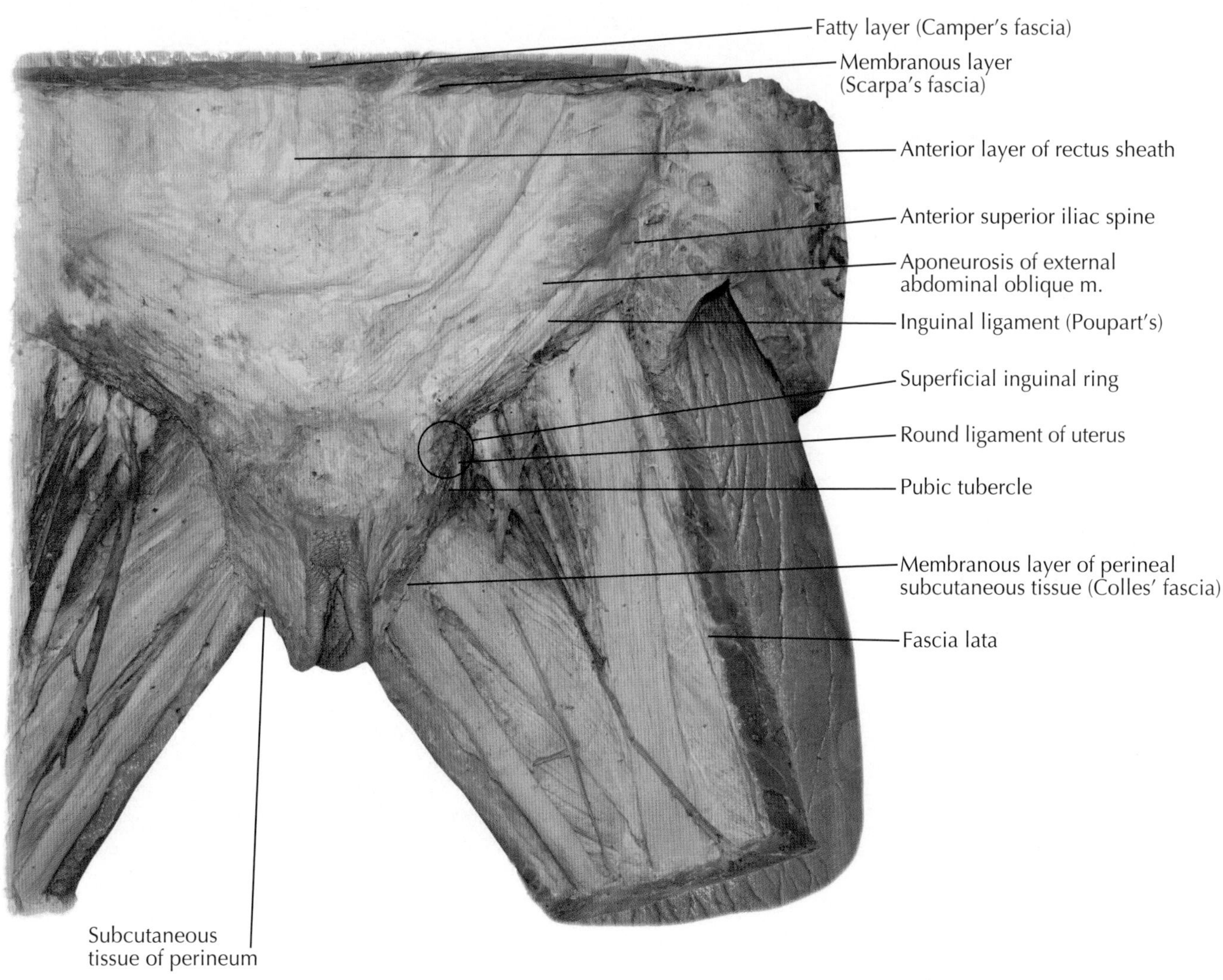
Fatty layer (Camper's fascia)
Membranous layer (Scarpa's fascia)
Anterior layer of rectus sheath
Anterior superior iliac spine
Aponeurosis of external abdominal oblique m.
Inguinal ligament (Poupart's)
Superficial inguinal ring
Round ligament of uterus
Pubic tubercle
Membranous layer of perineal subcutaneous tissue (Colles' fascia)
Fascia lata
Subcutaneous tissue of perineum

Fig. 5.12 Female Perineum (Superficial Dissection) (Photograph)

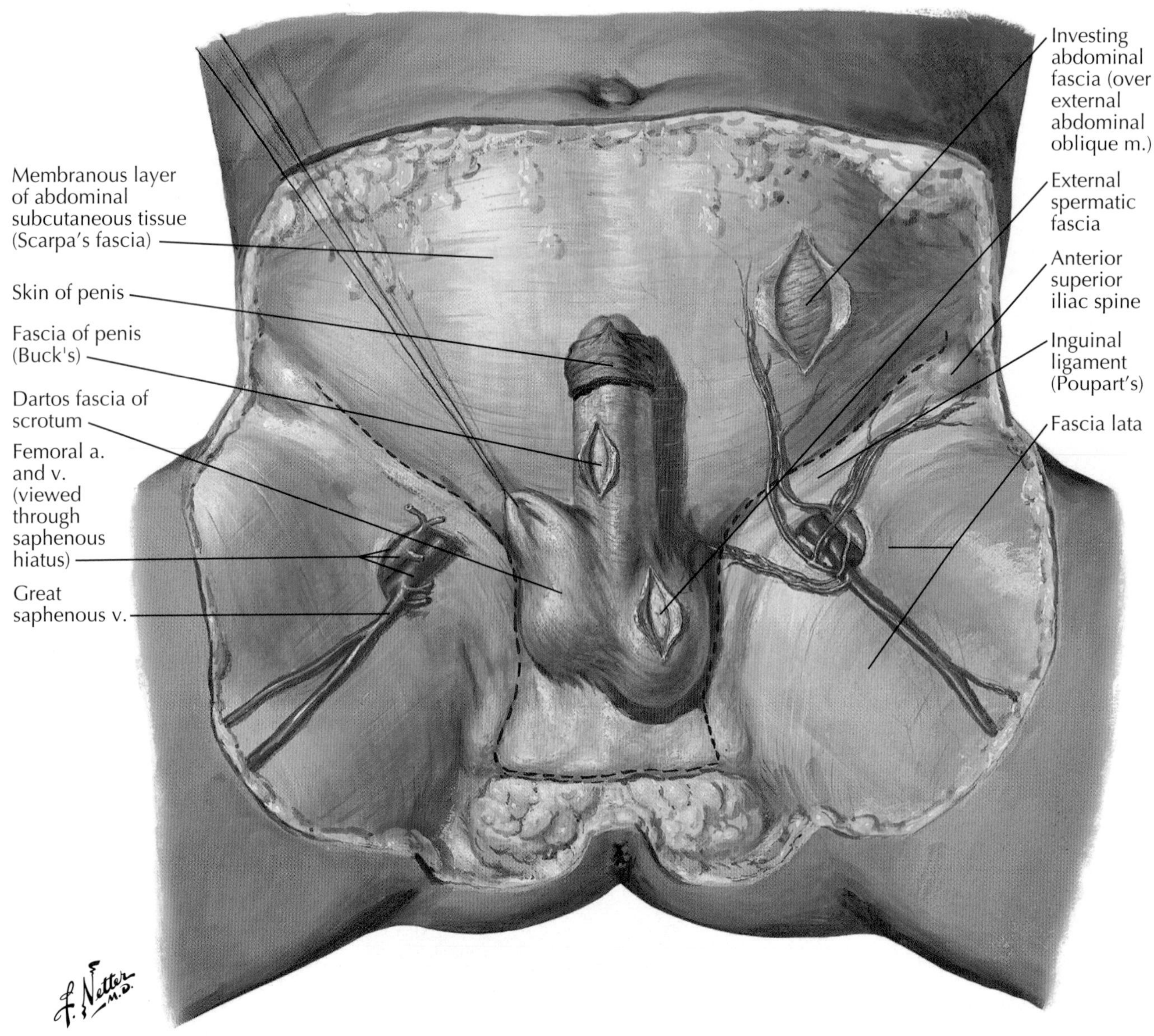
Membranous layer of abdominal subcutaneous tissue (Scarpa's fascia)
Skin of penis
Fascia of penis (Buck's)
Dartos fascia of scrotum
Femoral a. and v. (viewed through saphenous hiatus)
Great saphenous v.
Investing abdominal fascia (over external abdominal oblique m.)
External spermatic fascia
Anterior superior iliac spine
Inguinal ligament (Poupart's)
Fascia lata
F. Netter M.D.

Fig. 5.13 Male Perineum and External Genitalia (Superficial Dissection) (Illustration)

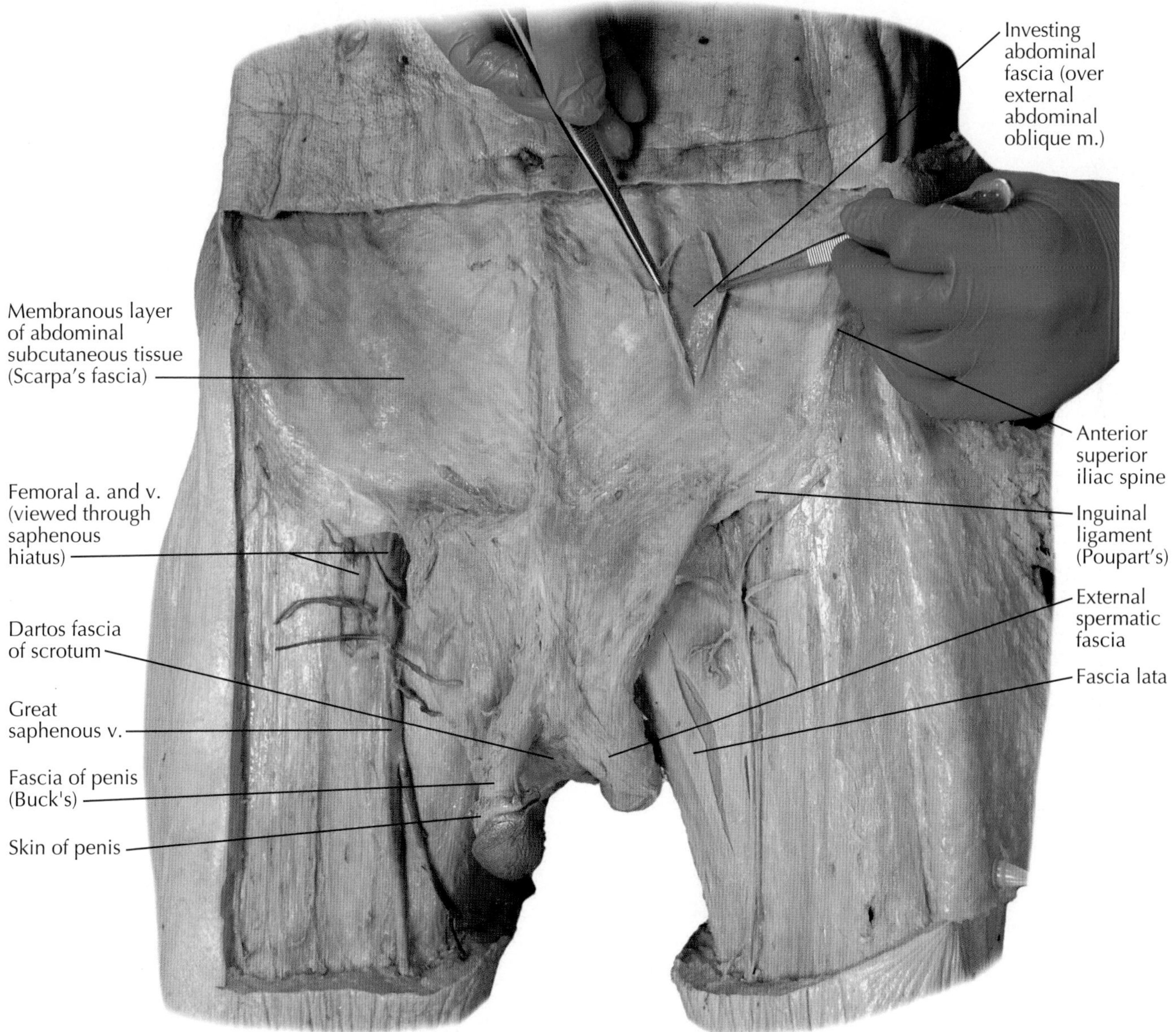
Investing
abdominal
fascia (over
external
abdominal
oblique m.)
Membranous layer
of abdominal
subcutaneous tissue
(Scarpa's fascia)
Anterior
superior
iliac spine
Femoral a. and v.
(viewed through
saphenous
hiatus)
Inguinal
ligament
(Poupart's)
External
spermatic
fascia
Dartos fascia
of scrotum
Fascia lata
Great
saphenous v.
Fascia of penis
(Buck's)
Skin of penis

Fig. 5.14 Male Perineum and External Genitalia (Superficial Dissection) (Photograph)

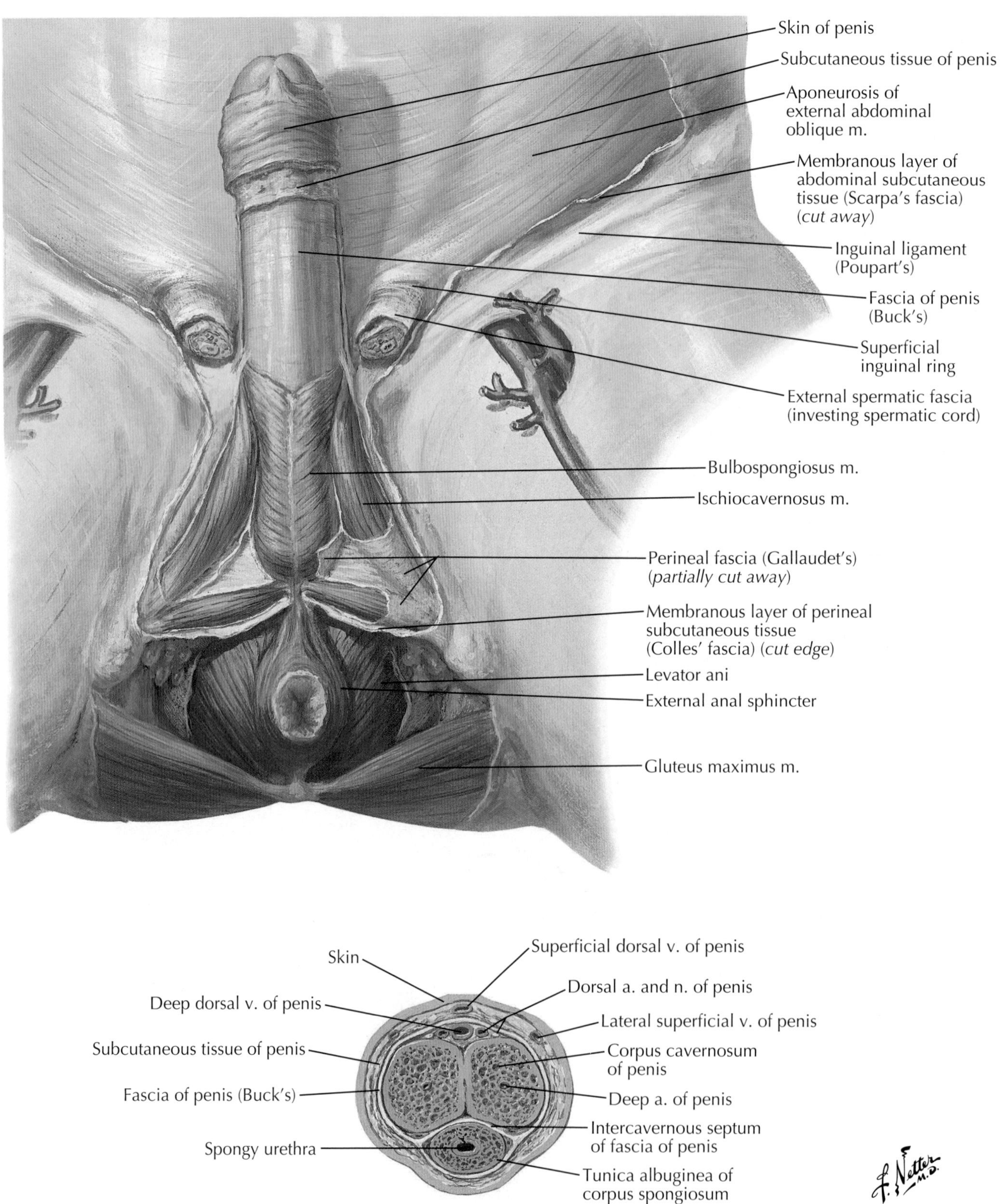
Skin of penis
Subcutaneous tissue of penis
Aponeurosis of external abdominal oblique m.
Membranous layer of abdominal subcutaneous tissue (Scarpa's fascia) (cut away)
Inguinal ligament (Poupart's)
Fascia of penis (Buck's)
Superficial inguinal ring
External spermatic fascia (investing spermatic cord)
Bulbospongiosus m.
Ischiocavernosus m.
Perineal fascia (Gallaudet's) (partially cut away)
Membranous layer of perineal subcutaneous tissue (Colles' fascia) (cut edge)
Levator ani
External anal sphincter
Gluteus maximus m.
Skin
Superficial dorsal v. of penis
Dorsal a. and n. of penis
Deep dorsal v. of penis
Lateral superficial v. of penis
Subcutaneous tissue of penis
Corpus cavernosum of penis
Fascia of penis (Buck's)
Deep a. of penis
Intercavernous septum of fascia of penis
Spongy urethra
Tunica albuginea of corpus spongiosum
F. Netter M.D.

Transverse section through body of penis

Fig. 5.15 Male Perineum and External Genitalia (Deeper Dissection) (Illustration)

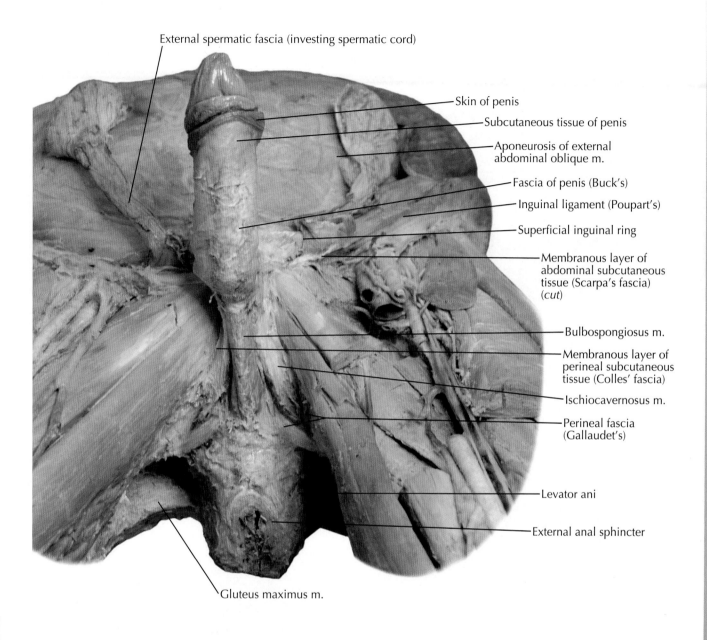

External spermatic fascia (investing spermatic cord)
Skin of penis
Subcutaneous tissue of penis
Aponeurosis of external abdominal oblique m.
Fascia of penis (Buck's)
Inguinal ligament (Poupart's)
Superficial inguinal ring
Membranous layer of abdominal subcutaneous tissue (Scarpa's fascia) (*cut*)
Bulbospongiosus m.
Membranous layer of perineal subcutaneous tissue (Colles' fascia)
Ischiocavernosus m.
Perineal fascia (Gallaudet's)
Levator ani
External anal sphincter
Gluteus maximus m.

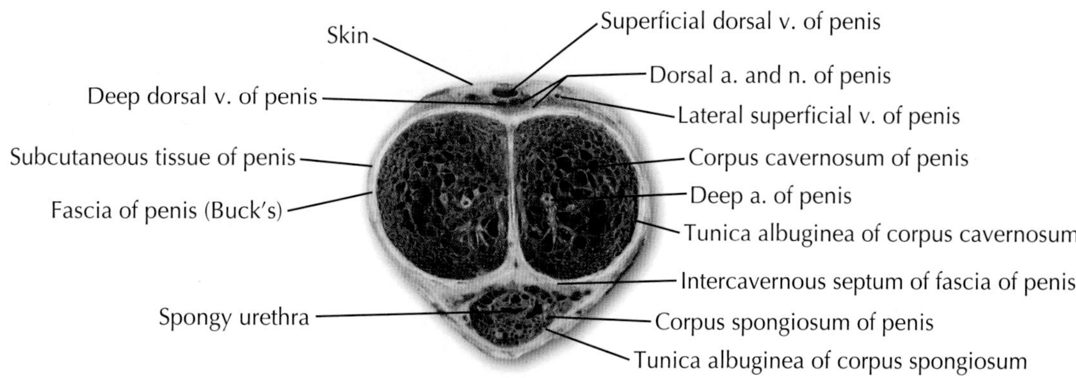
Skin
Superficial dorsal v. of penis
Dorsal a. and n. of penis
Deep dorsal v. of penis
Lateral superficial v. of penis
Subcutaneous tissue of penis
Corpus cavernosum of penis
Fascia of penis (Buck's)
Deep a. of penis
Tunica albuginea of corpus cavernosum
Intercavernous septum of fascia of penis
Spongy urethra
Corpus spongiosum of penis
Tunica albuginea of corpus spongiosum

Transverse section through body of penis

Fig. 5.16 Male Perineum and External Genitalia (Deeper Dissection) (Photograph)

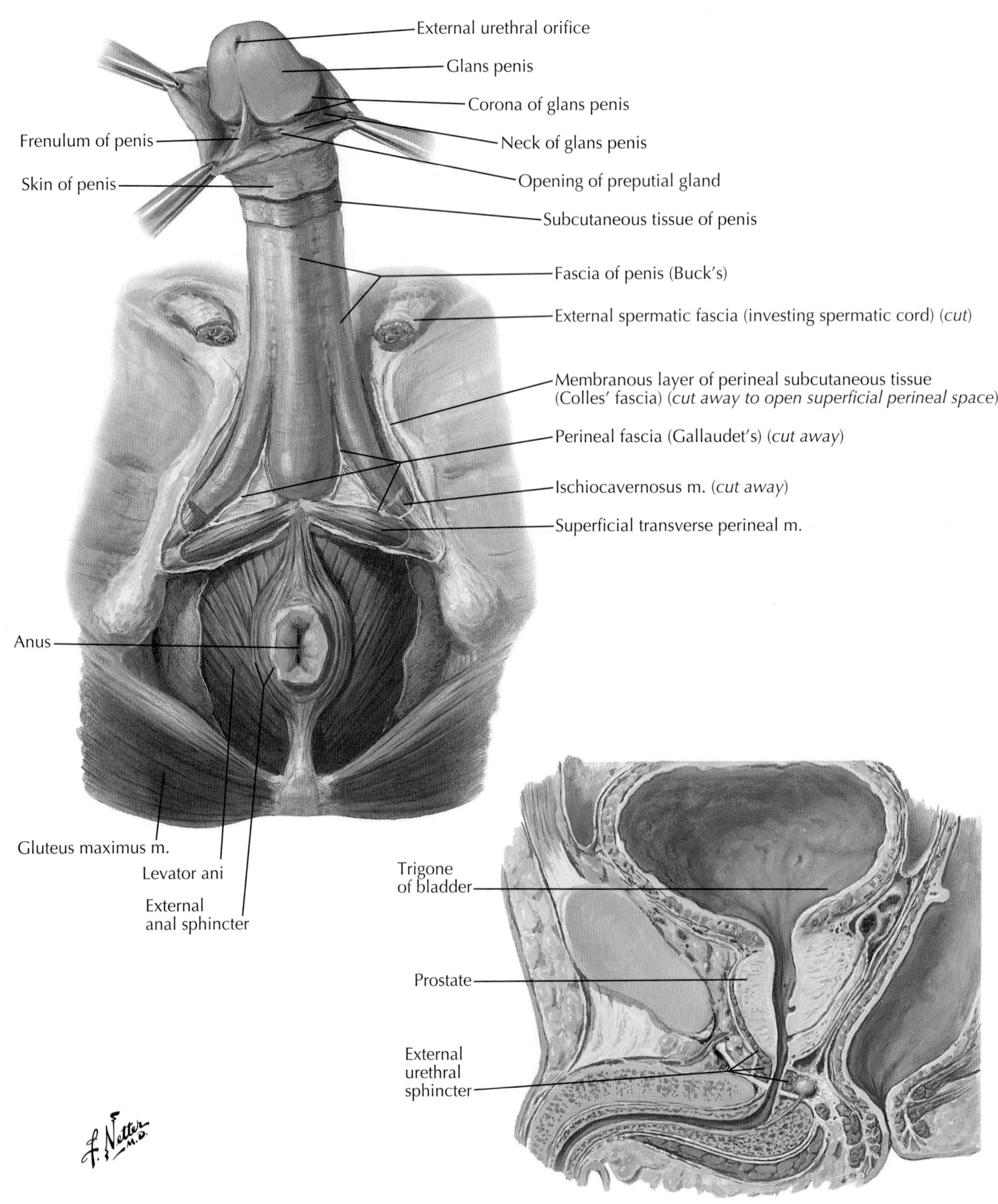
External urethral orifice
Glans penis
Corona of glans penis
Neck of glans penis
Frenulum of penis
Skin of penis
Opening of preputial gland
Subcutaneous tissue of penis
Fascia of penis (Buck's)
External spermatic fascia (investing spermatic cord) (cut)
Membranous layer of perineal subcutaneous tissue (Colles' fascia) (cut away to open superficial perineal space)
Perineal fascia (Gallaudet's) (cut away)
Ischiocavernosus m. (cut away)
Superficial transverse perineal m.
Anus
Gluteus maximus m.
Levator ani
External anal sphincter
Trigone of bladder
Prostate
External urethral sphincter

Fig. 5.17 Penis (Illustration)

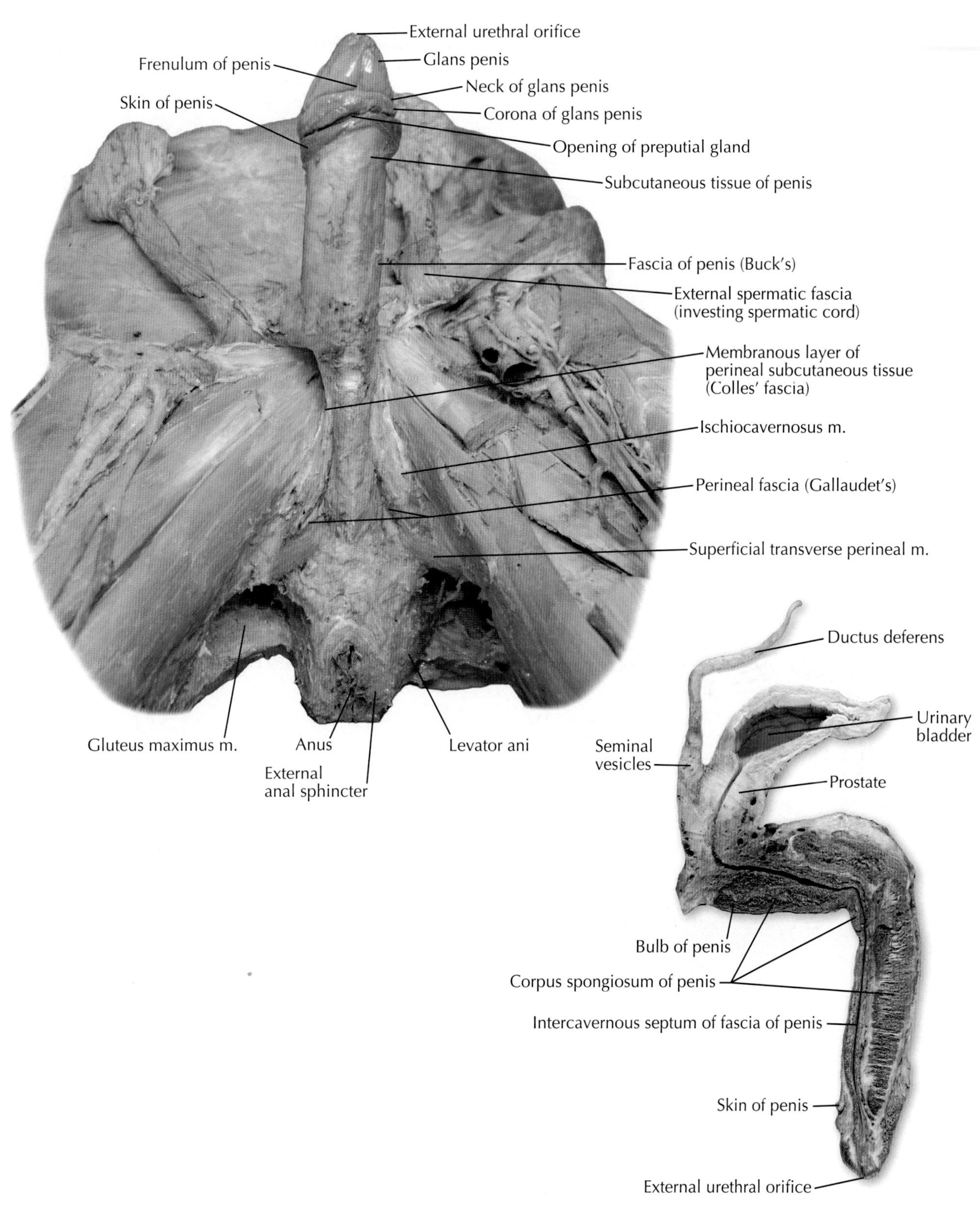
External urethral orifice
Glans penis
Frenulum of penis
Neck of glans penis
Skin of penis
Corona of glans penis
Opening of preputial gland
Subcutaneous tissue of penis
Fascia of penis (Buck's)
External spermatic fascia (investing spermatic cord)
Membranous layer of perineal subcutaneous tissue (Colles' fascia)
Ischiocavernosus m.
Perineal fascia (Gallaudet's)
Superficial transverse perineal m.
Gluteus maximus m.
Anus
External anal sphincter
Levator ani
Ductus deferens
Urinary bladder
Seminal vesicles
Prostate
Bulb of penis
Corpus spongiosum of penis
Intercavernous septum of fascia of penis
Skin of penis
External urethral orifice

Fig. 5.18 Penis (Photograph)

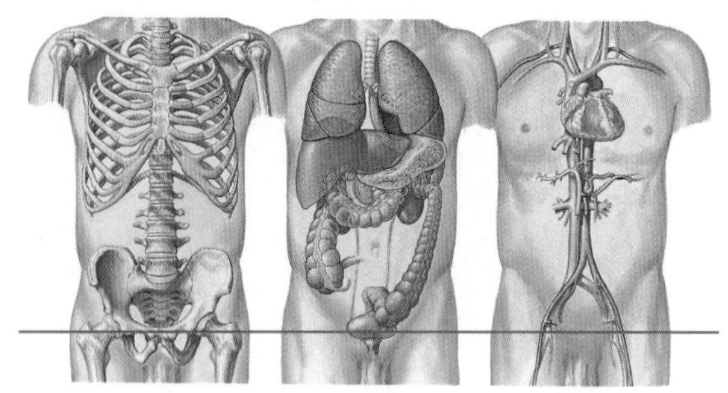

Pubic symphysis
Urinary bladder
Rectus abdominis m.
Spermatic cord
Body of pubis
Prostate
Pectineus m.
Psoas major
Femoral v., a. and n.
Internal pudendal vessels and n.
Sartorius m.
Iliacus m.
Iliopsoas
Head of femur
Rectus femoris m.
Tensor fasciae latae
Gluteus medius m.
Obturator a. and v.
Greater trochanter
Lunate surface of acetabulum
Ischium
Sciatic n.
Gluteus maximus m.
Inferior gluteal a. and v.
Obturator internus
Internal pudendal a. and v.
Adipose tissue
Pudendal n.
Prostatic urethra
Fat body of ischioanal fossa
Anorectal junction
Coccyx
Puboanalis m. (part of levator ani)
C. Machado M.D.

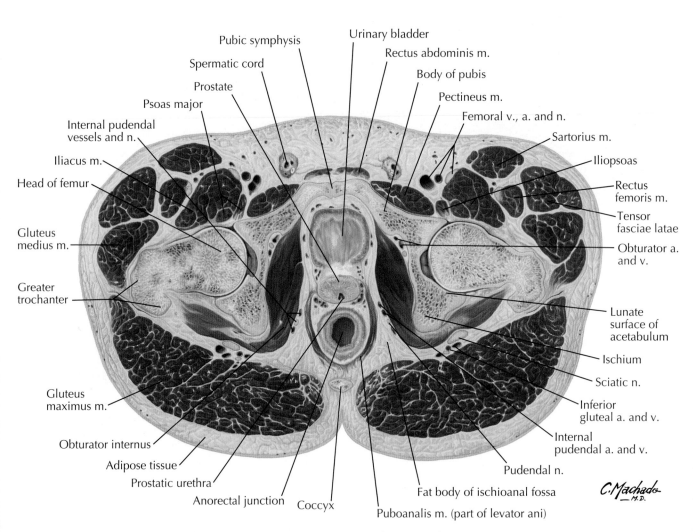

Fig. 5.19 Male Pelvis: Cross Section of Bladder-Prostate Junction (Illustration)

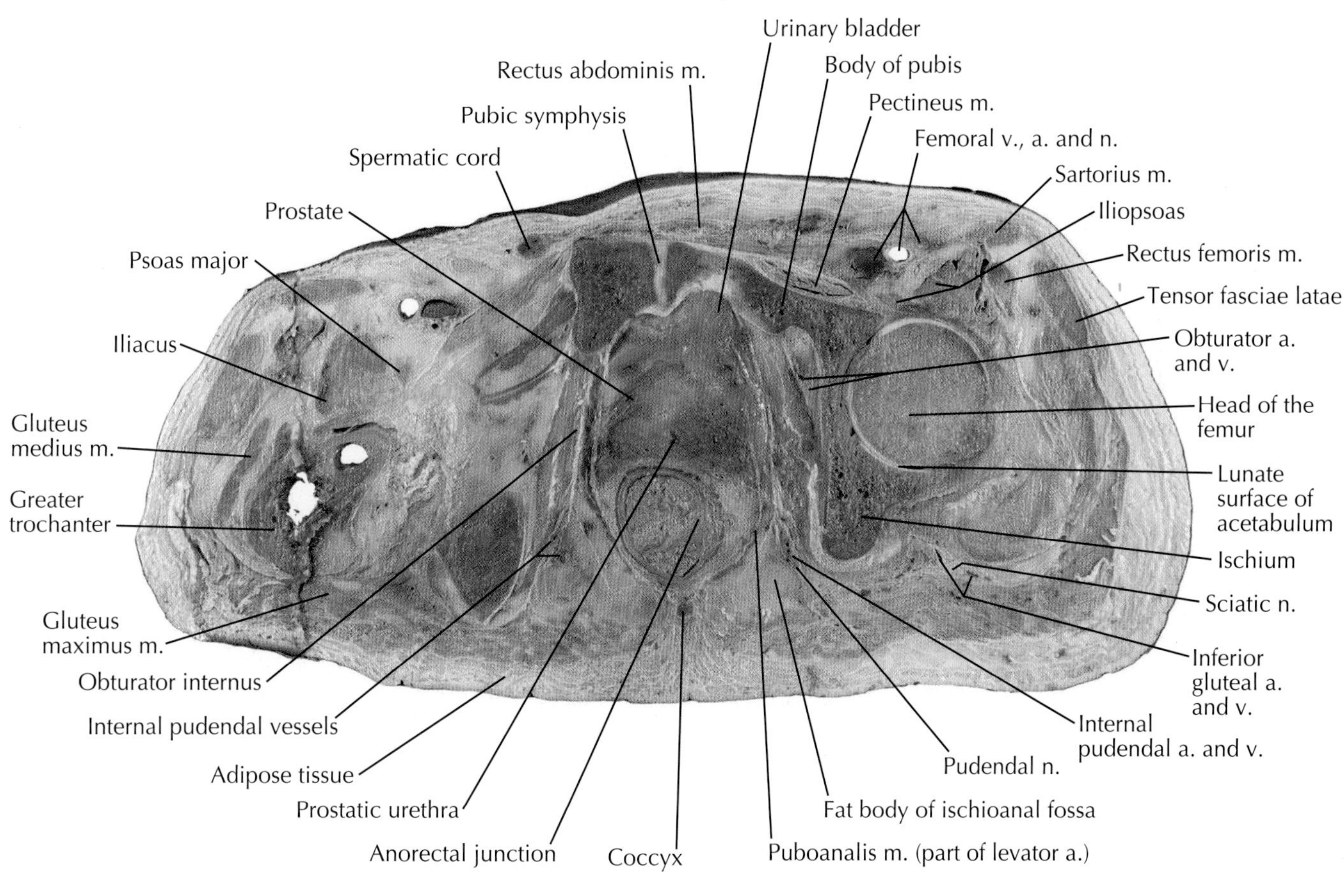
Urinary bladder
Body of pubis
Rectus abdominis m.
Pectineus m.
Pubic symphysis
Femoral v., a. and n.
Spermatic cord
Sartorius m.
Prostate
Iliopsoas
Psoas major
Rectus femoris m.
Tensor fasciae latae
Iliacus
Obturator a. and v.
Gluteus medius m.
Head of the femur
Greater trochanter
Lunate surface of acetabulum
Ischium
Sciatic n.
Gluteus maximus m.
Inferior gluteal a. and v.
Obturator internus
Internal pudendal vessels
Internal pudendal a. and v.
Pudendal n.
Adipose tissue
Prostatic urethra
Fat body of ischioanal fossa
Anorectal junction
Coccyx
Puboanalis m. (part of levator a.)

Fig. 5.20 Male Pelvis: Cross Section of Bladder-Prostate Junction (Photograph)

UPPER LIMB

CHAPTER 6

Alternate Version Available in Appendix

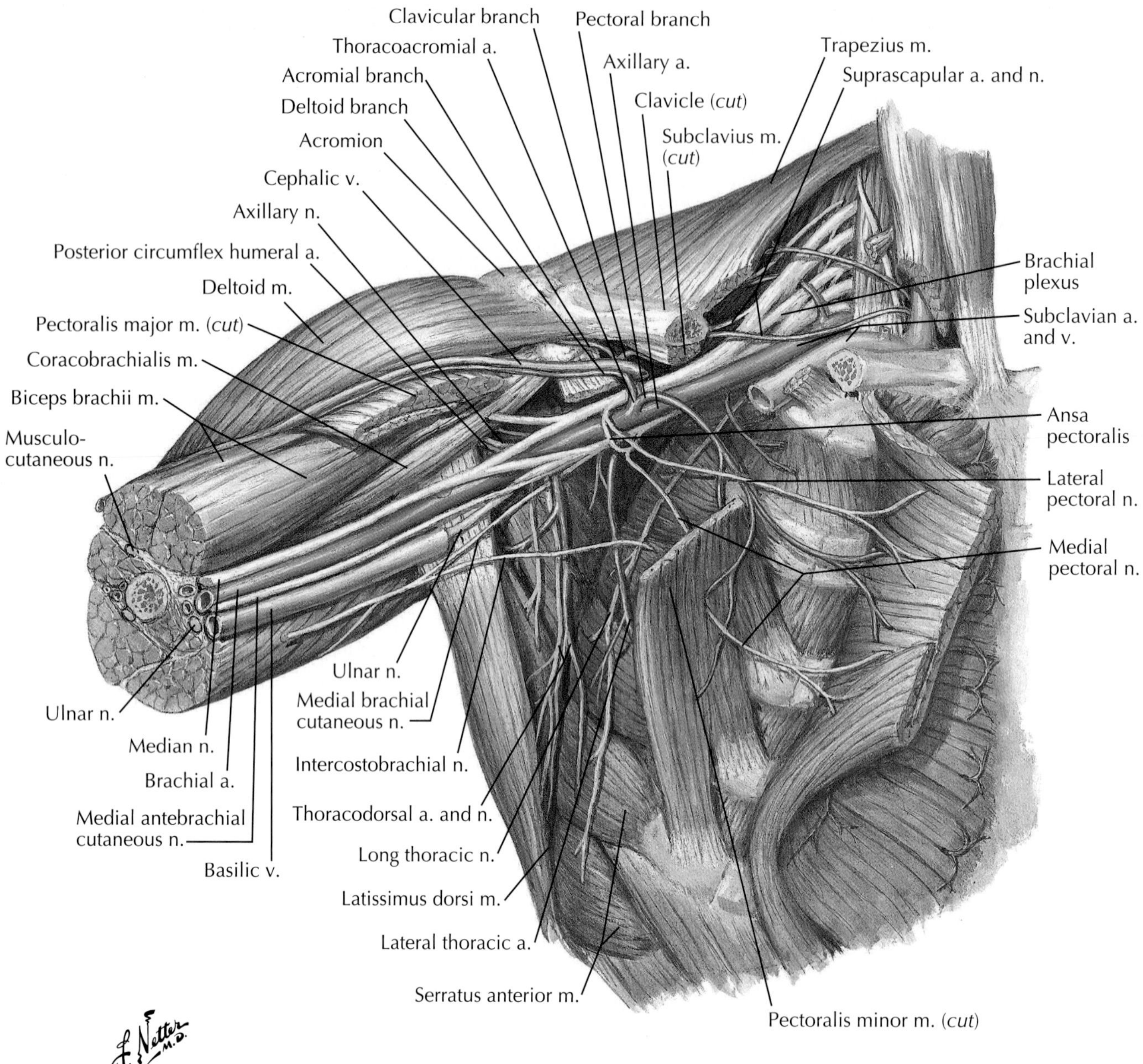
Clavicular branch
Pectoral branch
Thoracoacromial a.
Axillary a.
Trapezius m.
Suprascapular a. and n.
Acromial branch
Deltoid branch
Clavicle (cut)
Subclavius m. (cut)
Acromion
Cephalic v.
Axillary n.
Posterior circumflex humeral a.
Deltoid m.
Pectoralis major m. (cut)
Coracobrachialis m.
Biceps brachii m.
Musculo-cutaneous n.
Brachial plexus
Subclavian a. and v.
Ansa pectoralis
Lateral pectoral n.
Medial pectoral n.
Ulnar n.
Medial brachial cutaneous n.
Ulnar n.
Median n.
Brachial a.
Medial antebrachial cutaneous n.
Basilic v.
Intercostobrachial n.
Thoracodorsal a. and n.
Long thoracic n.
Latissimus dorsi m.
Lateral thoracic a.
Serratus anterior m.
Pectoralis minor m. (cut)

Fig. 6.1 Axilla: Anterior View (Illustration)

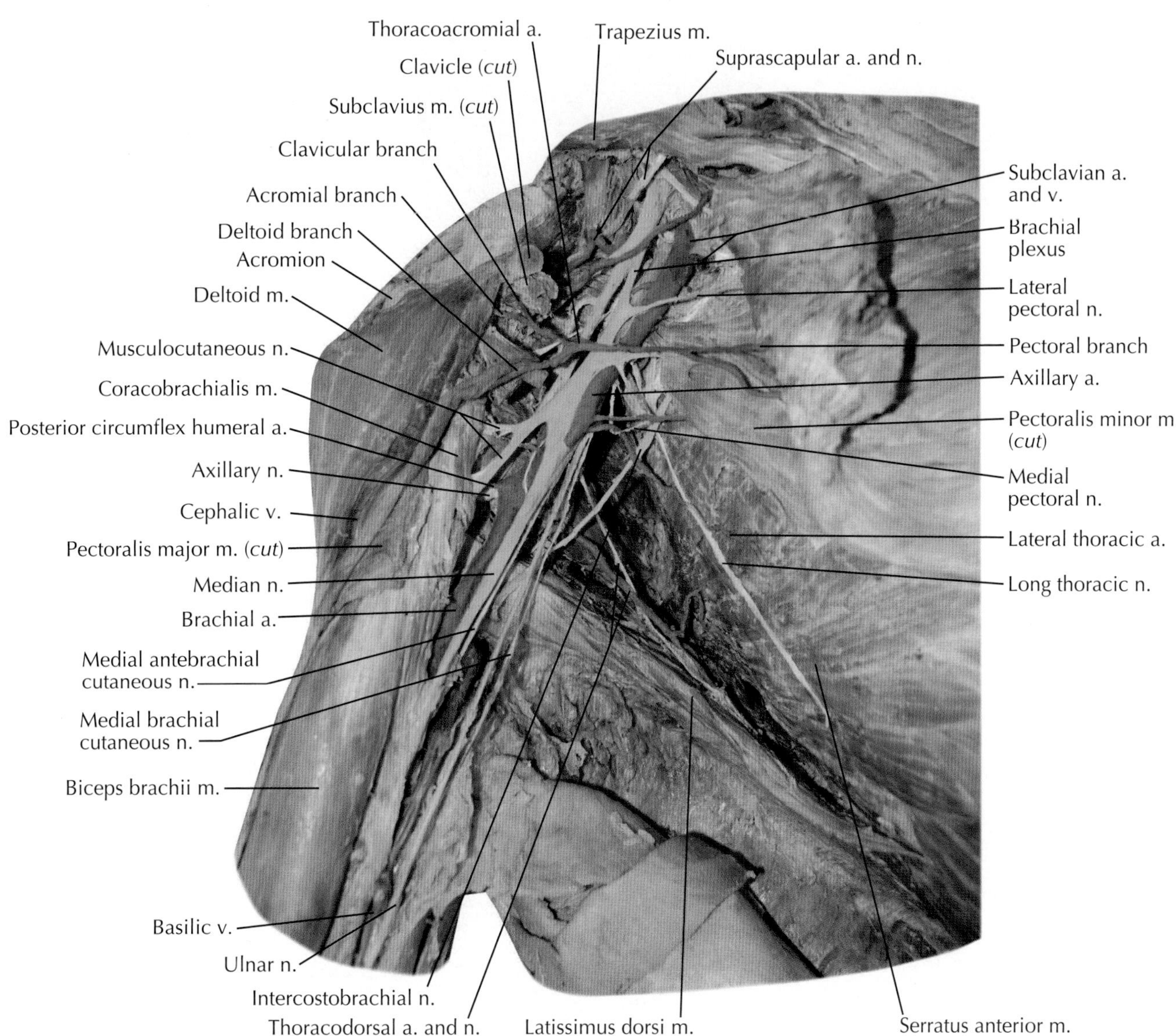
Thoracoacromial a.
Trapezius m.
Clavicle (*cut*)
Suprascapular a. and n.
Subclavius m. (*cut*)
Clavicular branch
Acromial branch
Deltoid branch
Acromion
Deltoid m.
Musculocutaneous n.
Coracobrachialis m.
Posterior circumflex humeral a.
Axillary n.
Cephalic v.
Pectoralis major m. (*cut*)
Median n.
Brachial a.
Medial antebrachial cutaneous n.
Medial brachial cutaneous n.
Biceps brachii m.
Basilic v.
Ulnar n.
Intercostobrachial n.
Thoracodorsal a. and n.
Latissimus dorsi m.
Serratus anterior m.
Subclavian a. and v.
Brachial plexus
Lateral pectoral n.
Pectoral branch
Axillary a.
Pectoralis minor m. (*cut*)
Medial pectoral n.
Lateral thoracic a.
Long thoracic n.

Fig. 6.2 Axilla: Anterior View (Photograph) (see Fig. A.13)

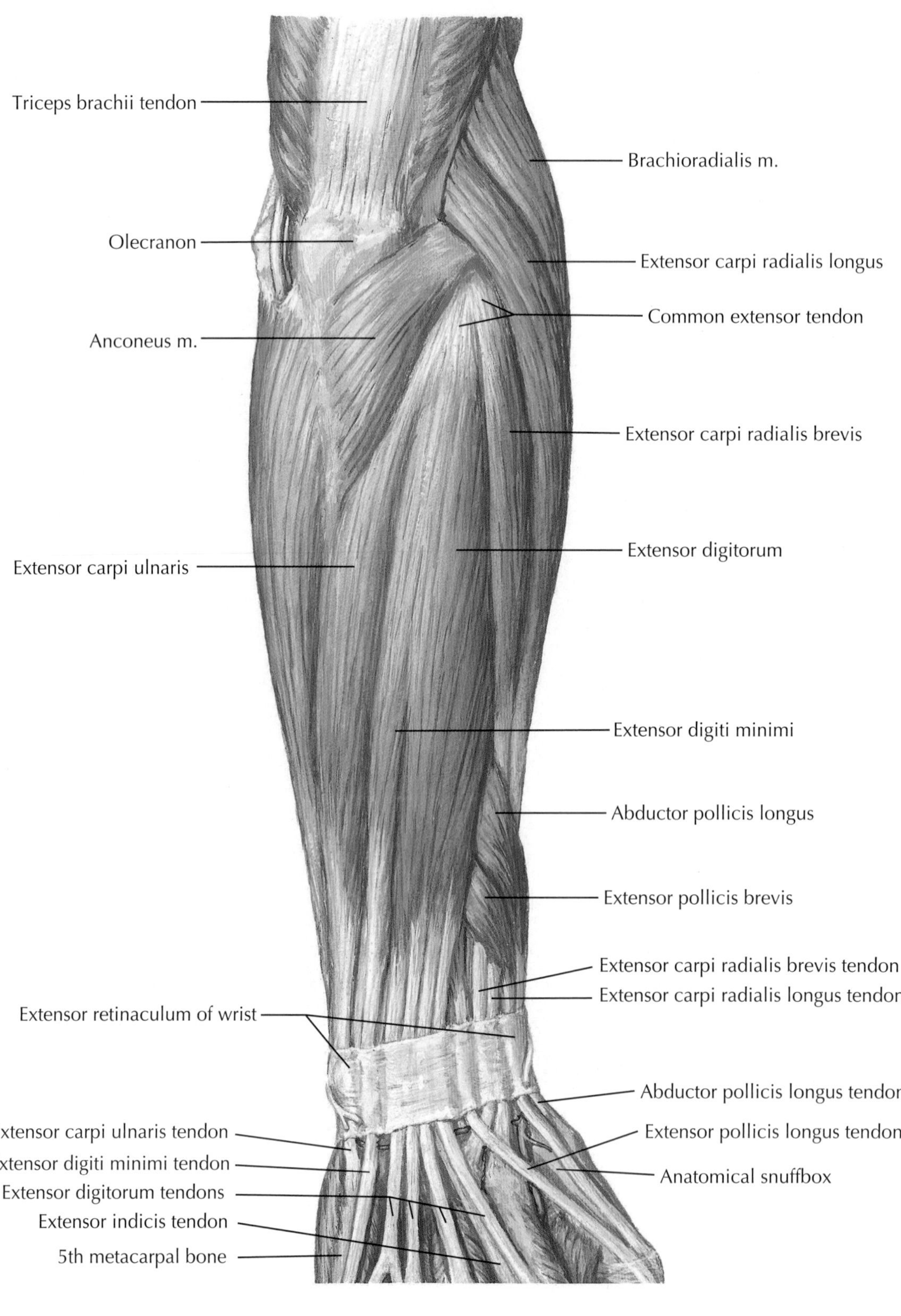
Triceps brachii tendon
Brachioradialis m.
Olecranon
Extensor carpi radialis longus
Common extensor tendon
Anconeus m.
Extensor carpi radialis brevis
Extensor carpi ulnaris
Extensor digitorum
Extensor digiti minimi
Abductor pollicis longus
Extensor pollicis brevis
Extensor carpi radialis brevis tendon
Extensor carpi radialis longus tendon
Extensor retinaculum of wrist
Abductor pollicis longus tendon
Extensor carpi ulnaris tendon
Extensor pollicis longus tendon
Extensor digiti minimi tendon
Anatomical snuffbox
Extensor digitorum tendons
Extensor indicis tendon
5th metacarpal bone
F. Netter M.D.

Fig. 6.3 Muscles of Forearm: Superficial Part of Posterior Compartment (Illustration)

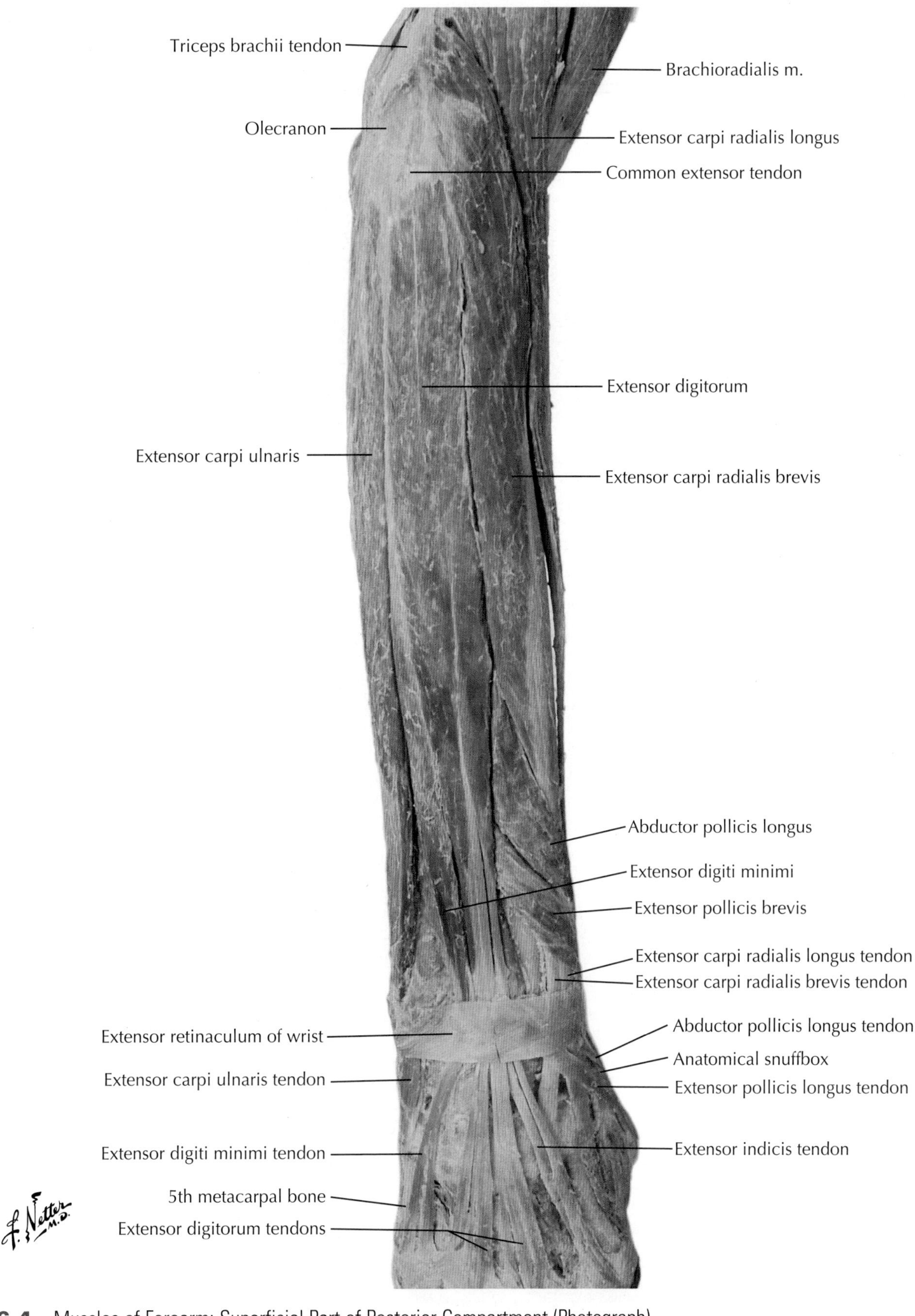
Triceps brachii tendon
Brachioradialis m.
Olecranon
Extensor carpi radialis longus
Common extensor tendon
Extensor digitorum
Extensor carpi ulnaris
Extensor carpi radialis brevis
Abductor pollicis longus
Extensor digiti minimi
Extensor pollicis brevis
Extensor carpi radialis longus tendon
Extensor carpi radialis brevis tendon
Extensor retinaculum of wrist
Abductor pollicis longus tendon
Anatomical snuffbox
Extensor carpi ulnaris tendon
Extensor pollicis longus tendon
Extensor digiti minimi tendon
Extensor indicis tendon
5th metacarpal bone
Extensor digitorum tendons
F. Netter M.D.

Fig. 6.4 Muscles of Forearm: Superficial Part of Posterior Compartment (Photograph)

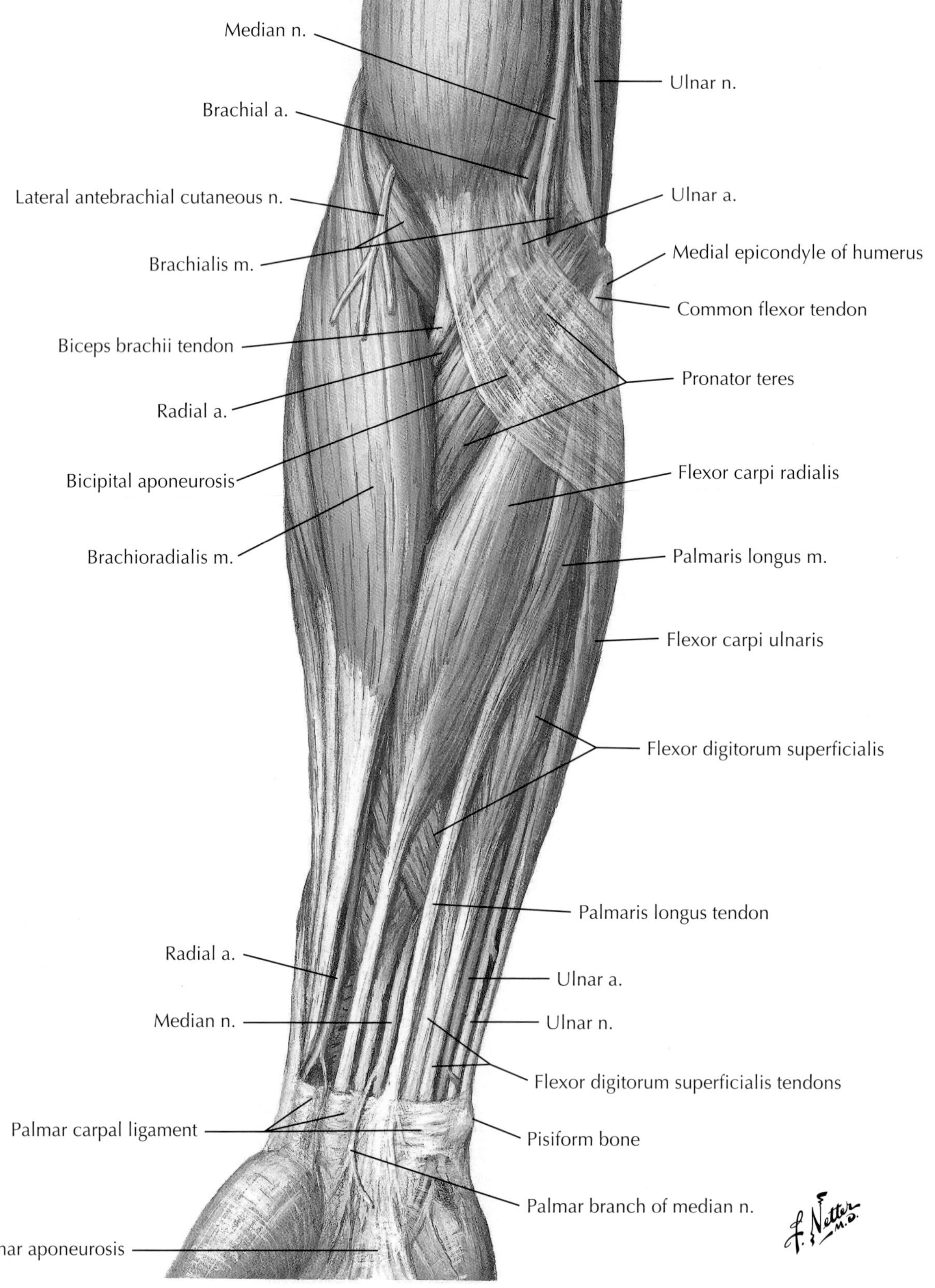
Median n.
Ulnar n.
Brachial a.
Lateral antebrachial cutaneous n.
Ulnar a.
Brachialis m.
Medial epicondyle of humerus
Common flexor tendon
Biceps brachii tendon
Pronator teres
Radial a.
Bicipital aponeurosis
Flexor carpi radialis
Brachioradialis m.
Palmaris longus m.
Flexor carpi ulnaris
Flexor digitorum superficialis
Palmaris longus tendon
Radial a.
Ulnar a.
Median n.
Ulnar n.
Flexor digitorum superficialis tendons
Palmar carpal ligament
Pisiform bone
Palmar branch of median n.
Palmar aponeurosis

Fig. 6.5 Muscles of Forearm: Superficial Part of Anterior Compartment (Illustration)

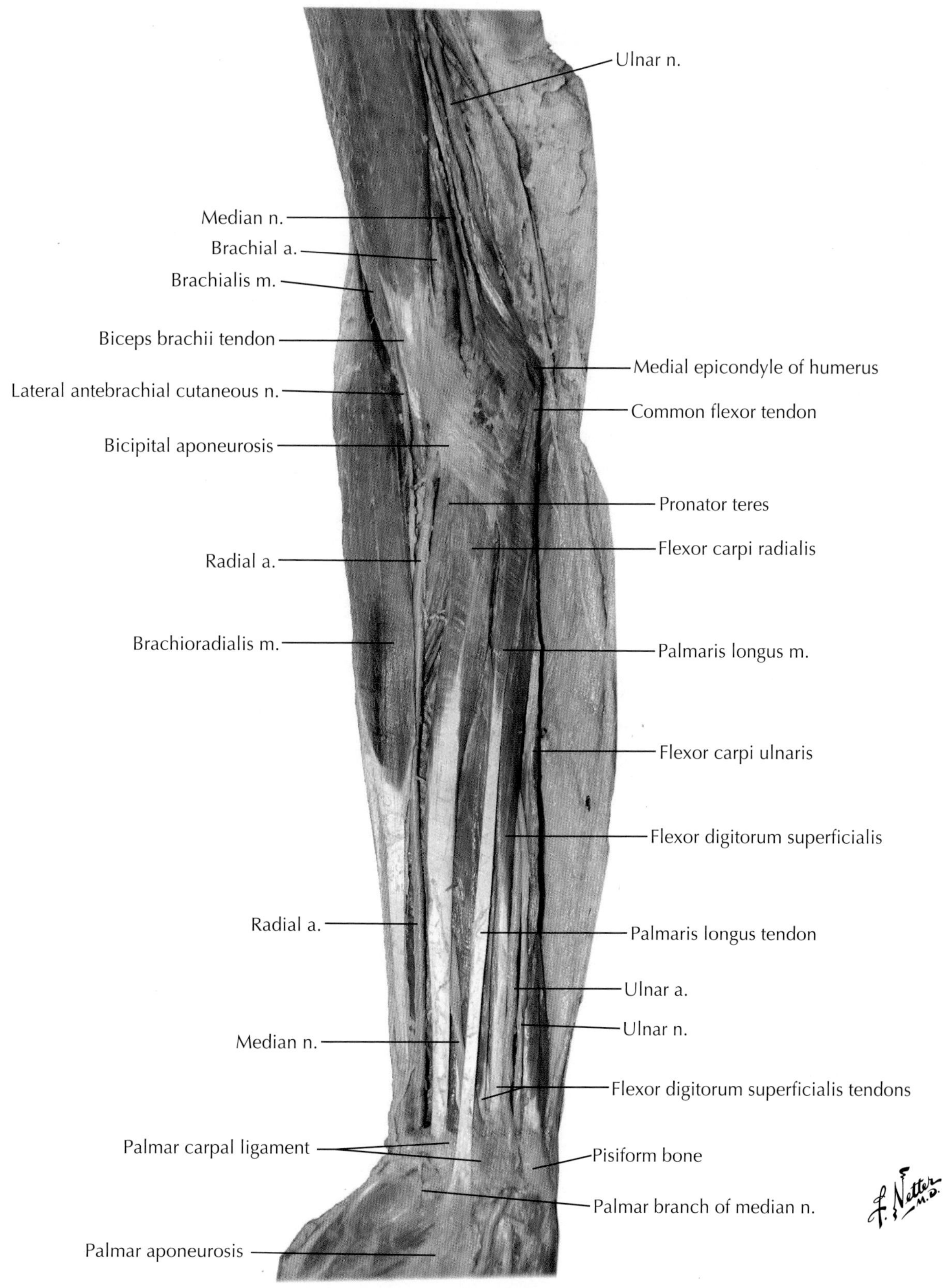
Ulnar n.
Median n.
Brachial a.
Brachialis m.
Biceps brachii tendon
Lateral antebrachial cutaneous n.
Bicipital aponeurosis
Medial epicondyle of humerus
Common flexor tendon
Pronator teres
Flexor carpi radialis
Radial a.
Brachioradialis m.
Palmaris longus m.
Flexor carpi ulnaris
Flexor digitorum superficialis
Radial a.
Palmaris longus tendon
Ulnar a.
Ulnar n.
Median n.
Flexor digitorum superficialis tendons
Palmar carpal ligament
Pisiform bone
Palmar branch of median n.
Palmar aponeurosis
F. Netter M.D.

Fig 6.6 Muscles of Forearm: Superficial Part of Anterior Compartment

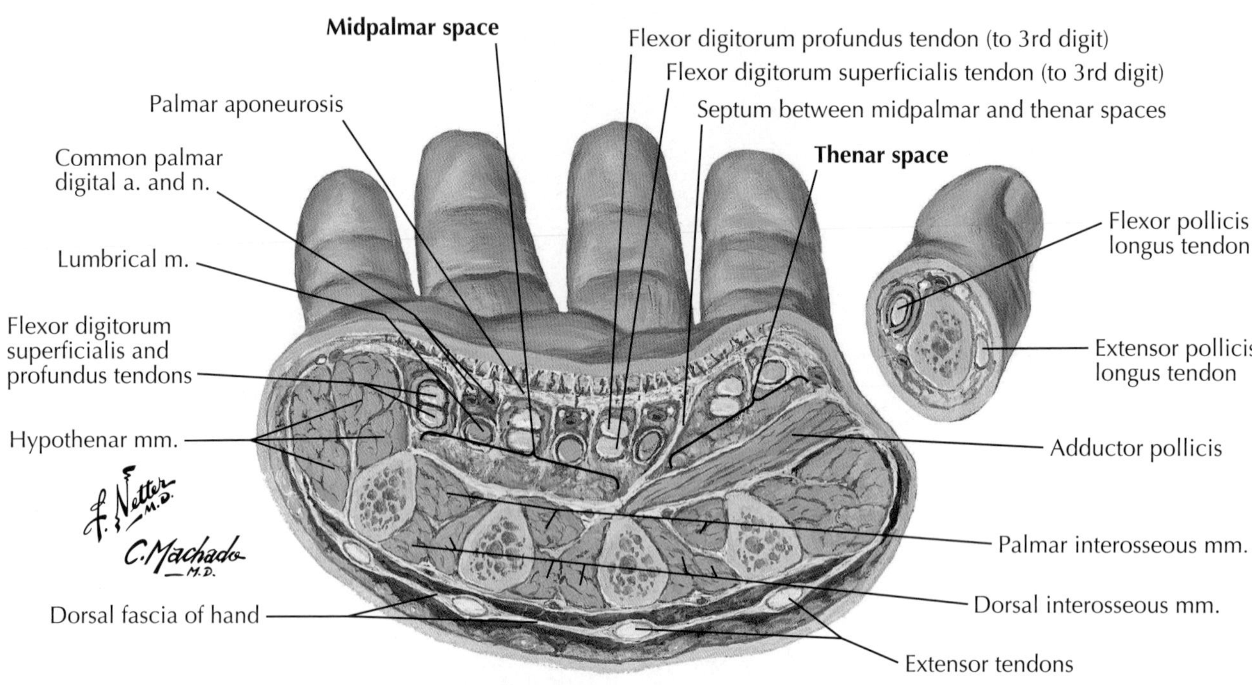
Midpalmar space
Flexor digitorum profundus tendon (to 3rd digit)
Flexor digitorum superficialis tendon (to 3rd digit)
Palmar aponeurosis
Septum between midpalmar and thenar spaces
Common palmar digital a. and n.
Thenar space
Flexor pollicis longus tendon
Lumbrical m.
Flexor digitorum superficialis and profundus tendons
Extensor pollicis longus tendon
Hypothenar mm.
Adductor pollicis
Palmar interosseous mm.
Dorsal interosseous mm.
Dorsal fascia of hand
Extensor tendons

Fig. 6.7 Spaces and Tendon Sheaths of Hand (Illustration)

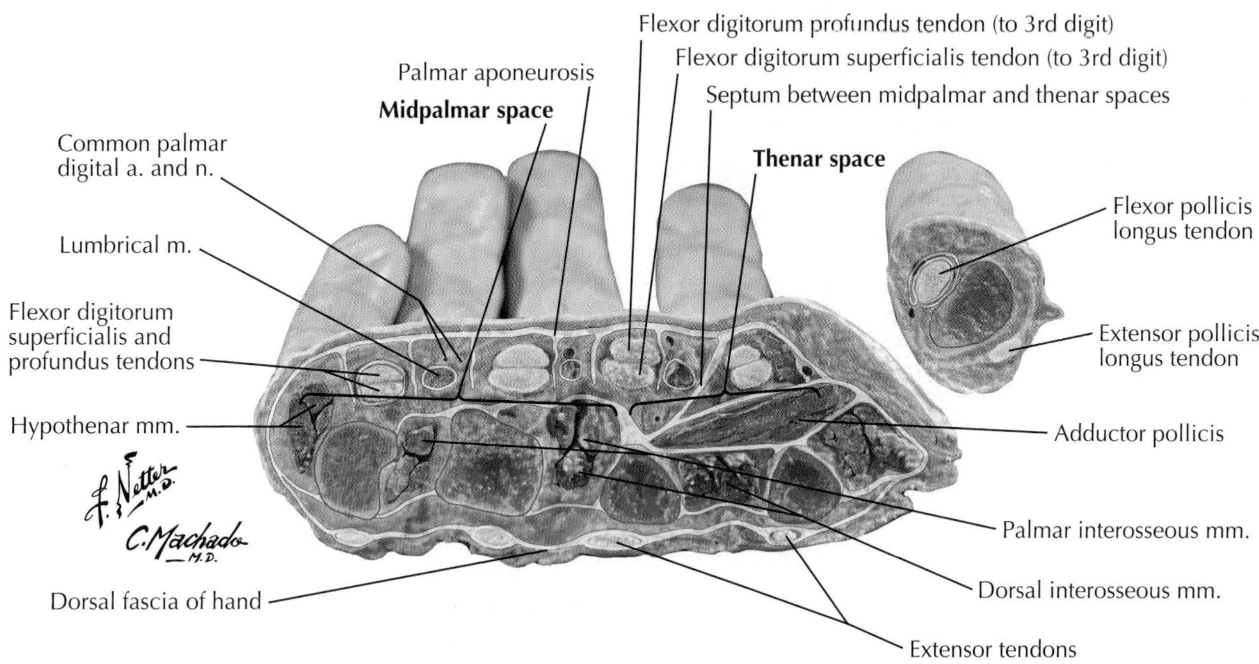
Flexor digitorum profundus tendon (to 3rd digit)
Flexor digitorum superficialis tendon (to 3rd digit)
Palmar aponeurosis
Septum between midpalmar and thenar spaces
Midpalmar space
Common palmar digital a. and n.
Thenar space
Flexor pollicis longus tendon
Lumbrical m.
Flexor digitorum superficialis and profundus tendons
Extensor pollicis longus tendon
Hypothenar mm.
Adductor pollicis
F. Netter M.D.
C.Machado M.D.
Palmar interosseous mm.
Dorsal interosseous mm.
Dorsal fascia of hand
Extensor tendons

Fig. 6.8 Spaces and Tendon Sheaths of Hand (Photograph) (see Fig. A.14)

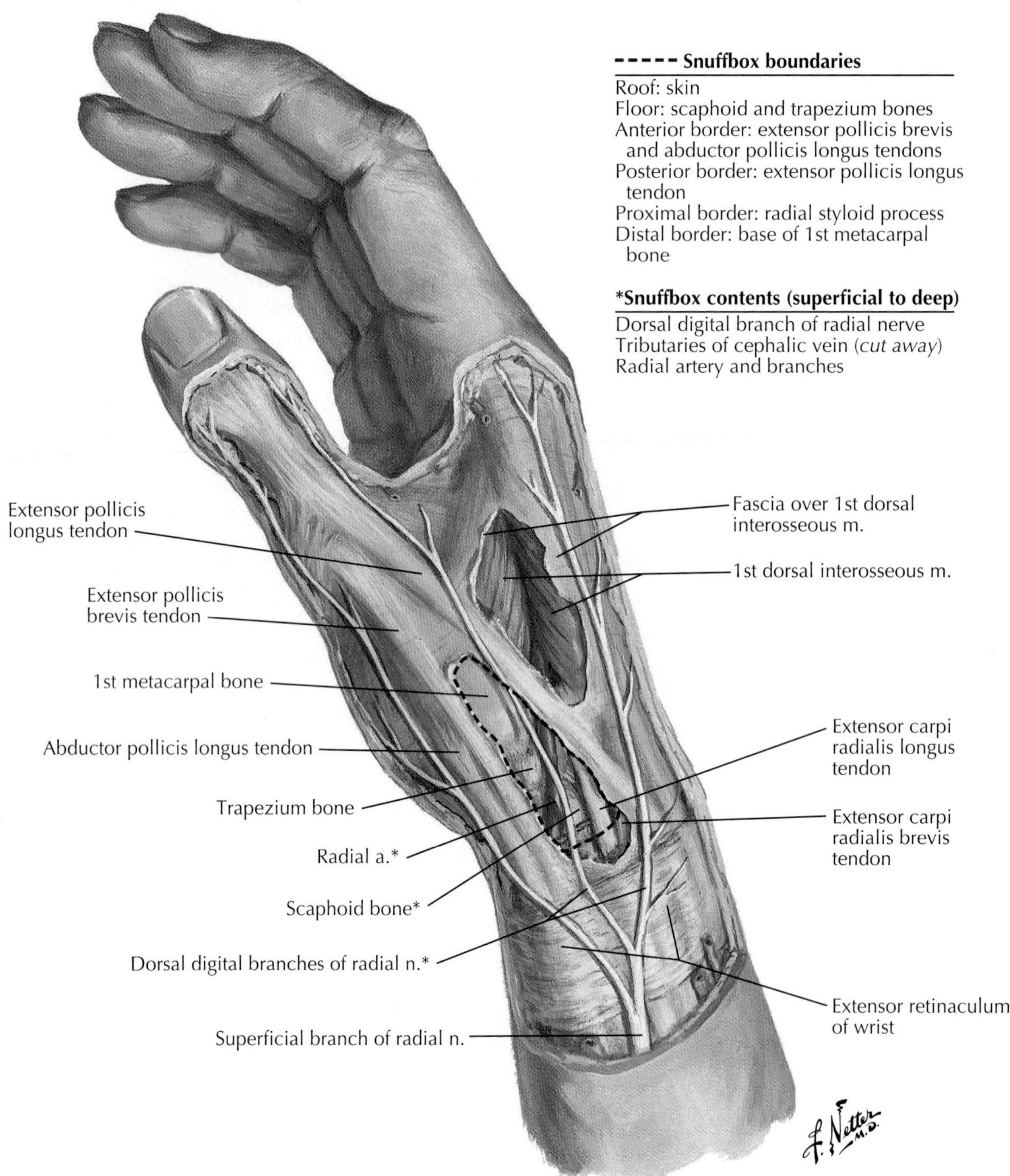
----- Snuffbox boundaries
Roof: skin
Floor: scaphoid and trapezium bones
Anterior border: extensor pollicis brevis and abductor pollicis longus tendons
Posterior border: extensor pollicis longus tendon
Proximal border: radial styloid process
Distal border: base of 1st metacarpal bone
*Snuffbox contents (superficial to deep)
Dorsal digital branch of radial nerve
Tributaries of cephalic vein (cut away)
Radial artery and branches
Extensor pollicis longus tendon
Extensor pollicis brevis tendon
1st metacarpal bone
Abductor pollicis longus tendon
Trapezium bone
Radial a.*
Scaphoid bone*
Dorsal digital branches of radial n.*
Superficial branch of radial n.
Fascia over 1st dorsal interosseous m.
1st dorsal interosseous m.
Extensor carpi radialis longus tendon
Extensor carpi radialis brevis tendon
Extensor retinaculum of wrist

Fig. 6.9 Wrist and Hand: Superficial Lateral Dissection (Illustration)

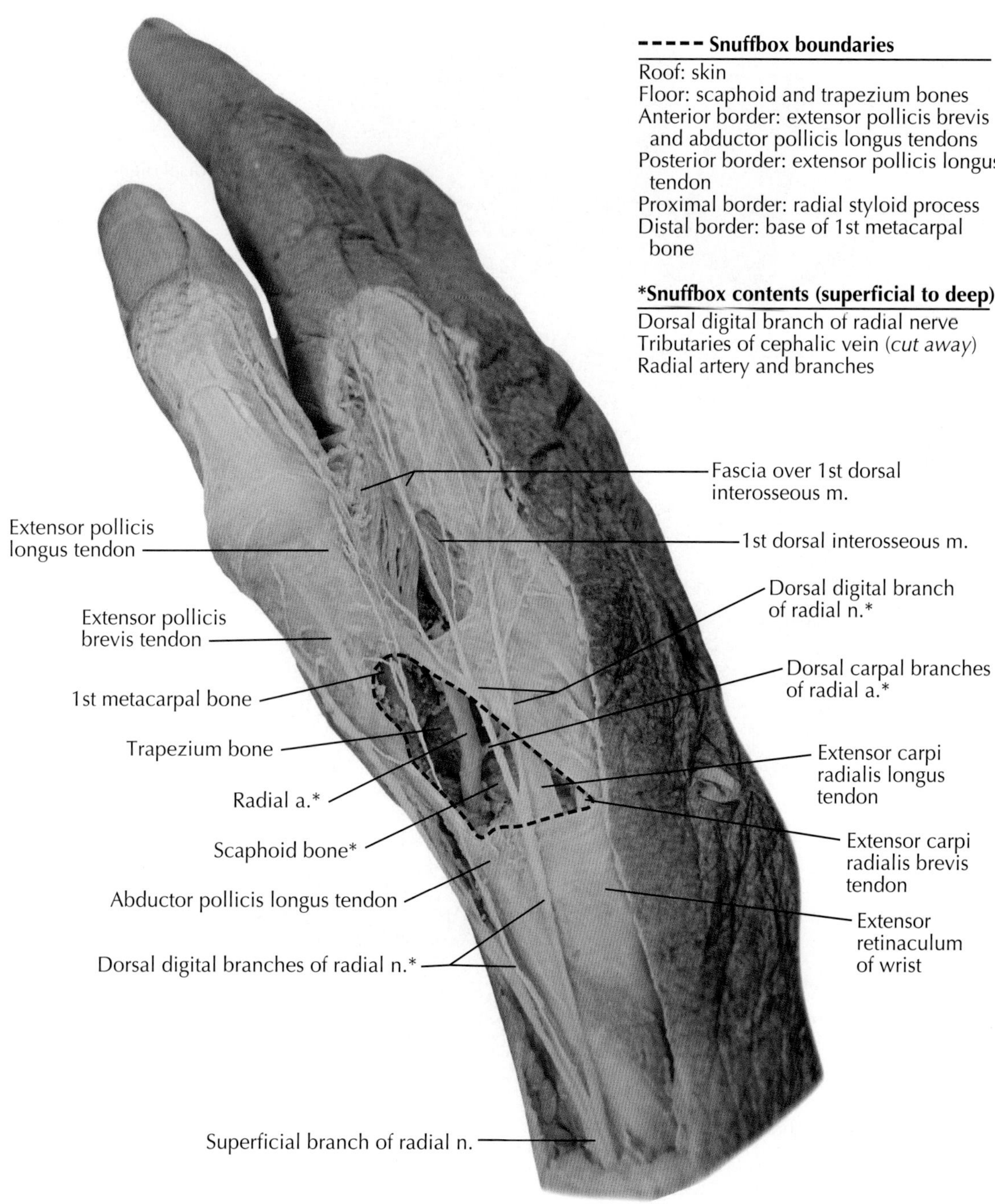
----- Snuffbox boundaries
Roof: skin
Floor: scaphoid and trapezium bones
Anterior border: extensor pollicis brevis and abductor pollicis longus tendons
Posterior border: extensor pollicis longus tendon
Proximal border: radial styloid process
Distal border: base of 1st metacarpal bone
*Snuffbox contents (superficial to deep)
Dorsal digital branch of radial nerve
Tributaries of cephalic vein (cut away)
Radial artery and branches
Fascia over 1st dorsal interosseous m.
1st dorsal interosseous m.
Dorsal digital branch of radial n.*
Dorsal carpal branches of radial a.*
Extensor carpi radialis longus tendon
Extensor carpi radialis brevis tendon
Extensor retinaculum of wrist
Extensor pollicis longus tendon
Extensor pollicis brevis tendon
1st metacarpal bone
Trapezium bone
Radial a.*
Scaphoid bone*
Abductor pollicis longus tendon
Dorsal digital branches of radial n.*
Superficial branch of radial n.

Fig. 6.10 Wrist and Hand: Superficial Lateral Dissection (Photograph)

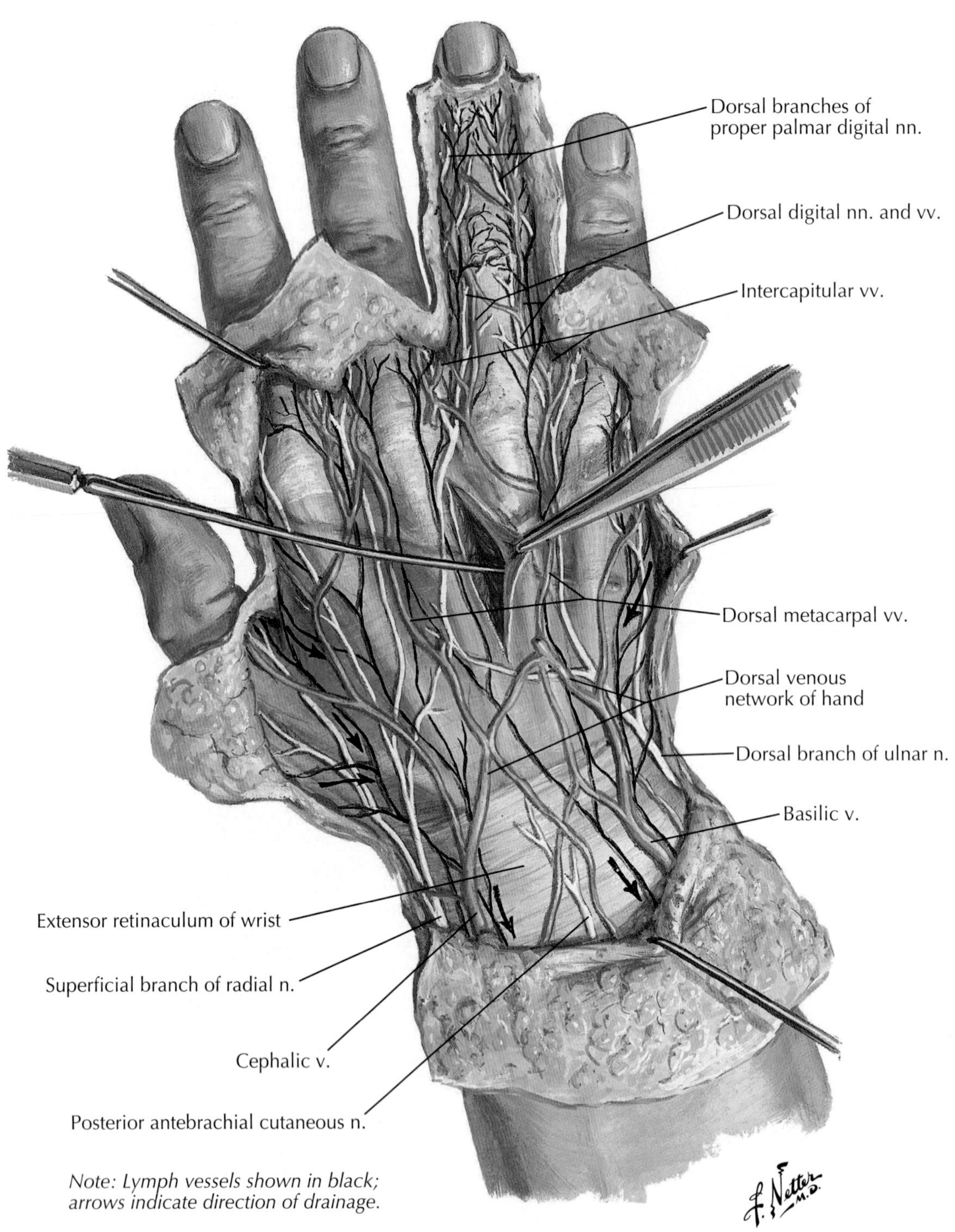
Dorsal branches of
proper palmar digital nn.
Dorsal digital nn. and vv.
Intercapitular vv.
Dorsal metacarpal vv.
Dorsal venous
network of hand
Dorsal branch of ulnar n.
Basilic v.
Extensor retinaculum of wrist
Superficial branch of radial n.
Cephalic v.
Posterior antebrachial cutaneous n.
Note: Lymph vessels shown in black;
arrows indicate direction of drainage.

Fig. 6.11 Wrist and Hand: Superficial Dorsal Dissection (Illustration)

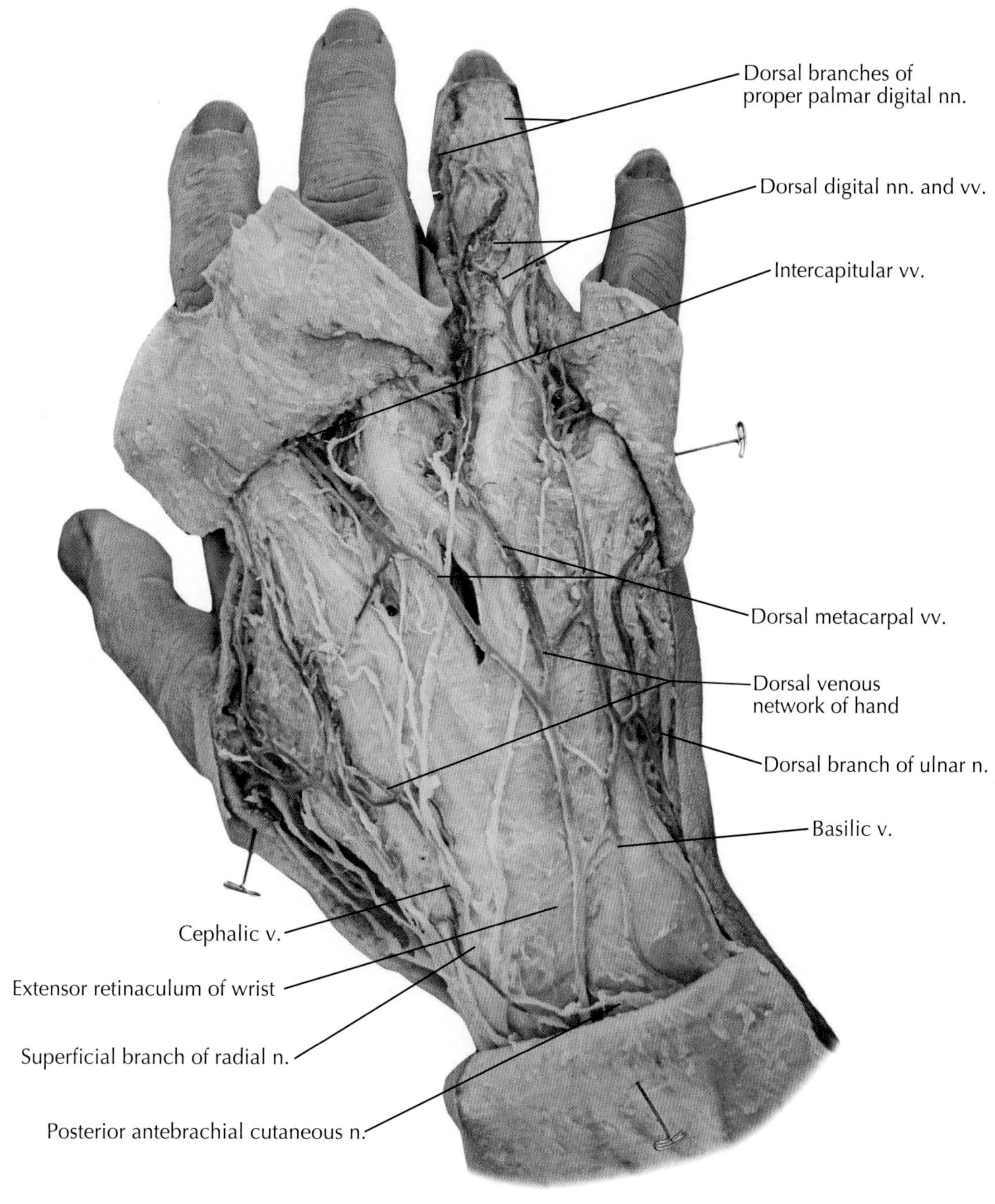
Dorsal branches of proper palmar digital nn.
Dorsal digital nn. and vv.
Intercapitular vv.
Dorsal metacarpal vv.
Dorsal venous network of hand
Dorsal branch of ulnar n.
Basilic v.
Cephalic v.
Extensor retinaculum of wrist
Superficial branch of radial n.
Posterior antebrachial cutaneous n.

Fig. 6.12 Wrist and Hand: Superficial Dorsal Dissection (Photograph)

LOWER LIMB

CHAPTER 7

Alternate Version Available in Appendix

Superficial dissections

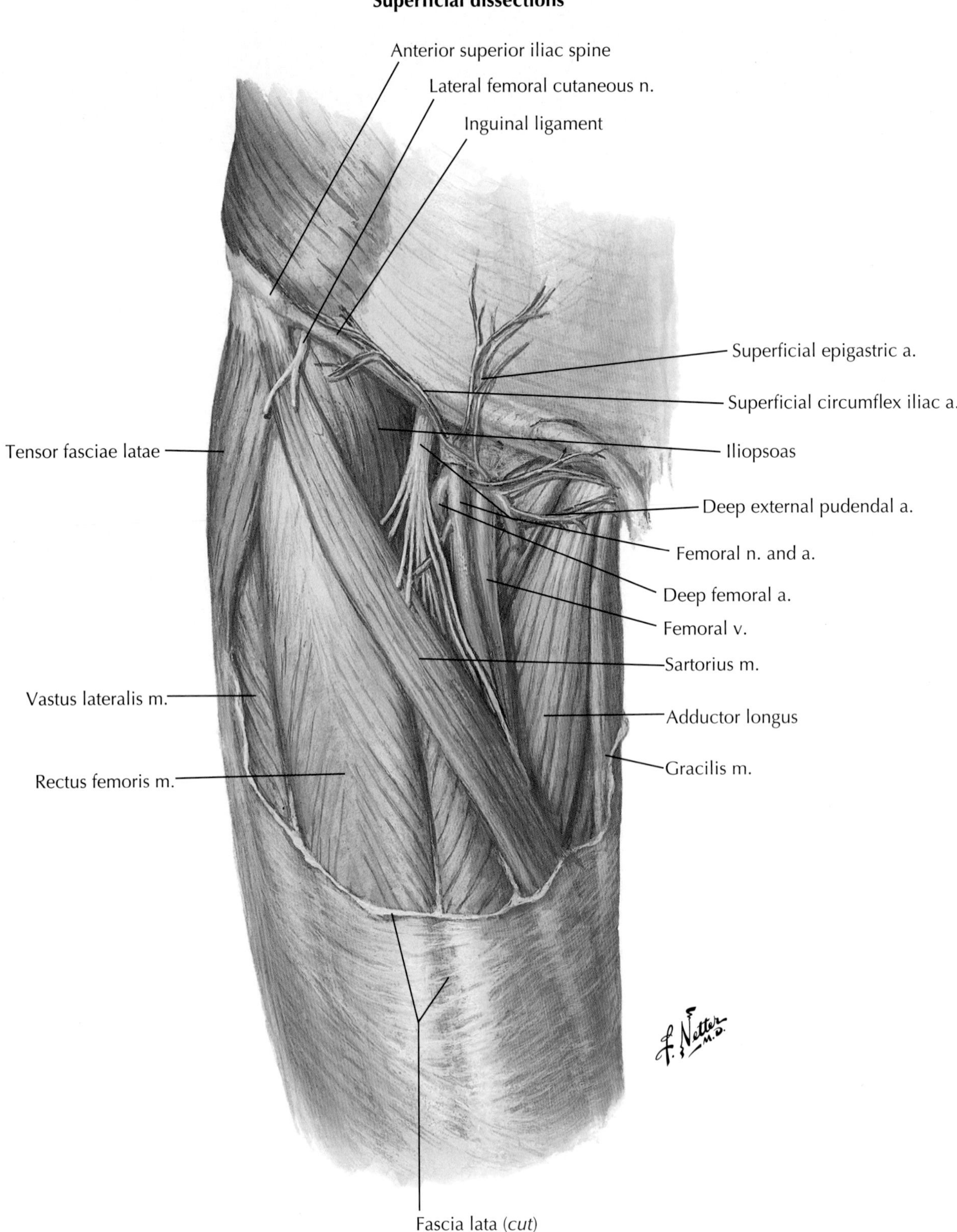
Anterior superior iliac spine
Lateral femoral cutaneous n.
Inguinal ligament
Superficial epigastric a.
Superficial circumflex iliac a.
Tensor fasciae latae
Iliopsoas
Deep external pudendal a.
Femoral n. and a.
Deep femoral a.
Femoral v.
Sartorius m.
Vastus lateralis m.
Adductor longus
Gracilis m.
Rectus femoris m.
Fascia lata (*cut*)

Fig. 7.1 Arteries of Thigh: Anterior Views (Illustration)

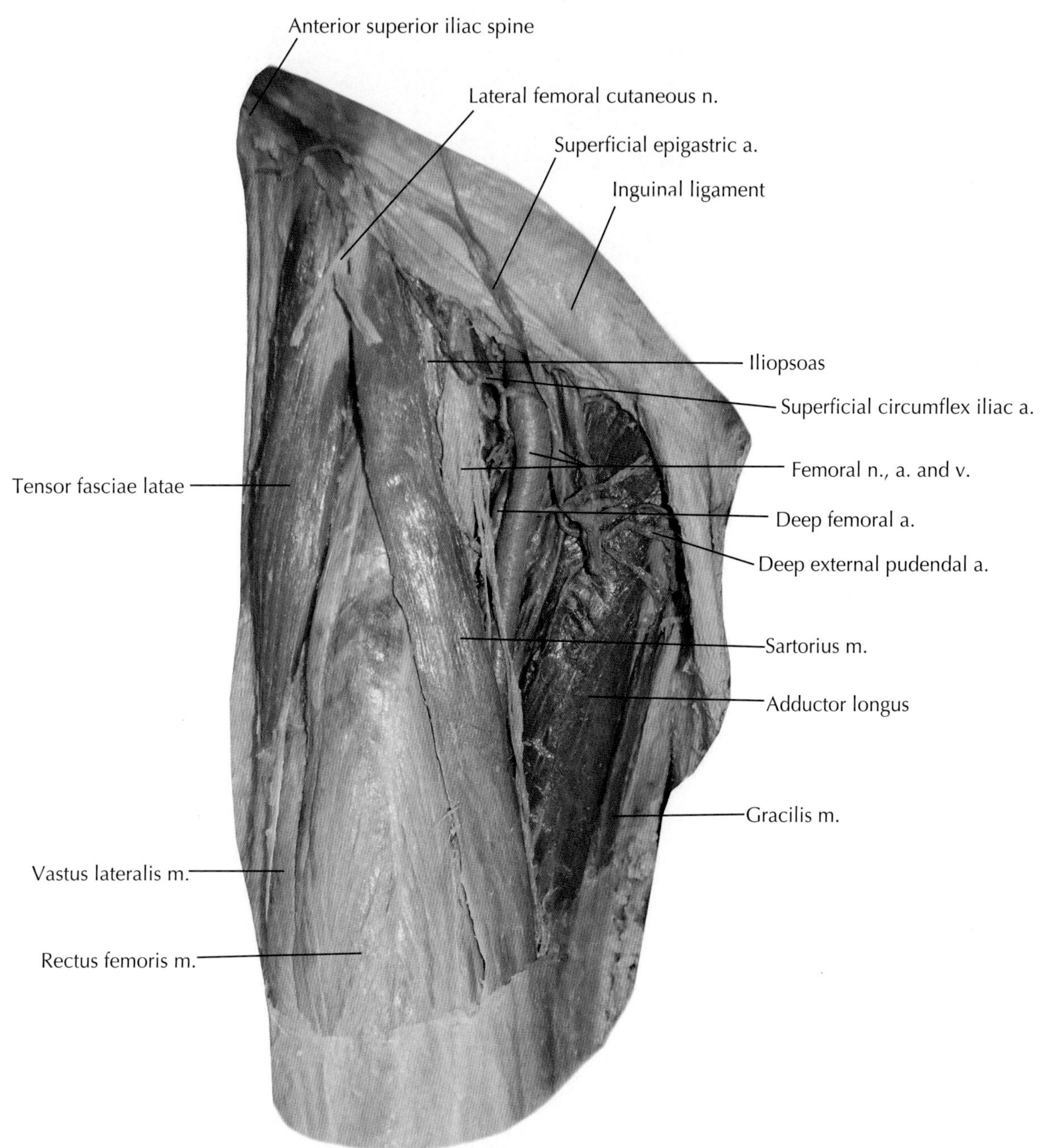
Superficial dissections
Anterior superior iliac spine
Lateral femoral cutaneous n.
Superficial epigastric a.
Inguinal ligament
Iliopsoas
Superficial circumflex iliac a.
Femoral n., a. and v.
Deep femoral a.
Deep external pudendal a.
Tensor fasciae latae
Sartorius m.
Adductor longus
Gracilis m.
Vastus lateralis m.
Rectus femoris m.

Fig. 7.2 Arteries of Thigh: Anterior Views (Photograph) (see Fig. A.15)

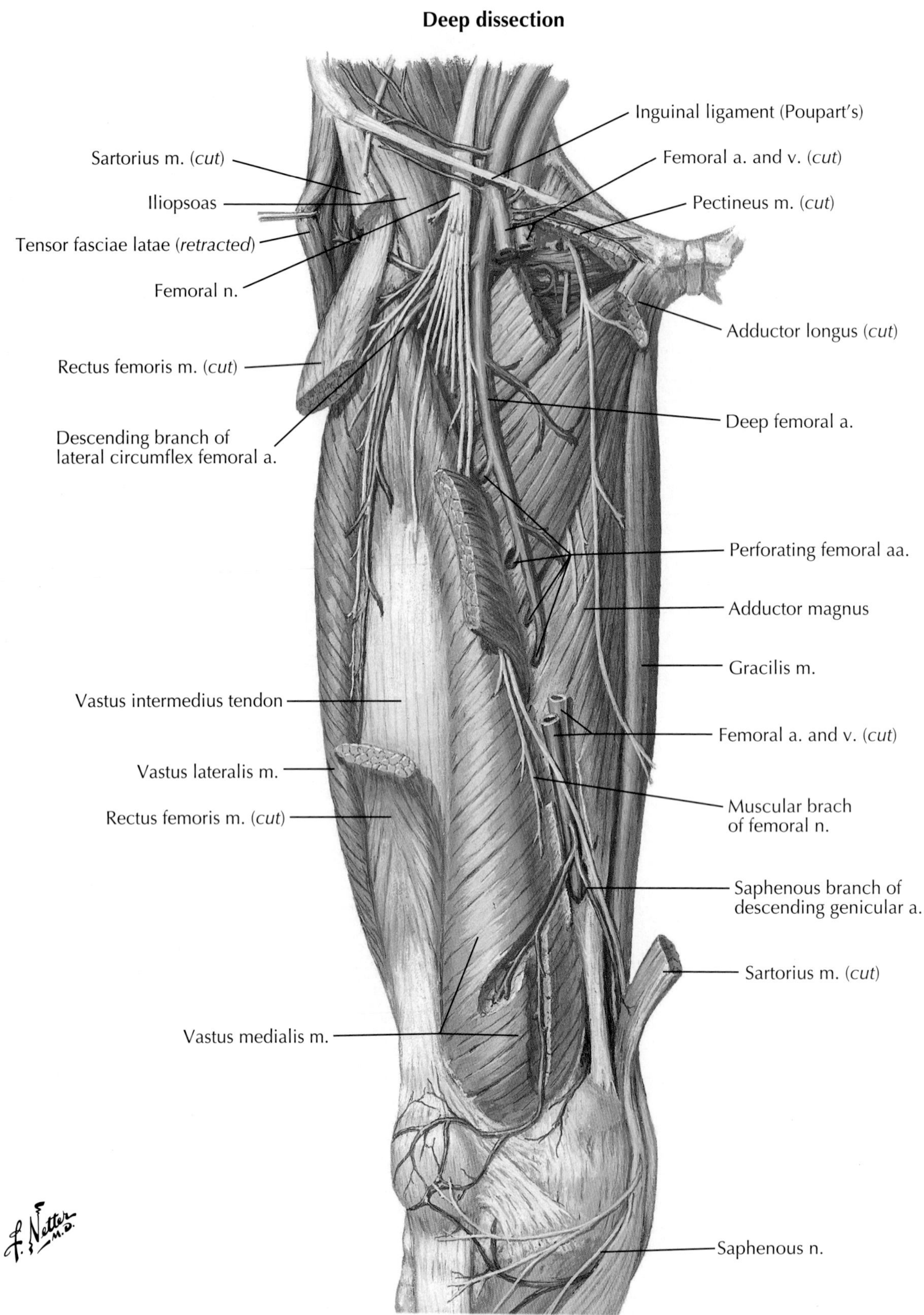
Deep dissection
Inguinal ligament (Poupart's)
Femoral a. and v. (cut)
Pectineus m. (cut)
Sartorius m. (cut)
Iliopsoas
Tensor fasciae latae (retracted)
Femoral n.
Adductor longus (cut)
Rectus femoris m. (cut)
Deep femoral a.
Descending branch of
lateral circumflex femoral a.
Perforating femoral aa.
Adductor magnus
Gracilis m.
Vastus intermedius tendon
Femoral a. and v. (cut)
Vastus lateralis m.
Rectus femoris m. (cut)
Muscular brach
of femoral n.
Saphenous branch of
descending genicular a.
Sartorius m. (cut)
Vastus medialis m.
Saphenous n.

Fig. 7.3 Arteries of Thigh: Anterior View of Deeper Dissection (Illustration)

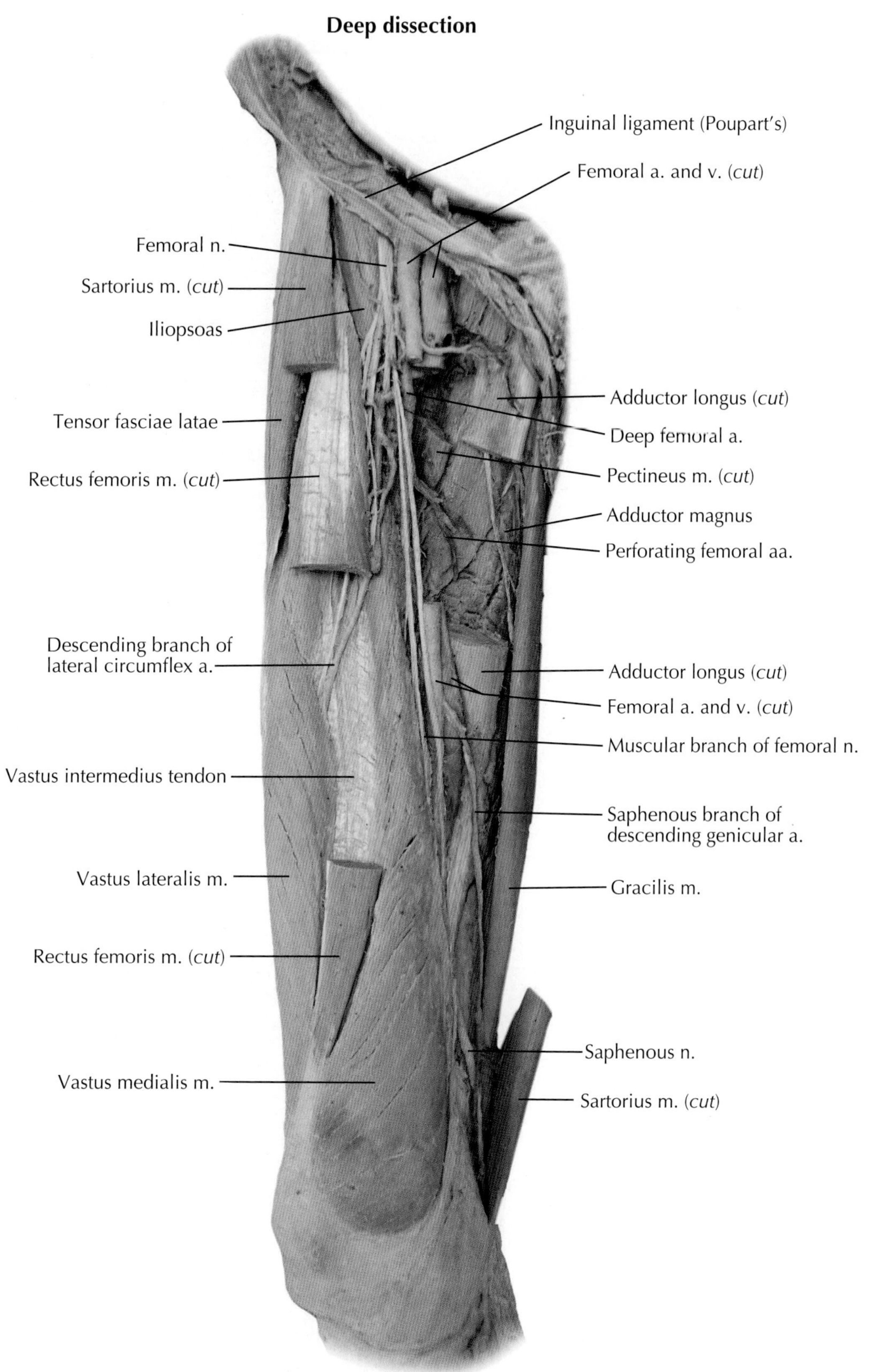
Deep dissection
Inguinal ligament (Poupart's)
Femoral a. and v. (cut)
Femoral n.
Sartorius m. (cut)
Iliopsoas
Adductor longus (cut)
Deep femoral a.
Tensor fasciae latae
Rectus femoris m. (cut)
Pectineus m. (cut)
Adductor magnus
Perforating femoral aa.
Descending branch of lateral circumflex a.
Adductor longus (cut)
Femoral a. and v. (cut)
Muscular branch of femoral n.
Vastus intermedius tendon
Saphenous branch of descending genicular a.
Vastus lateralis m.
Gracilis m.
Rectus femoris m. (cut)
Saphenous n.
Vastus medialis m.
Sartorius m. (cut)

Fig. 7.4 Arteries of Thigh: Anterior View of Deeper Dissection (Photograph) (see Fig. A.16)

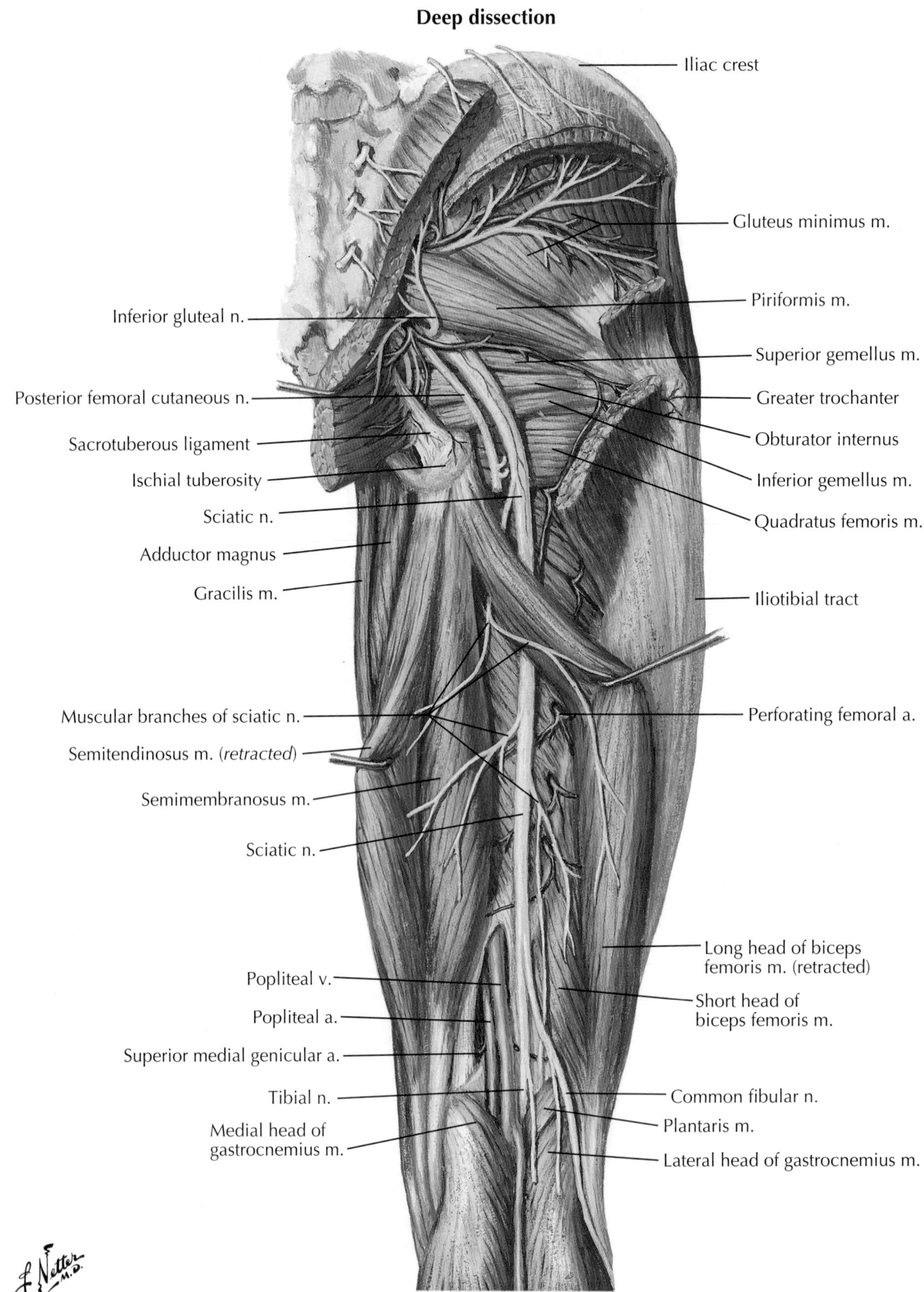
Deep dissection
Iliac crest
Gluteus minimus m.
Piriformis m.
Inferior gluteal n.
Superior gemellus m.
Posterior femoral cutaneous n.
Greater trochanter
Obturator internus
Sacrotuberous ligament
Ischial tuberosity
Inferior gemellus m.
Sciatic n.
Quadratus femoris m.
Adductor magnus
Gracilis m.
Iliotibial tract
Muscular branches of sciatic n.
Perforating femoral a.
Semitendinosus m. (retracted)
Semimembranosus m.
Sciatic n.
Long head of biceps femoris m. (retracted)
Popliteal v.
Short head of biceps femoris m.
Popliteal a.
Superior medial genicular a.
Tibial n.
Common fibular n.
Plantaris m.
Medial head of gastrocnemius m.
Lateral head of gastrocnemius m.
F. Netter M.D.

Fig. 7.5 Arteries of Thigh: Posterior View (Illustration)

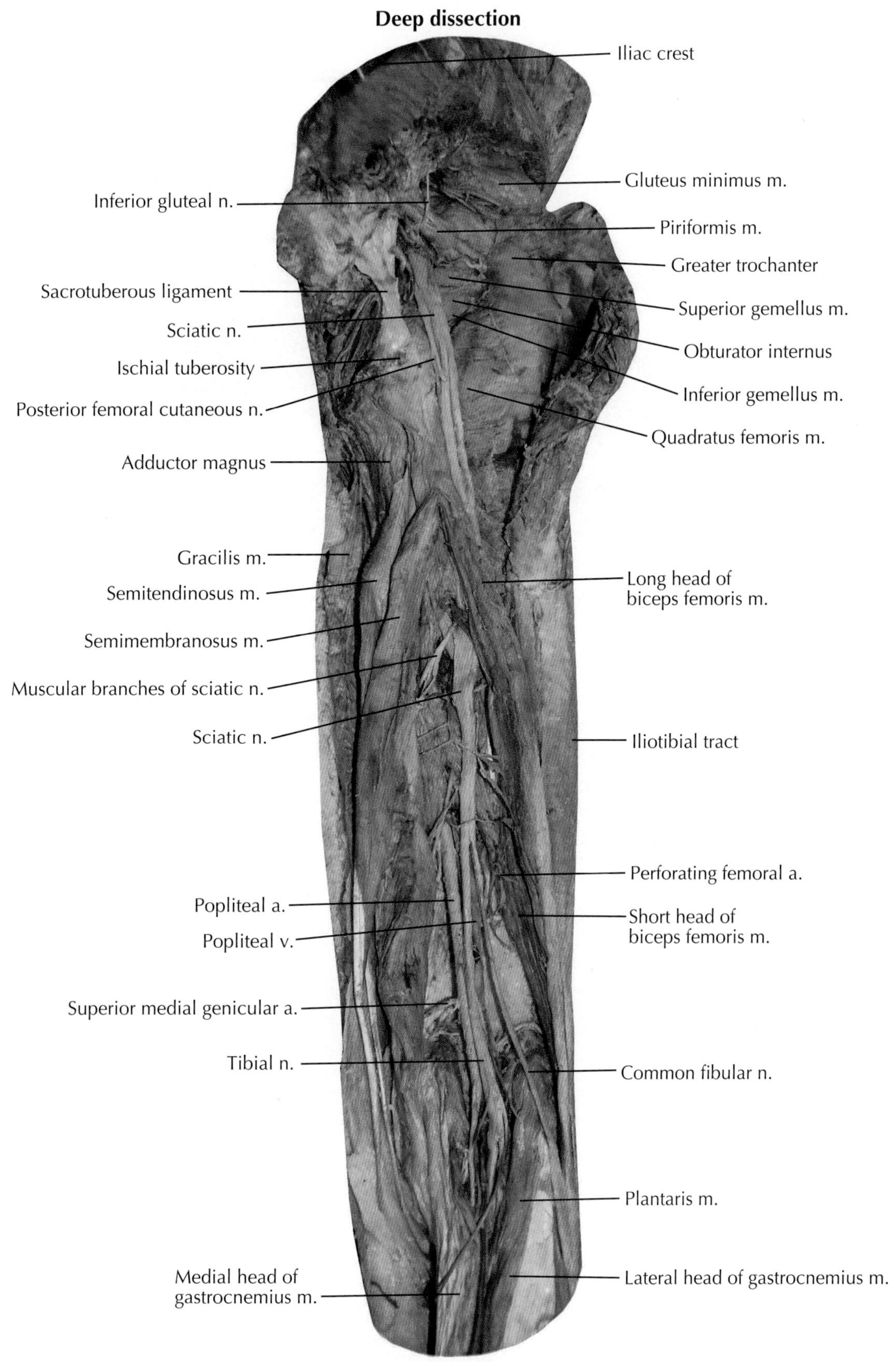
Deep dissection
Iliac crest
Gluteus minimus m.
Inferior gluteal n.
Piriformis m.
Greater trochanter
Sacrotuberous ligament
Superior gemellus m.
Sciatic n.
Obturator internus
Ischial tuberosity
Inferior gemellus m.
Posterior femoral cutaneous n.
Quadratus femoris m.
Adductor magnus
Gracilis m.
Long head of biceps femoris m.
Semitendinosus m.
Semimembranosus m.
Muscular branches of sciatic n.
Sciatic n.
Iliotibial tract
Perforating femoral a.
Popliteal a.
Short head of biceps femoris m.
Popliteal v.
Superior medial genicular a.
Tibial n.
Common fibular n.
Plantaris m.
Medial head of gastrocnemius m.
Lateral head of gastrocnemius m.

Fig. 7.6 Arteries of Thigh. Posterior View (Photograph)

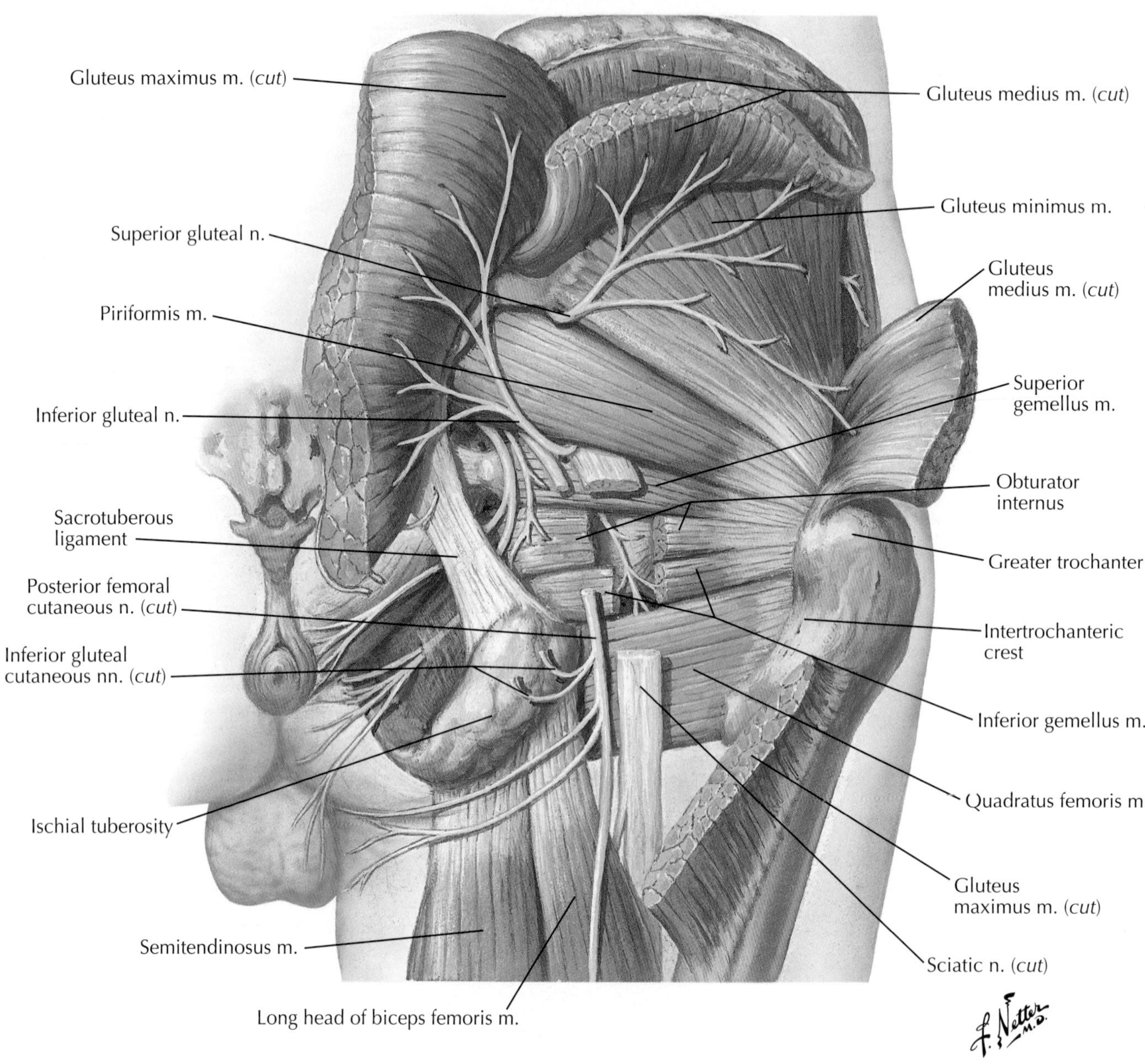

Gluteus maximus m. (*cut*)
Gluteus medius m. (*cut*)
Gluteus minimus m.
Superior gluteal n.
Gluteus medius m. (*cut*)
Piriformis m.
Superior gemellus m.
Inferior gluteal n.
Obturator internus
Sacrotuberous ligament
Greater trochanter
Posterior femoral cutaneous n. (*cut*)
Intertrochanteric crest
Inferior gluteal cutaneous nn. (*cut*)
Inferior gemellus m.
Quadratus femoris m.
Ischial tuberosity
Gluteus maximus m. (*cut*)
Semitendinosus m.
Sciatic n. (*cut*)
Long head of biceps femoris m.
F. Netter M.D.

Fig. 7.7 Nerves of Buttock (Illustration)

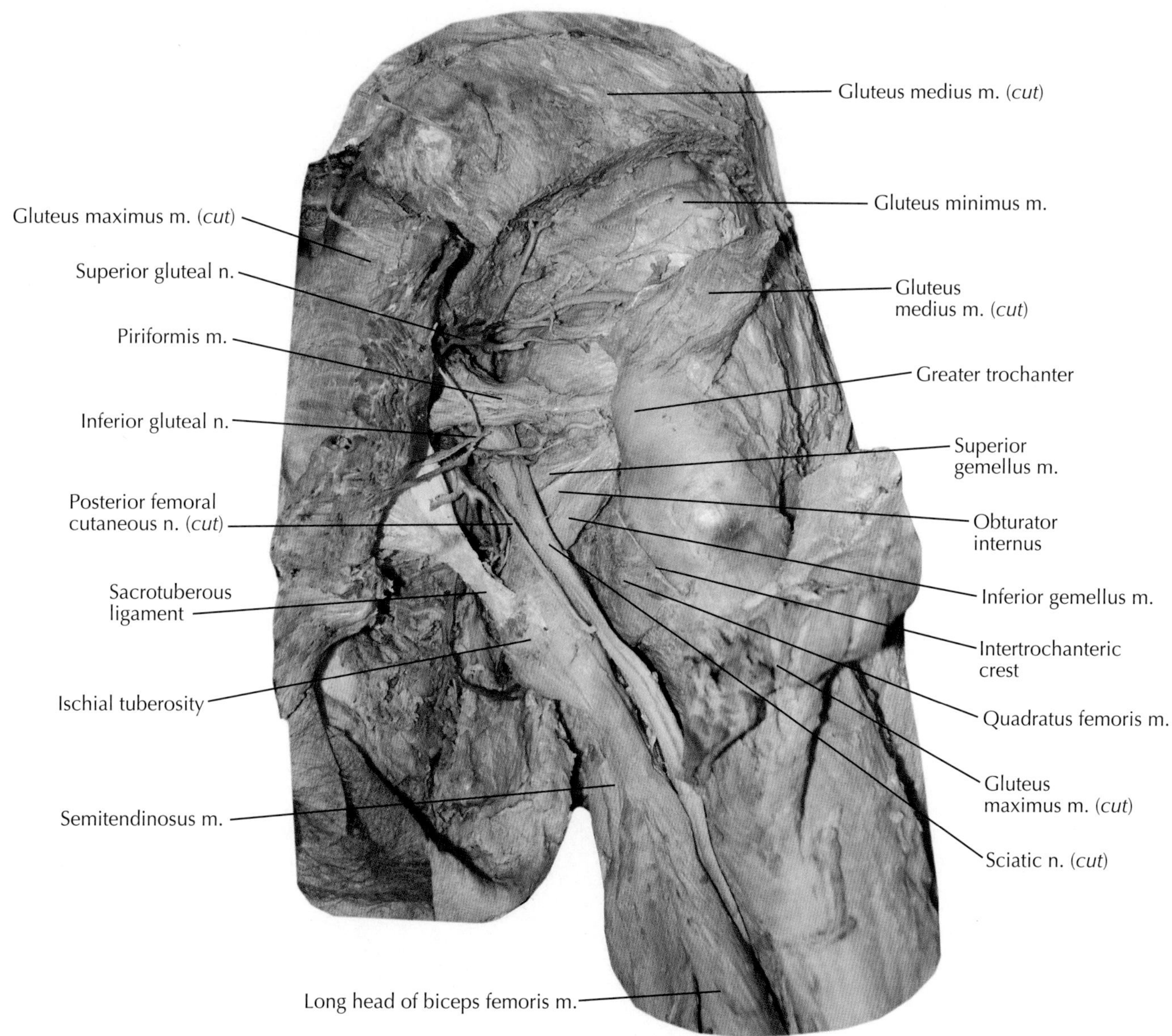
Gluteus medius m. (*cut*)
Gluteus maximus m. (*cut*)
Gluteus minimus m.
Superior gluteal n.
Gluteus
medius m. (*cut*)
Piriformis m.
Greater trochanter
Inferior gluteal n.
Superior
gemellus m.
Posterior femoral
cutaneous n. (*cut*)
Obturator
internus
Inferior gemellus m.
Sacrotuberous
ligament
Intertrochanteric
crest
Ischial tuberosity
Quadratus femoris m.
Gluteus
maximus m. (*cut*)
Semitendinosus m.
Sciatic n. (*cut*)
Long head of biceps femoris m.

Fig. 7.8 Nerves of Buttock (Photograph)

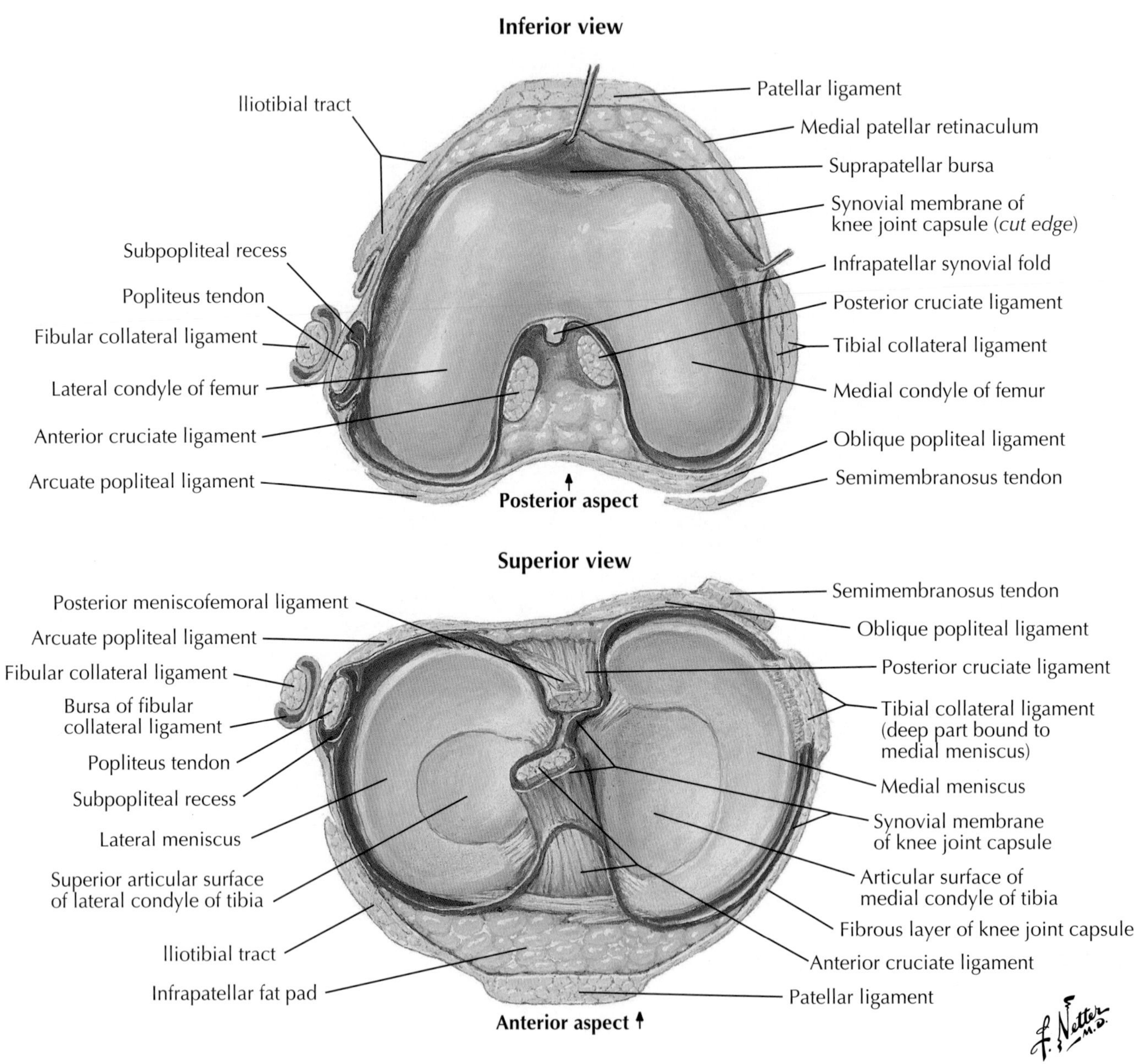
Inferior view
Iliotibial tract
Patellar ligament
Medial patellar retinaculum
Suprapatellar bursa
Synovial membrane of knee joint capsule (cut edge)
Subpopliteal recess
Infrapatellar synovial fold
Popliteus tendon
Posterior cruciate ligament
Fibular collateral ligament
Tibial collateral ligament
Lateral condyle of femur
Medial condyle of femur
Anterior cruciate ligament
Oblique popliteal ligament
Arcuate popliteal ligament
Semimembranosus tendon
Posterior aspect
Superior view
Posterior meniscofemoral ligament
Semimembranosus tendon
Arcuate popliteal ligament
Oblique popliteal ligament
Fibular collateral ligament
Posterior cruciate ligament
Bursa of fibular collateral ligament
Tibial collateral ligament (deep part bound to medial meniscus)
Popliteus tendon
Medial meniscus
Subpopliteal recess
Synovial membrane of knee joint capsule
Lateral meniscus
Articular surface of medial condyle of tibia
Superior articular surface of lateral condyle of tibia
Fibrous layer of knee joint capsule
Iliotibial tract
Anterior cruciate ligament
Infrapatellar fat pad
Patellar ligament
Anterior aspect

Fig. 7.9 Knee: Interior Views (Illustration)

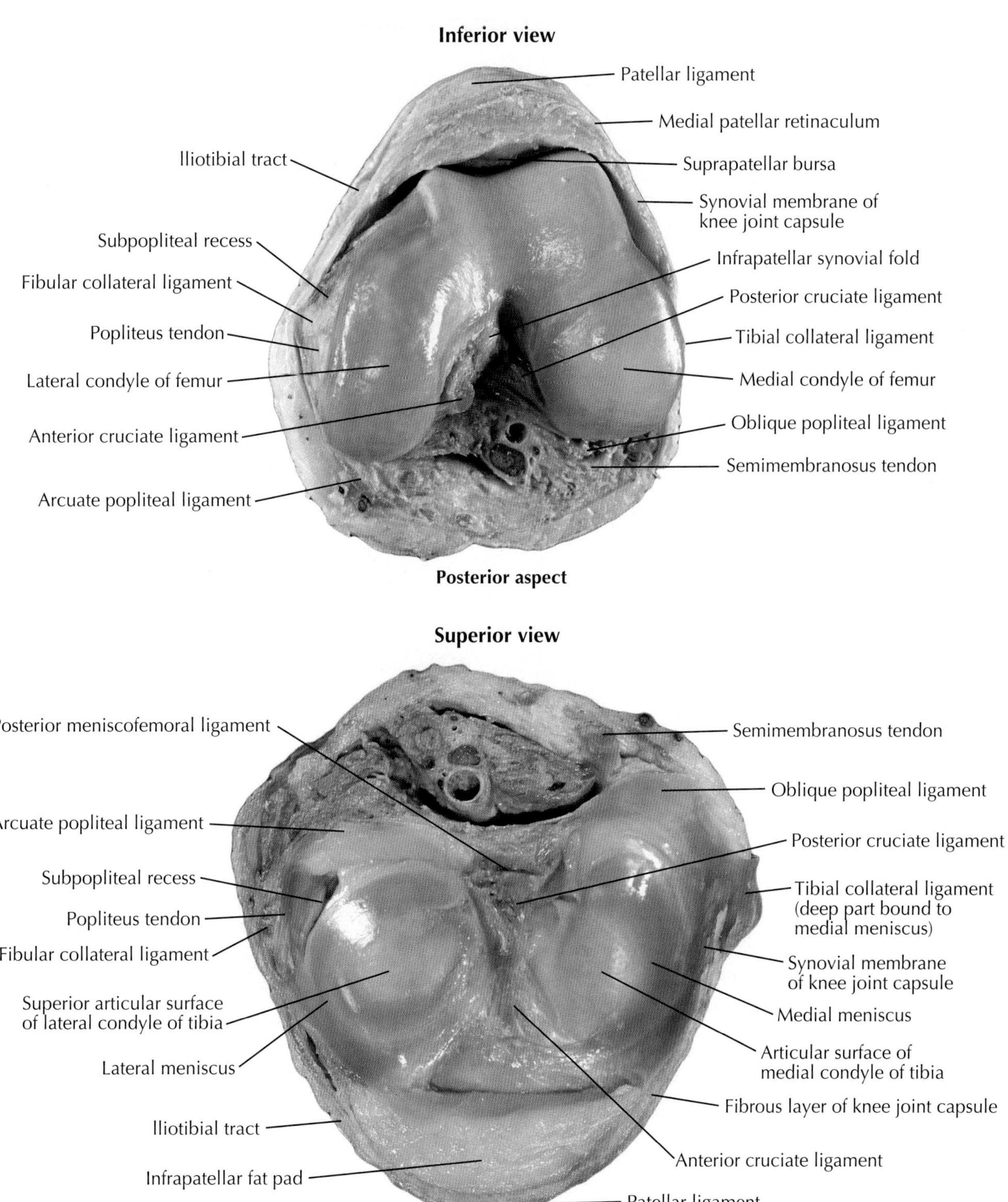
Inferior view
Patellar ligament
Medial patellar retinaculum
Iliotibial tract
Suprapatellar bursa
Synovial membrane of knee joint capsule
Subpopliteal recess
Infrapatellar synovial fold
Fibular collateral ligament
Posterior cruciate ligament
Popliteus tendon
Tibial collateral ligament
Lateral condyle of femur
Medial condyle of femur
Anterior cruciate ligament
Oblique popliteal ligament
Semimembranosus tendon
Arcuate popliteal ligament
Posterior aspect
Superior view
Posterior meniscofemoral ligament
Semimembranosus tendon
Oblique popliteal ligament
Arcuate popliteal ligament
Posterior cruciate ligament
Subpopliteal recess
Tibial collateral ligament (deep part bound to medial meniscus)
Popliteus tendon
Fibular collateral ligament
Synovial membrane of knee joint capsule
Superior articular surface of lateral condyle of tibia
Medial meniscus
Lateral meniscus
Articular surface of medial condyle of tibia
Fibrous layer of knee joint capsule
Iliotibial tract
Anterior cruciate ligament
Infrapatellar fat pad
Patellar ligament
Anterior aspect

Fig. 7.10 Knee: Interior Views (Photograph)

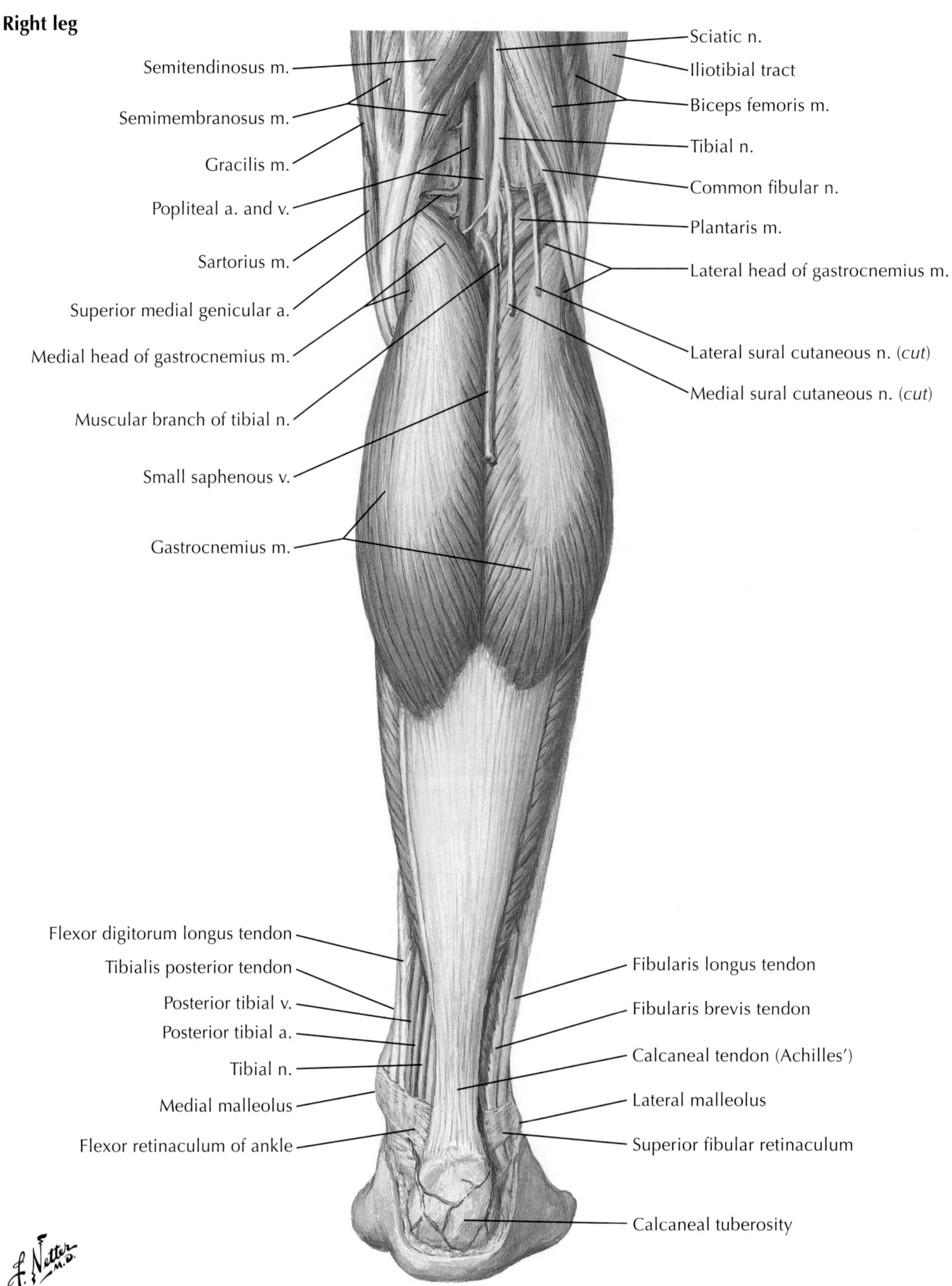
Right leg
Semitendinosus m.
Semimembranosus m.
Gracilis m.
Popliteal a. and v.
Sartorius m.
Superior medial genicular a.
Medial head of gastrocnemius m.
Muscular branch of tibial n.
Small saphenous v.
Gastrocnemius m.
Sciatic n.
Iliotibial tract
Biceps femoris m.
Tibial n.
Common fibular n.
Plantaris m.
Lateral head of gastrocnemius m.
Lateral sural cutaneous n. (cut)
Medial sural cutaneous n. (cut)
Flexor digitorum longus tendon
Tibialis posterior tendon
Posterior tibial v.
Posterior tibial a.
Tibial n.
Medial malleolus
Flexor retinaculum of ankle
Fibularis longus tendon
Fibularis brevis tendon
Calcaneal tendon (Achilles')
Lateral malleolus
Superior fibular retinaculum
Calcaneal tuberosity
F. Netter M.D.

Fig. 7.11 Muscles of Leg: Superficial Part of Posterior Compartment (Illustration)

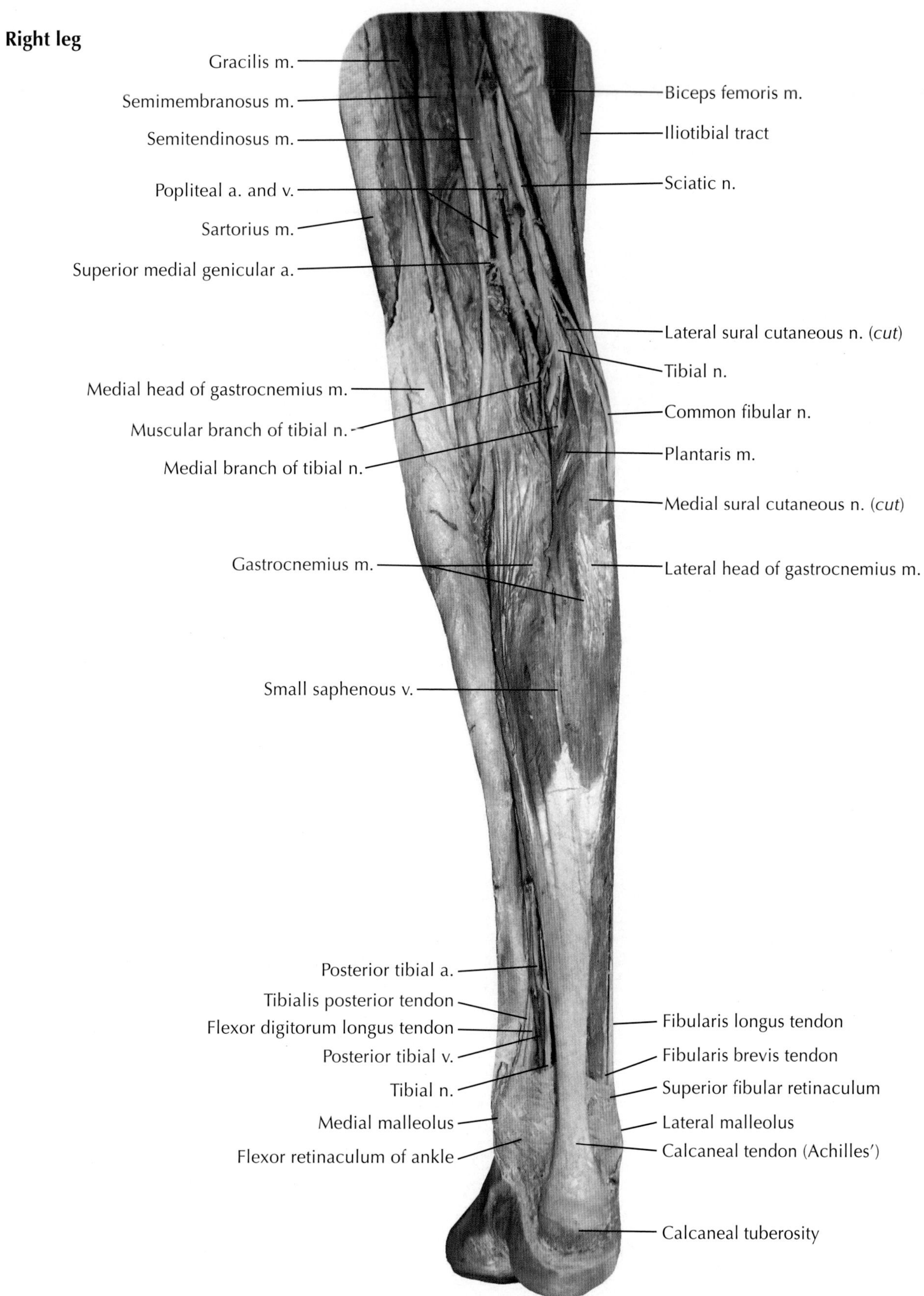
Right leg
Gracilis m.
Semimembranosus m.
Semitendinosus m.
Popliteal a. and v.
Sartorius m.
Superior medial genicular a.
Medial head of gastrocnemius m.
Muscular branch of tibial n.
Medial branch of tibial n.
Gastrocnemius m.
Small saphenous v.
Posterior tibial a.
Tibialis posterior tendon
Flexor digitorum longus tendon
Posterior tibial v.
Tibial n.
Medial malleolus
Flexor retinaculum of ankle
Biceps femoris m.
Iliotibial tract
Sciatic n.
Lateral sural cutaneous n. (cut)
Tibial n.
Common fibular n.
Plantaris m.
Medial sural cutaneous n. (cut)
Lateral head of gastrocnemius m.
Fibularis longus tendon
Fibularis brevis tendon
Superior fibular retinaculum
Lateral malleolus
Calcaneal tendon (Achilles')
Calcaneal tuberosity

Fig. 7.12 Muscles of Leg: Superficial Part of Posterior Compartment (Photograph) (see Fig. A.17)

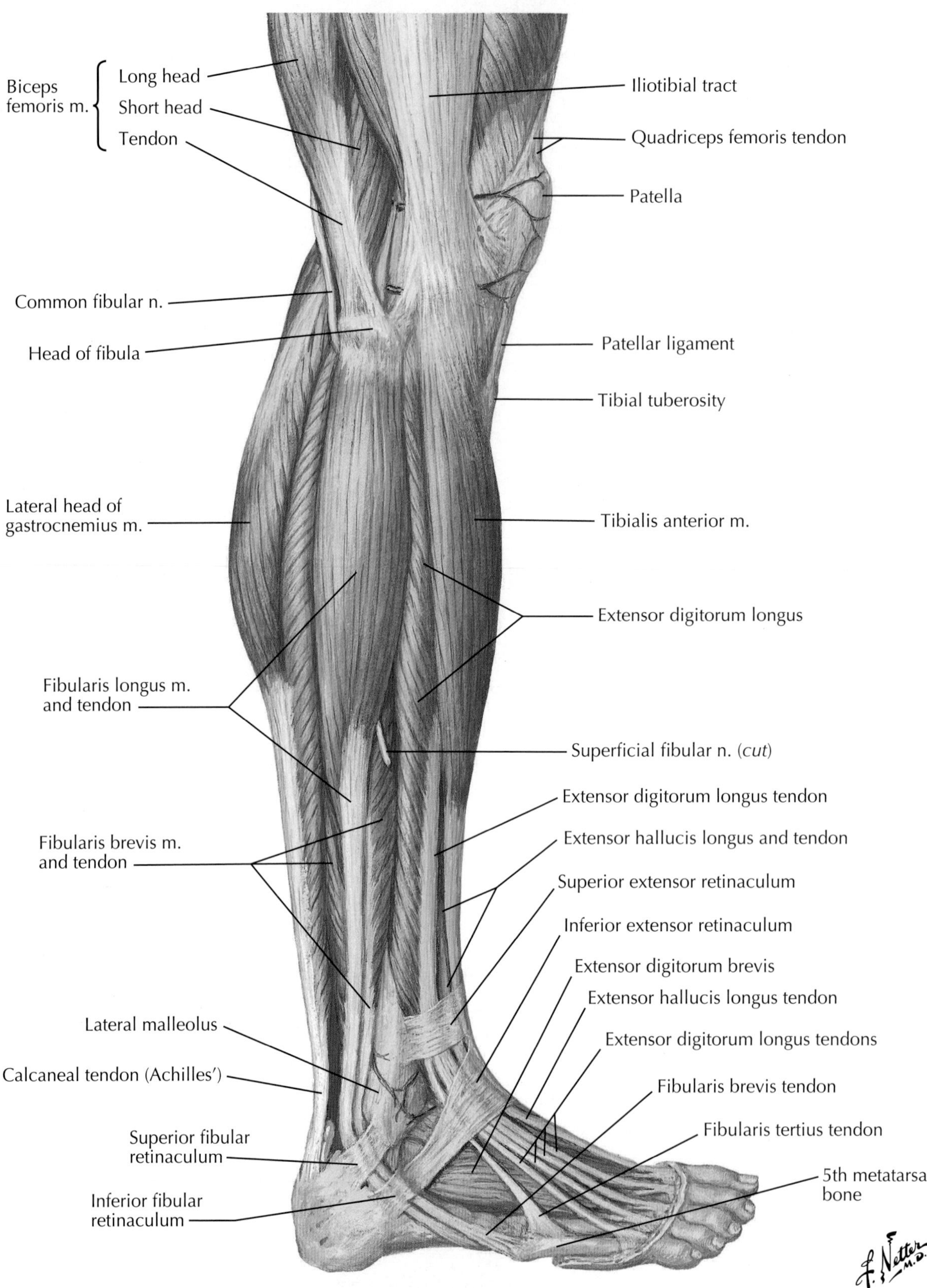
Biceps femoris m.
Long head
Short head
Tendon
Iliotibial tract
Quadriceps femoris tendon
Patella
Common fibular n.
Head of fibula
Patellar ligament
Tibial tuberosity
Lateral head of gastrocnemius m.
Tibialis anterior m.
Extensor digitorum longus
Fibularis longus m. and tendon
Superficial fibular n. (cut)
Extensor digitorum longus tendon
Fibularis brevis m. and tendon
Extensor hallucis longus and tendon
Superior extensor retinaculum
Inferior extensor retinaculum
Extensor digitorum brevis
Extensor hallucis longus tendon
Lateral malleolus
Extensor digitorum longus tendons
Calcaneal tendon (Achilles')
Fibularis brevis tendon
Superior fibular retinaculum
Fibularis tertius tendon
Inferior fibular retinaculum
5th metatarsal bone
F. Netter M.D.

Fig. 7.13 Muscles of Leg: Lateral Compartment (Illustration)

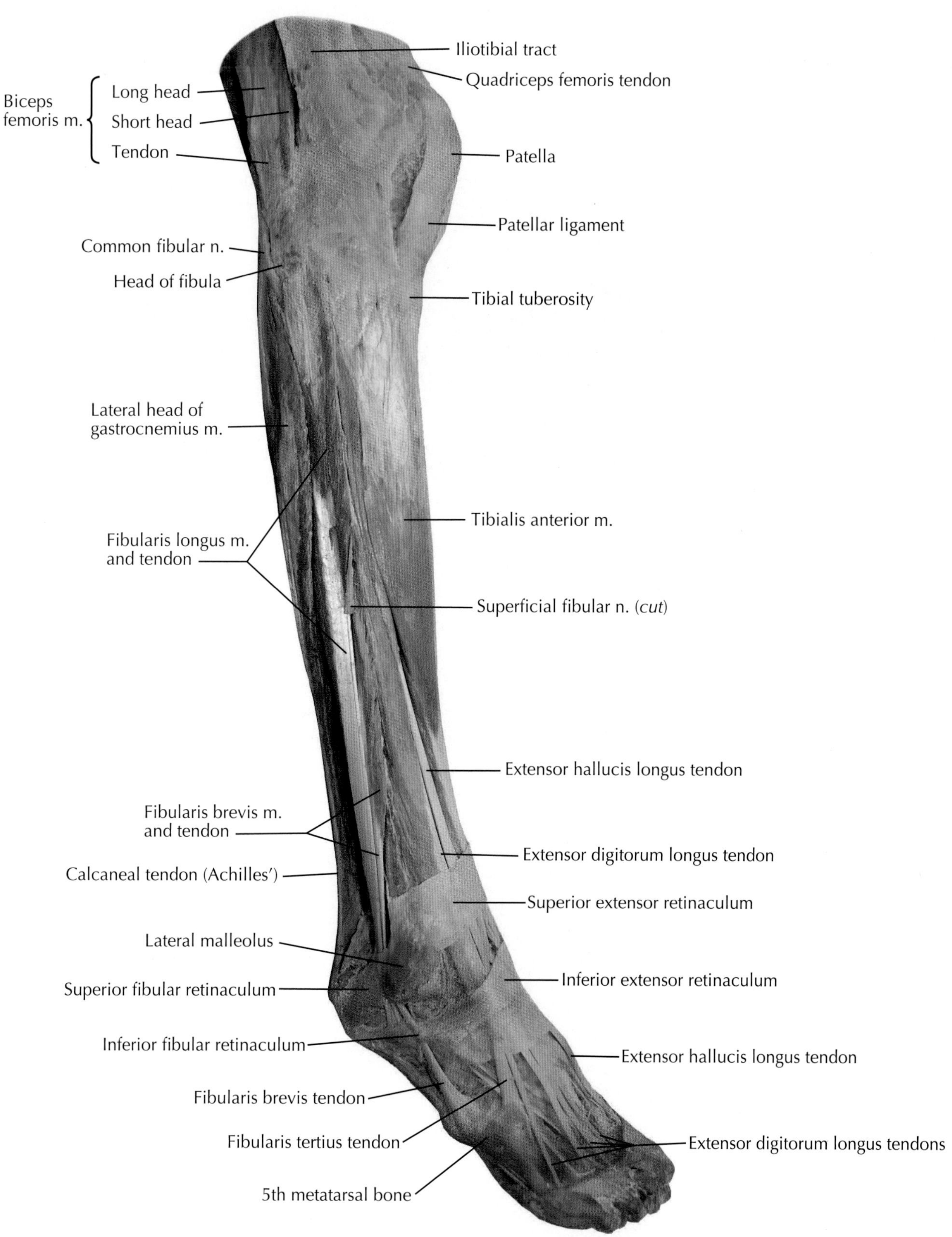
Iliotibial tract
Quadriceps femoris tendon
Biceps femoris m.
Long head
Short head
Tendon
Patella
Patellar ligament
Common fibular n.
Head of fibula
Tibial tuberosity
Lateral head of gastrocnemius m.
Tibialis anterior m.
Fibularis longus m. and tendon
Superficial fibular n. (cut)
Extensor hallucis longus tendon
Fibularis brevis m. and tendon
Extensor digitorum longus tendon
Calcaneal tendon (Achilles')
Superior extensor retinaculum
Lateral malleolus
Inferior extensor retinaculum
Superior fibular retinaculum
Inferior fibular retinaculum
Extensor hallucis longus tendon
Fibularis brevis tendon
Fibularis tertius tendon
Extensor digitorum longus tendons
5th metatarsal bone

Fig. 7.14 Muscles of Leg: Lateral Compartment (Photograph)

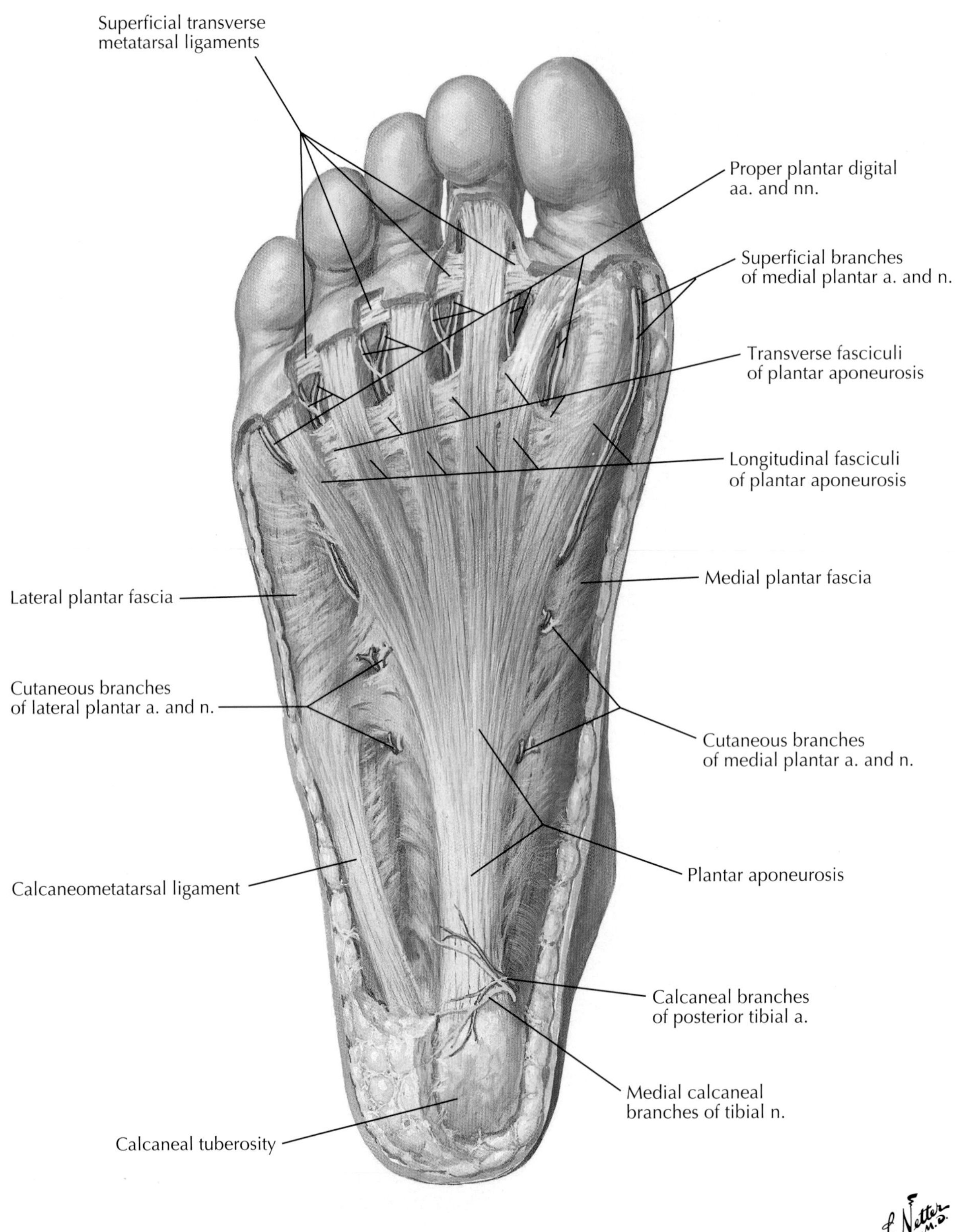
Superficial transverse metatarsal ligaments
Proper plantar digital aa. and nn.
Superficial branches of medial plantar a. and n.
Transverse fasciculi of plantar aponeurosis
Longitudinal fasciculi of plantar aponeurosis
Medial plantar fascia
Lateral plantar fascia
Cutaneous branches of lateral plantar a. and n.
Cutaneous branches of medial plantar a. and n.
Plantar aponeurosis
Calcaneometatarsal ligament
Calcaneal branches of posterior tibial a.
Medial calcaneal branches of tibial n.
Calcaneal tuberosity

Fig. 7.15 Sole of Foot: Superficial Dissection (Illustration)

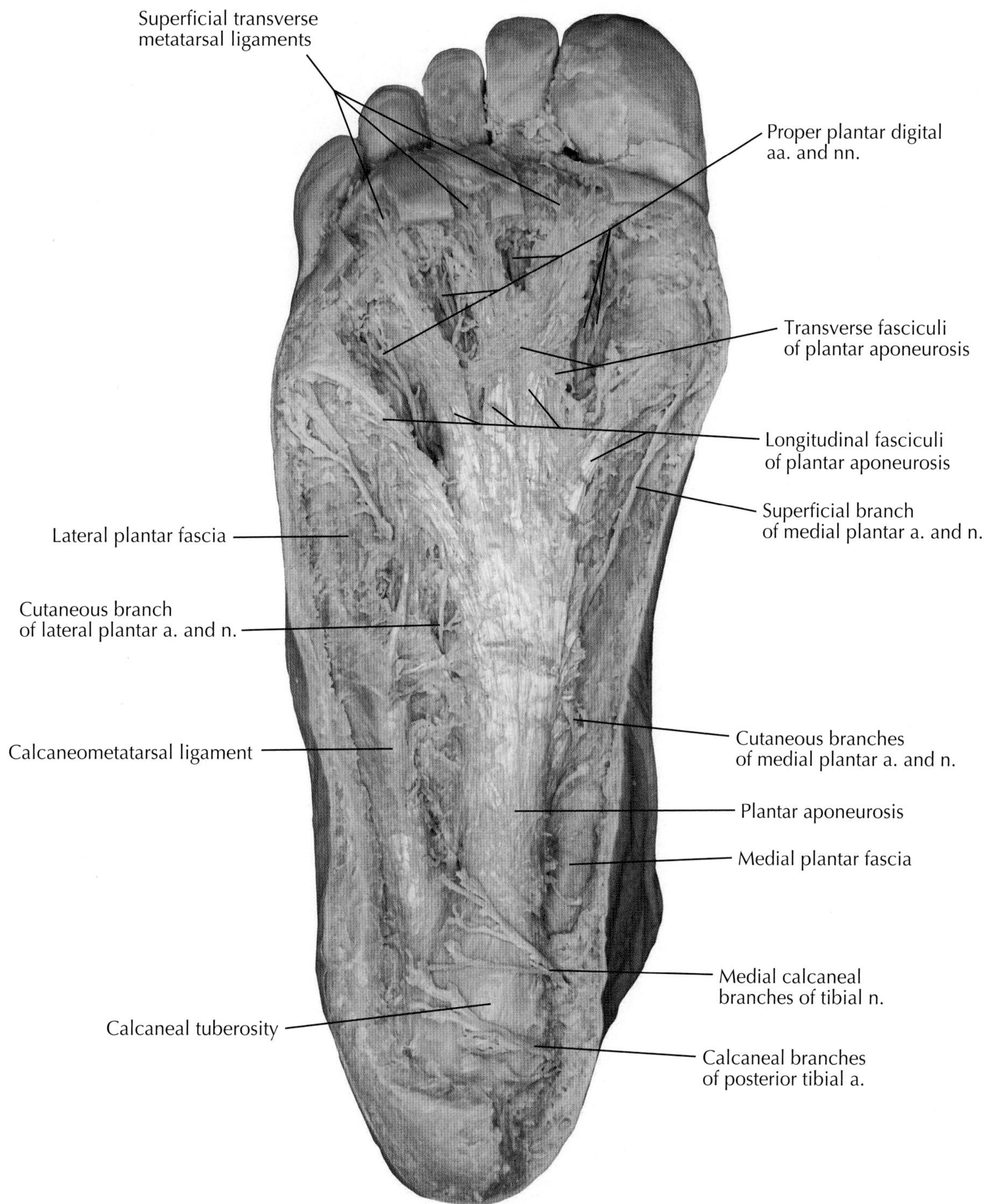
Superficial transverse metatarsal ligaments
Proper plantar digital aa. and nn.
Transverse fasciculi of plantar aponeurosis
Longitudinal fasciculi of plantar aponeurosis
Superficial branch of medial plantar a. and n.
Lateral plantar fascia
Cutaneous branch of lateral plantar a. and n.
Calcaneometatarsal ligament
Cutaneous branches of medial plantar a. and n.
Plantar aponeurosis
Medial plantar fascia
Medial calcaneal branches of tibial n.
Calcaneal tuberosity
Calcaneal branches of posterior tibial a.

Fig. 7.16 Sole of Foot: Superficial Dissection (Photograph)

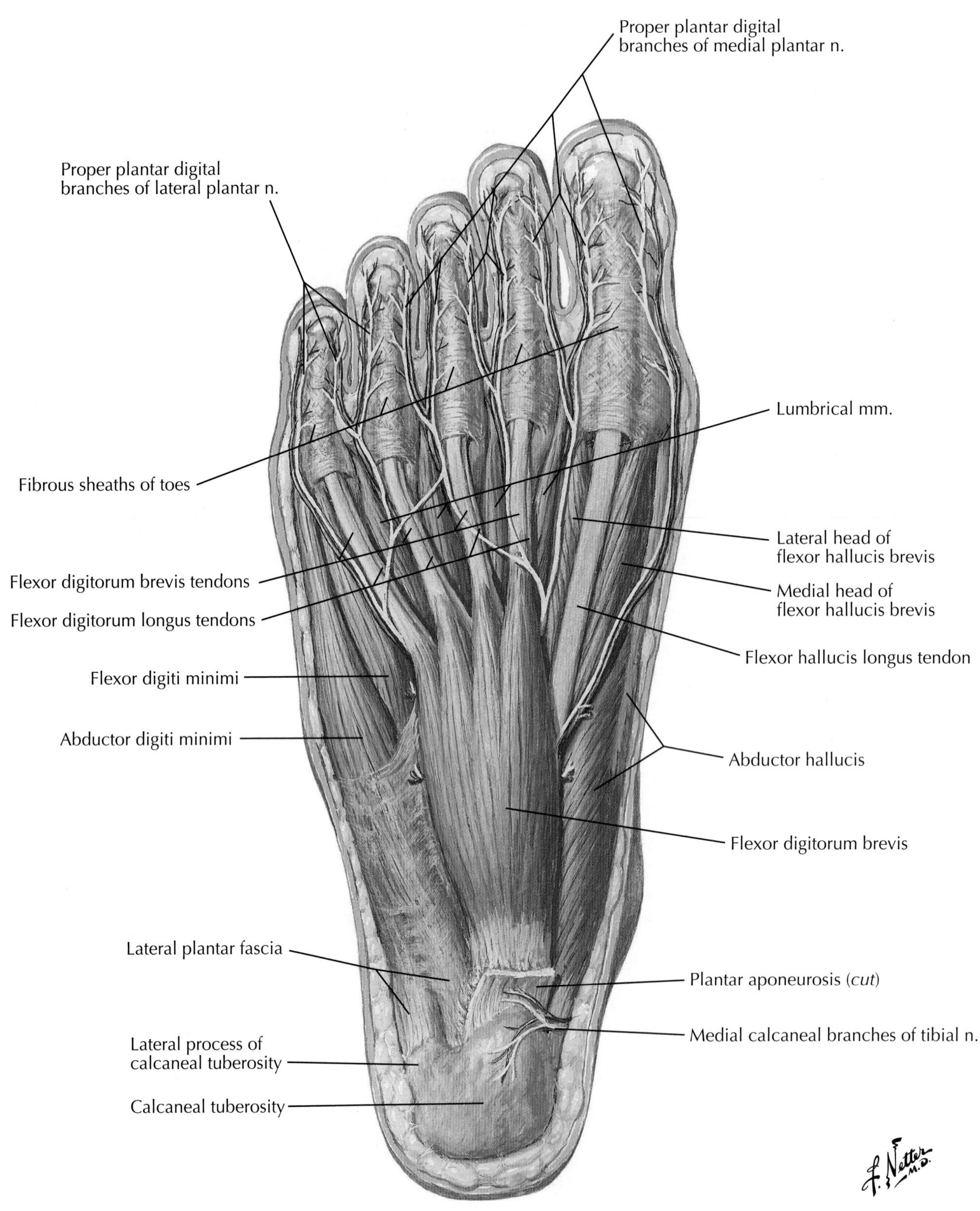

Proper plantar digital branches of medial plantar n.
Proper plantar digital branches of lateral plantar n.
Lumbrical mm.
Fibrous sheaths of toes
Lateral head of flexor hallucis brevis
Flexor digitorum brevis tendons
Medial head of flexor hallucis brevis
Flexor digitorum longus tendons
Flexor hallucis longus tendon
Flexor digiti minimi
Abductor digiti minimi
Abductor hallucis
Flexor digitorum brevis
Lateral plantar fascia
Plantar aponeurosis (cut)
Medial calcaneal branches of tibial n.
Lateral process of calcaneal tuberosity
Calcaneal tuberosity
F. Netter M.D.

Fig. 7.17 Muscles of Sole of Foot: First Layer (Illustration)

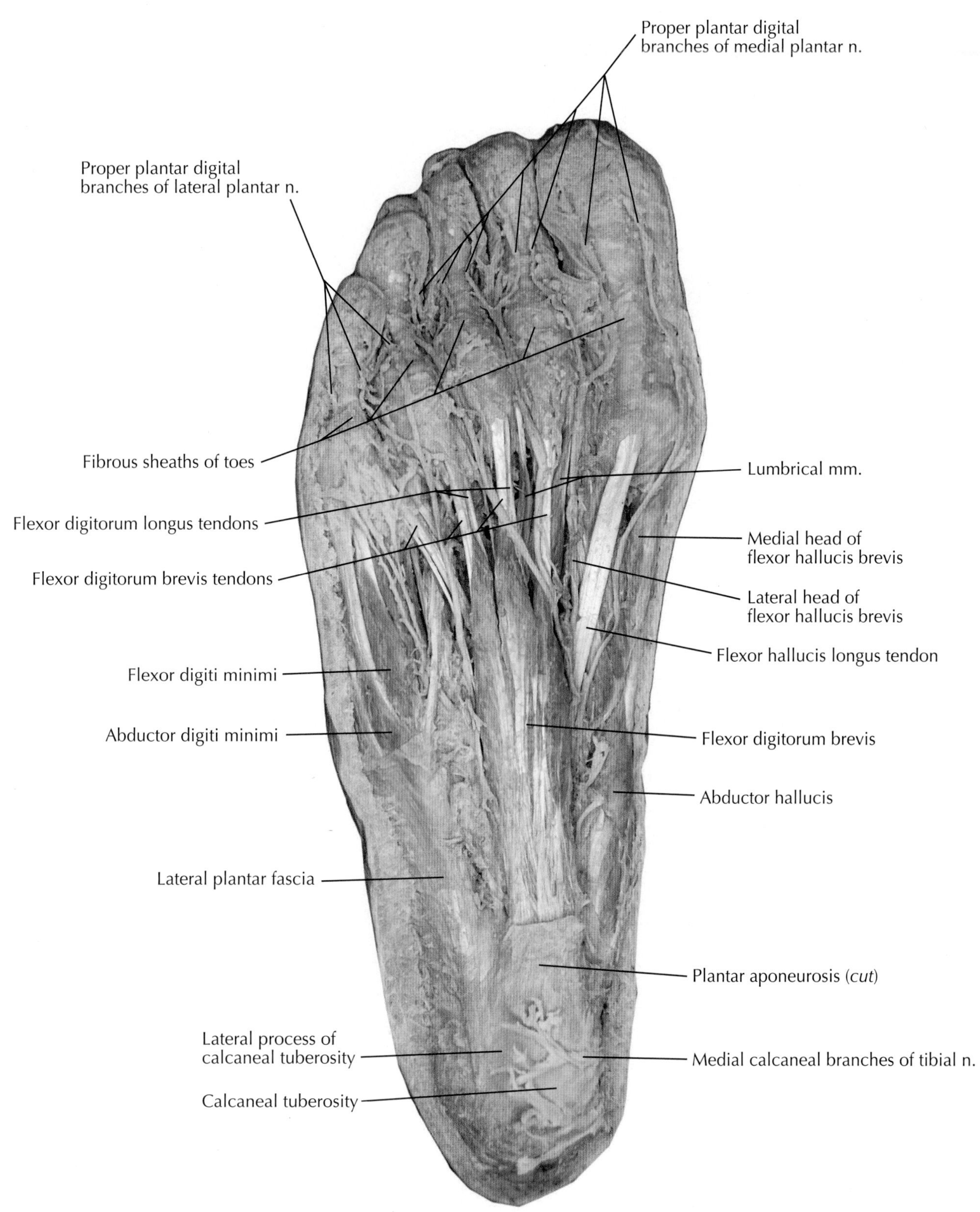
Proper plantar digital branches of medial plantar n.
Proper plantar digital branches of lateral plantar n.
Fibrous sheaths of toes
Lumbrical mm.
Flexor digitorum longus tendons
Medial head of flexor hallucis brevis
Flexor digitorum brevis tendons
Lateral head of flexor hallucis brevis
Flexor hallucis longus tendon
Flexor digiti minimi
Abductor digiti minimi
Flexor digitorum brevis
Abductor hallucis
Lateral plantar fascia
Plantar aponeurosis (*cut*)
Lateral process of calcaneal tuberosity
Medial calcaneal branches of tibial n.
Calcaneal tuberosity

Fig. 7.18 Muscles of Sole of Foot: First Layer (Photograph)

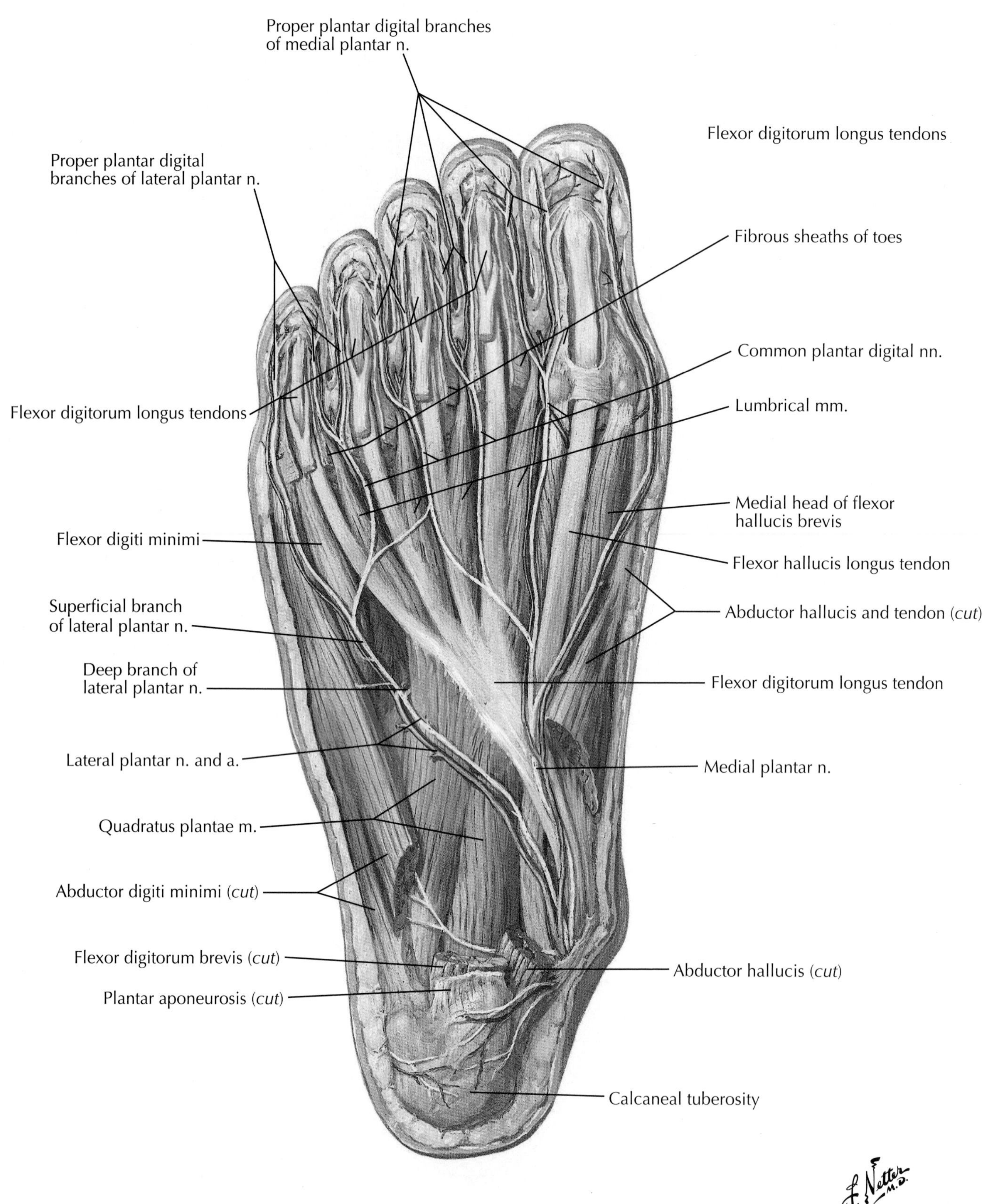
Proper plantar digital branches of medial plantar n.
Flexor digitorum longus tendons
Proper plantar digital branches of lateral plantar n.
Fibrous sheaths of toes
Common plantar digital nn.
Lumbrical mm.
Flexor digitorum longus tendons
Medial head of flexor hallucis brevis
Flexor digiti minimi
Flexor hallucis longus tendon
Superficial branch of lateral plantar n.
Abductor hallucis and tendon (cut)
Deep branch of lateral plantar n.
Flexor digitorum longus tendon
Lateral plantar n. and a.
Medial plantar n.
Quadratus plantae m.
Abductor digiti minimi (cut)
Flexor digitorum brevis (cut)
Abductor hallucis (cut)
Plantar aponeurosis (cut)
Calcaneal tuberosity
F. Netter M.D.

Fig. 7.19 Muscles of Sole of Foot: Second Layer (Illustration)

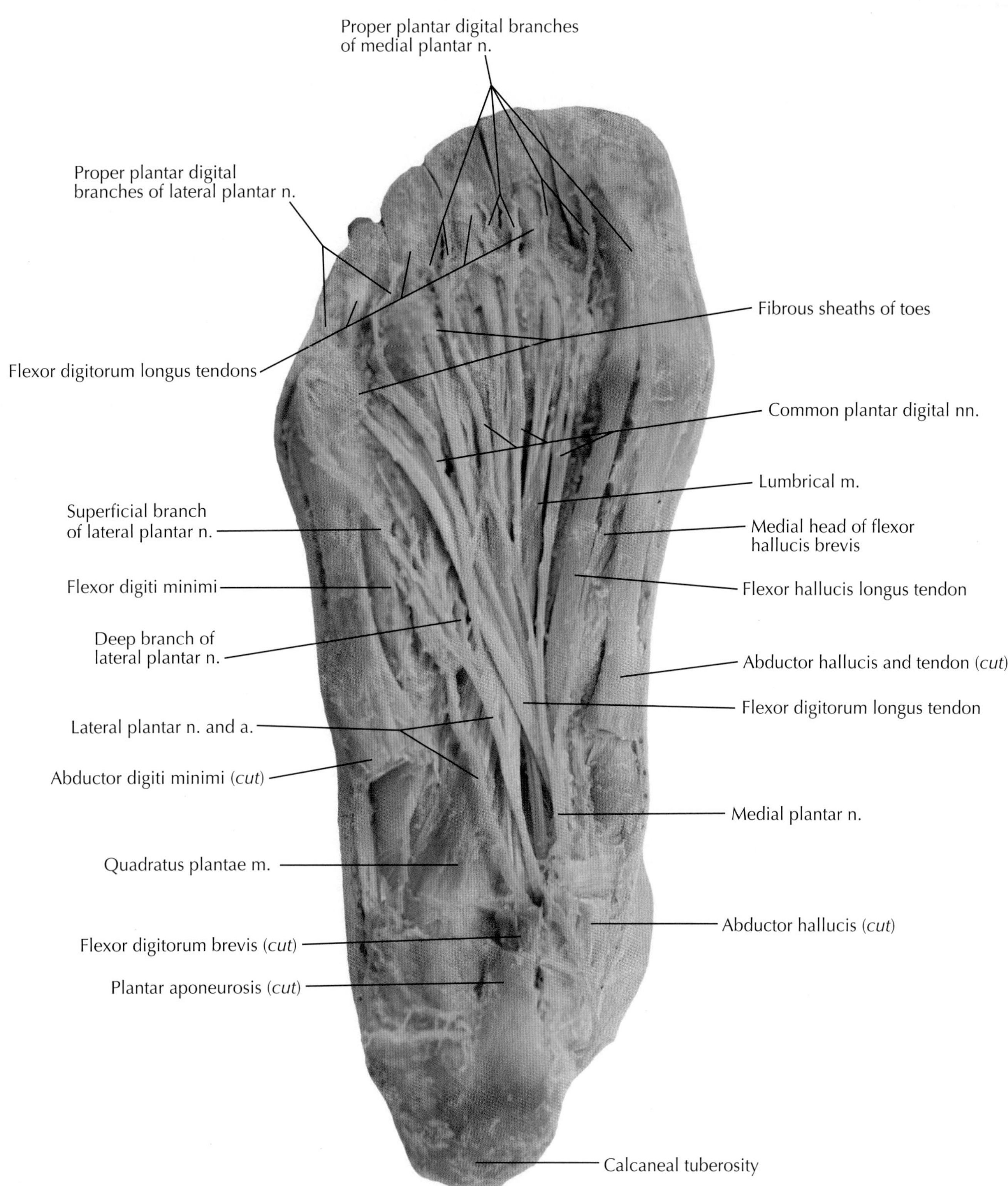
Proper plantar digital branches of medial plantar n.
Proper plantar digital branches of lateral plantar n.
Fibrous sheaths of toes
Flexor digitorum longus tendons
Common plantar digital nn.
Lumbrical m.
Superficial branch of lateral plantar n.
Medial head of flexor hallucis brevis
Flexor digiti minimi
Flexor hallucis longus tendon
Deep branch of lateral plantar n.
Abductor hallucis and tendon (cut)
Flexor digitorum longus tendon
Lateral plantar n. and a.
Abductor digiti minimi (cut)
Medial plantar n.
Quadratus plantae m.
Abductor hallucis (cut)
Flexor digitorum brevis (cut)
Plantar aponeurosis (cut)
Calcaneal tuberosity

Fig. 7.20 Muscles of Sole of Foot: Second Layer (Photograph)

Appendix Non-Colorized Photographs

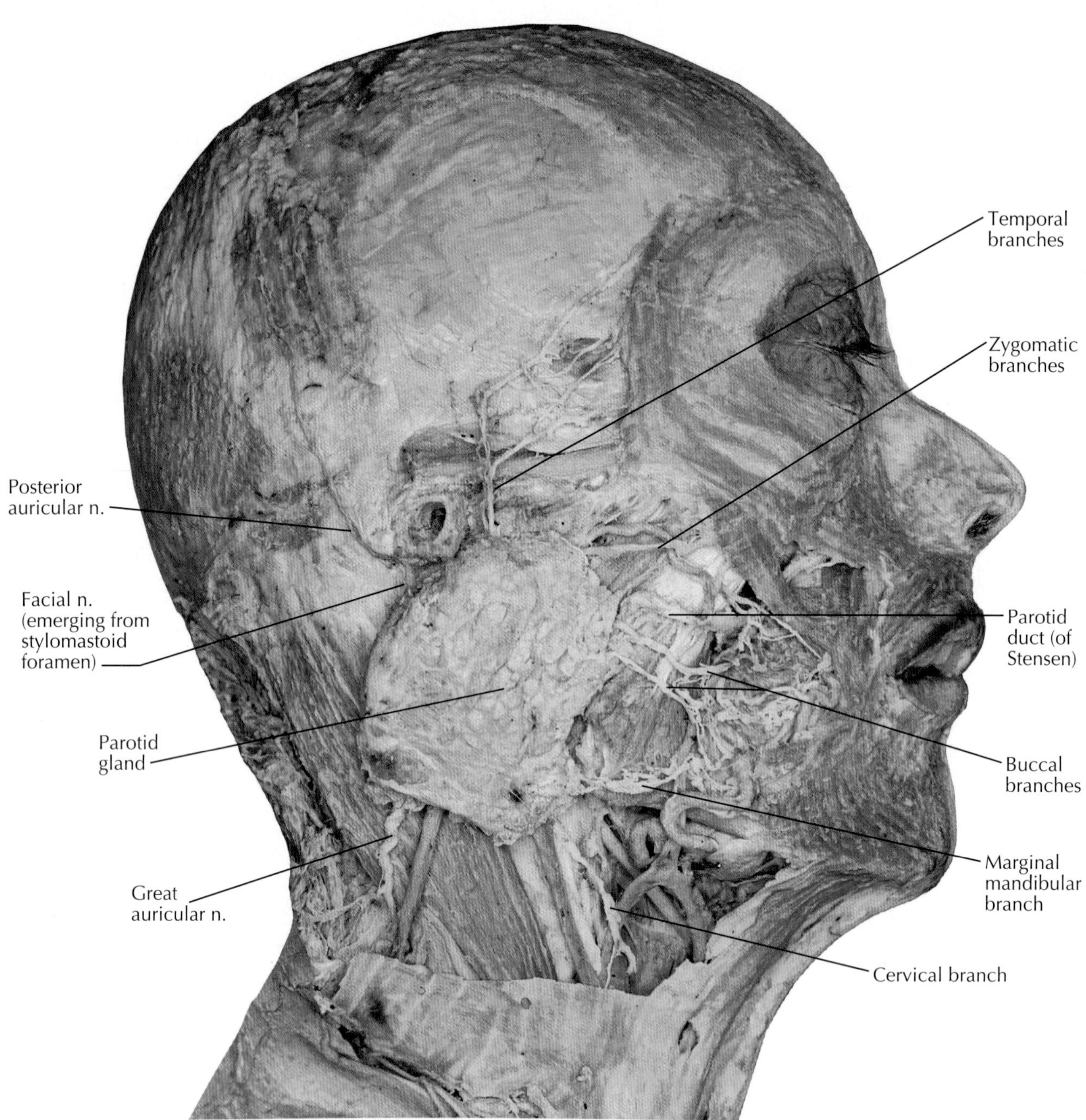
Temporal branches
Zygomatic branches
Posterior auricular n.
Facial n. (emerging from stylomastoid foramen)
Parotid duct (of Stensen)
Parotid gland
Buccal branches
Marginal mandibular branch
Great auricular n.
Cervical branch

Fig. A.1 Facial Nerve Branches and Parotid Gland (Photograph) (see Figs. 1.15 and 1.16)

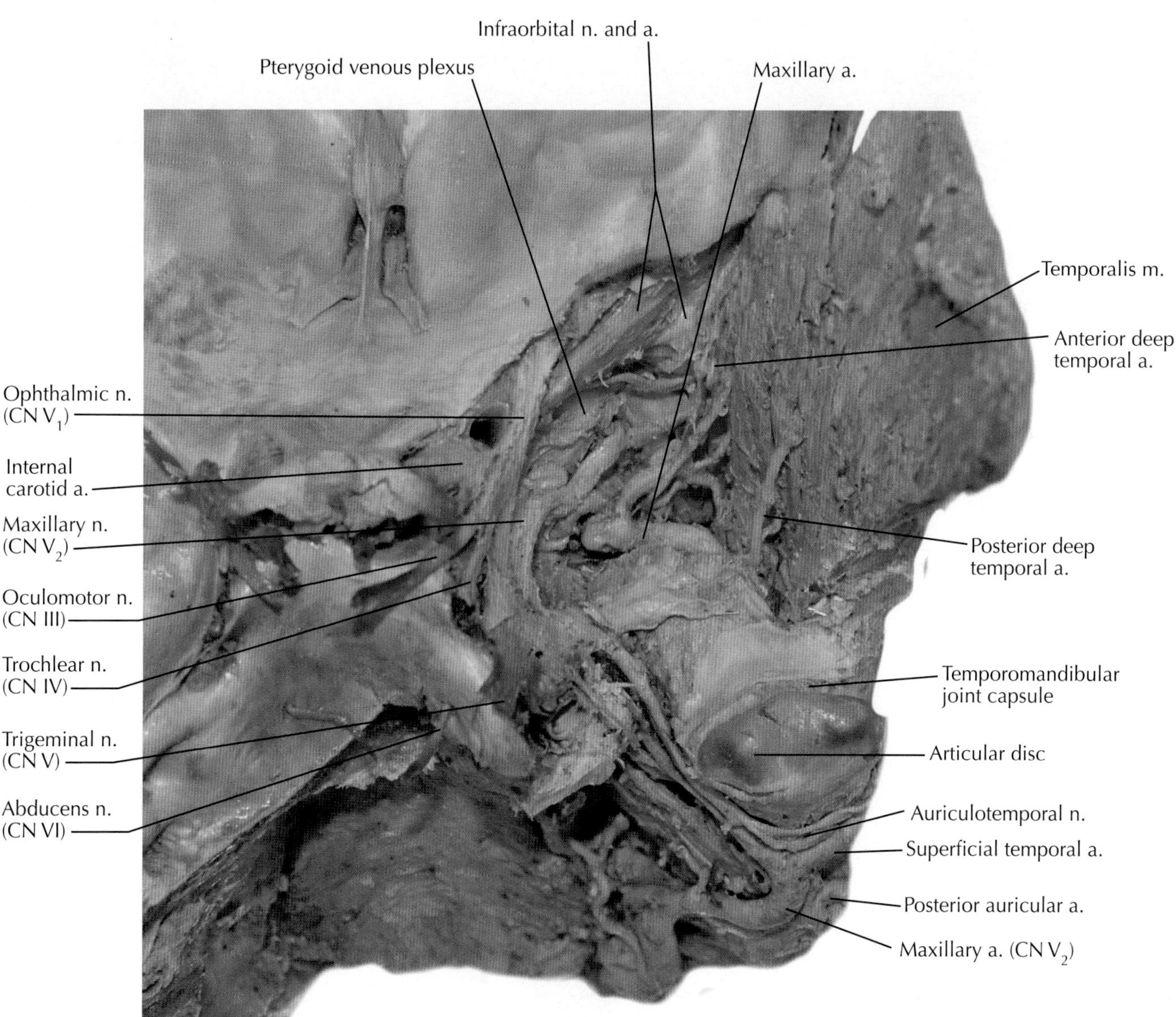
Infraorbital n. and a.
Pterygoid venous plexus
Maxillary a.
Temporalis m.
Anterior deep temporal a.
Ophthalmic n. (CN V_1)
Internal carotid a.
Maxillary n. (CN V_2)
Oculomotor n. (CN III)
Trochlear n. (CN IV)
Trigeminal n. (CN V)
Abducens n. (CN VI)
Posterior deep temporal a.
Temporomandibular joint capsule
Articular disc
Auriculotemporal n.
Superficial temporal a.
Posterior auricular a.
Maxillary a. (CN V_2)

Fig. A.2 Infratemporal Fossa (Photograph) (see Figs. 1.19 and 1.20)

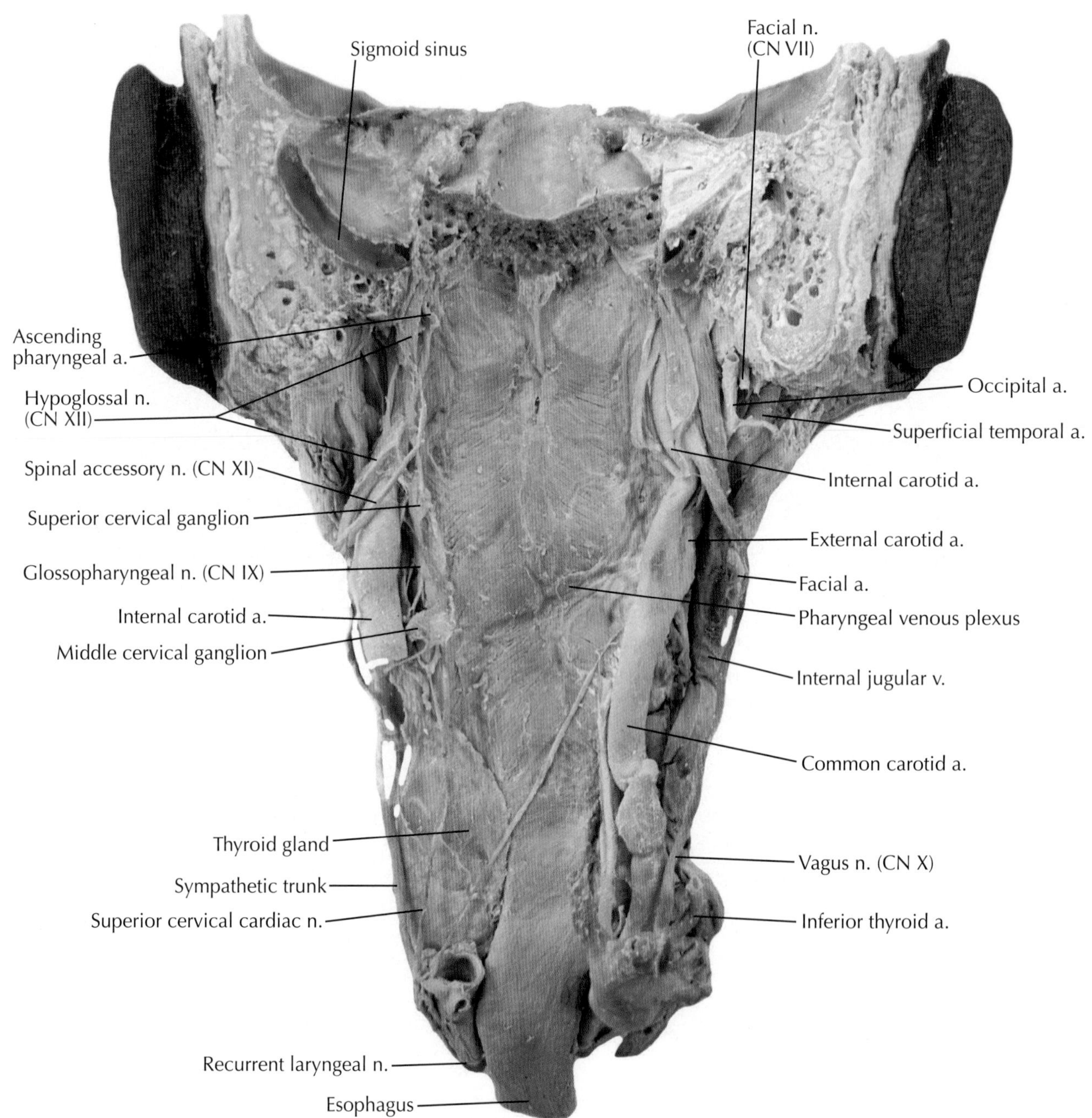
Sigmoid sinus
Facial n. (CN VII)
Ascending pharyngeal a.
Hypoglossal n. (CN XII)
Spinal accessory n. (CN XI)
Superior cervical ganglion
Glossopharyngeal n. (CN IX)
Internal carotid a.
Middle cervical ganglion
Occipital a.
Superficial temporal a.
Internal carotid a.
External carotid a.
Facial a.
Pharyngeal venous plexus
Internal jugular v.
Common carotid a.
Thyroid gland
Sympathetic trunk
Superior cervical cardiac n.
Vagus n. (CN X)
Inferior thyroid a.
Recurrent laryngeal n.
Esophagus

Fig. A.3 Posterior View of Pharynx: Nerves and Vessels (Photograph) (see Figs. 1.23 and 1.24)

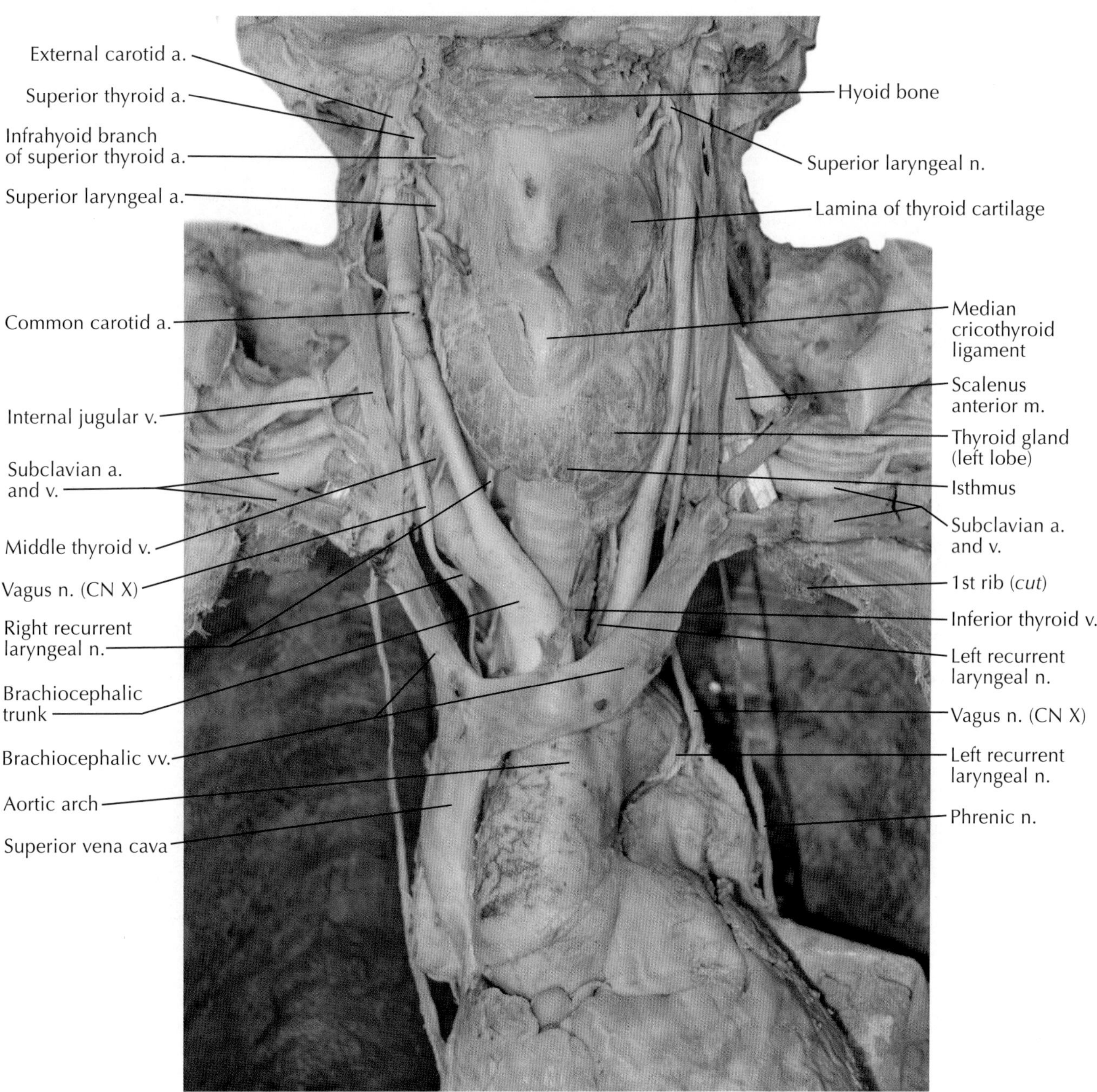
External carotid a.
Superior thyroid a.
Infrahyoid branch of superior thyroid a.
Superior laryngeal a.
Common carotid a.
Internal jugular v.
Subclavian a. and v.
Middle thyroid v.
Vagus n. (CN X)
Right recurrent laryngeal n.
Brachiocephalic trunk
Brachiocephalic vv.
Aortic arch
Superior vena cava
Hyoid bone
Superior laryngeal n.
Lamina of thyroid cartilage
Median cricothyroid ligament
Scalenus anterior m.
Thyroid gland (left lobe)
Isthmus
Subclavian a. and v.
1st rib (cut)
Inferior thyroid v.
Left recurrent laryngeal n.
Vagus n. (CN X)
Left recurrent laryngeal n.
Phrenic n.

Fig. A.4 Thyroid Gland: Anterior View (Photograph) (see Figs. 1.27 and 1.28)

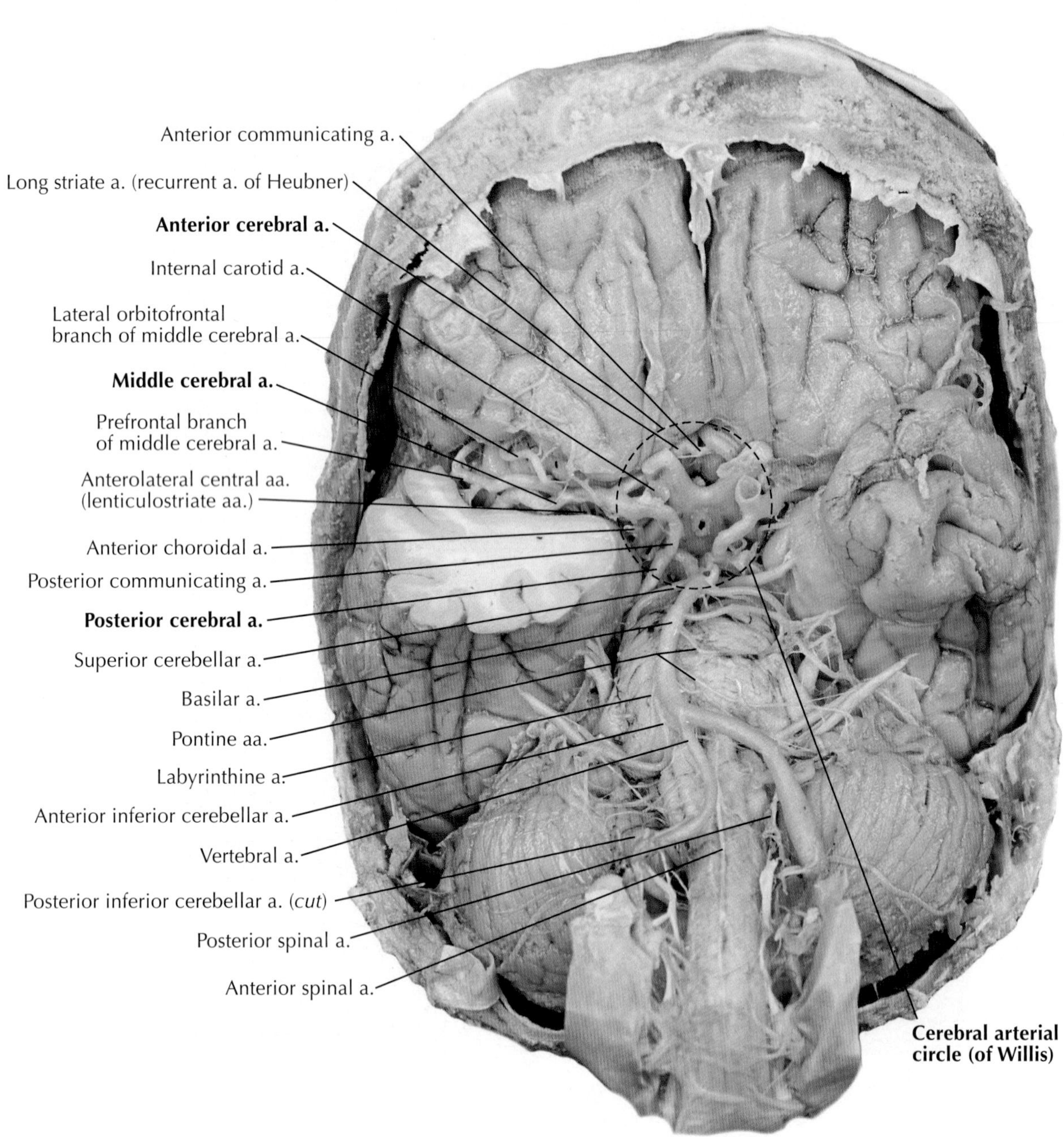
Anterior communicating a.
Long striate a. (recurrent a. of Heubner)
Anterior cerebral a.
Internal carotid a.
Lateral orbitofrontal branch of middle cerebral a.
Middle cerebral a.
Prefrontal branch of middle cerebral a.
Anterolateral central aa. (lenticulostriate aa.)
Anterior choroidal a.
Posterior communicating a.
Posterior cerebral a.
Superior cerebellar a.
Basilar a.
Pontine aa.
Labyrinthine a.
Anterior inferior cerebellar a.
Vertebral a.
Posterior inferior cerebellar a. (cut)
Posterior spinal a.
Anterior spinal a.
Cerebral arterial circle (of Willis)

Fig. A.5 Arteries of Brain: Inferior Views (Photograph) (see Figs. 1.47 and 1.48)

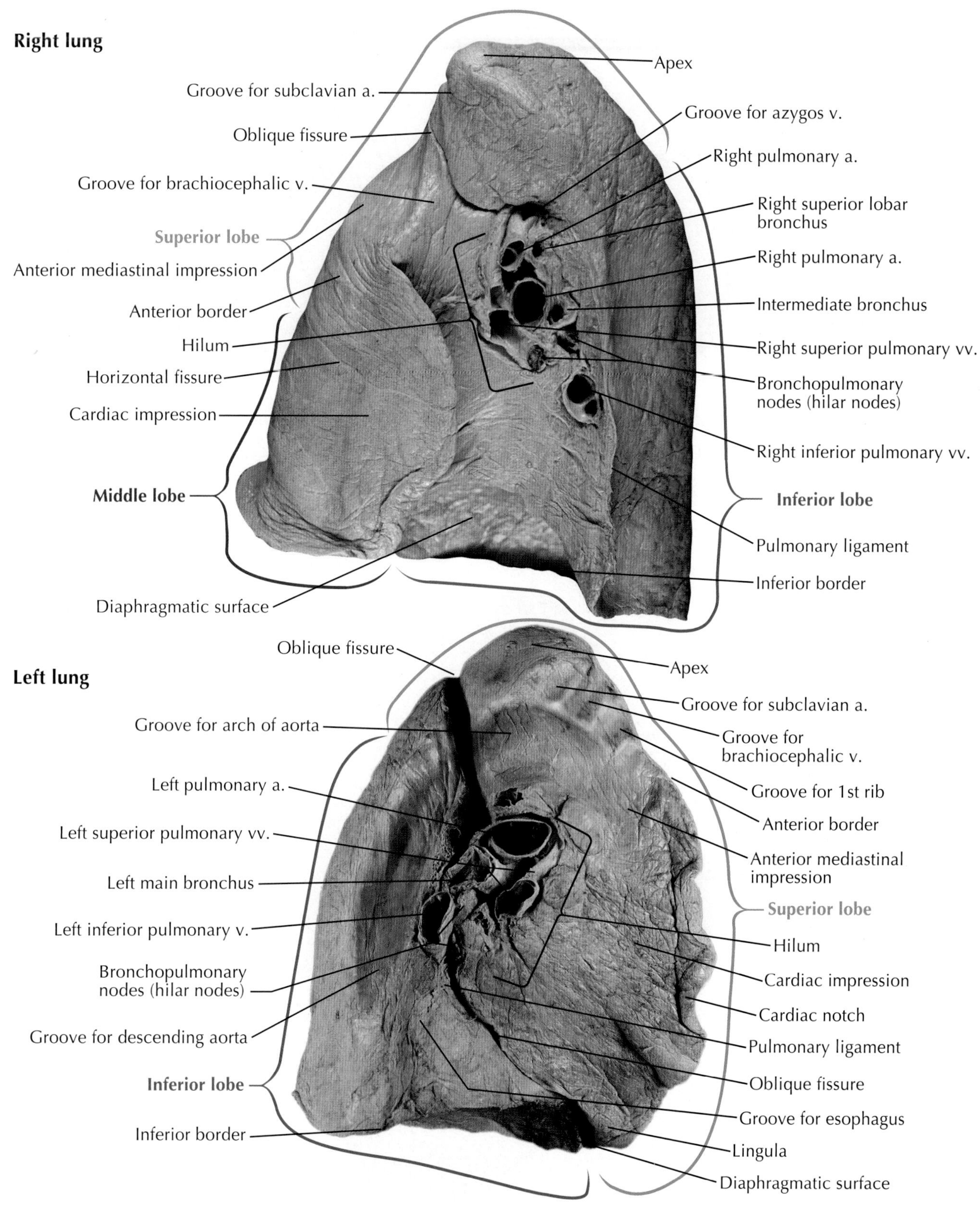
Right lung
Apex
Groove for subclavian a.
Groove for azygos v.
Oblique fissure
Right pulmonary a.
Groove for brachiocephalic v.
Right superior lobar bronchus
Superior lobe
Anterior mediastinal impression
Right pulmonary a.
Anterior border
Intermediate bronchus
Hilum
Right superior pulmonary vv.
Horizontal fissure
Bronchopulmonary nodes (hilar nodes)
Cardiac impression
Right inferior pulmonary vv.
Middle lobe
Inferior lobe
Pulmonary ligament
Inferior border
Diaphragmatic surface
Oblique fissure
Apex
Left lung
Groove for subclavian a.
Groove for arch of aorta
Groove for brachiocephalic v.
Left pulmonary a.
Groove for 1st rib
Anterior border
Left superior pulmonary vv.
Anterior mediastinal impression
Left main bronchus
Superior lobe
Left inferior pulmonary v.
Hilum
Bronchopulmonary nodes (hilar nodes)
Cardiac impression
Cardiac notch
Groove for descending aorta
Pulmonary ligament
Inferior lobe
Oblique fissure
Groove for esophagus
Inferior border
Lingula
Diaphragmatic surface

Fig. A.6 Lungs: Medial Views (Photograph) (see Figs. 3.7 and 3.8)

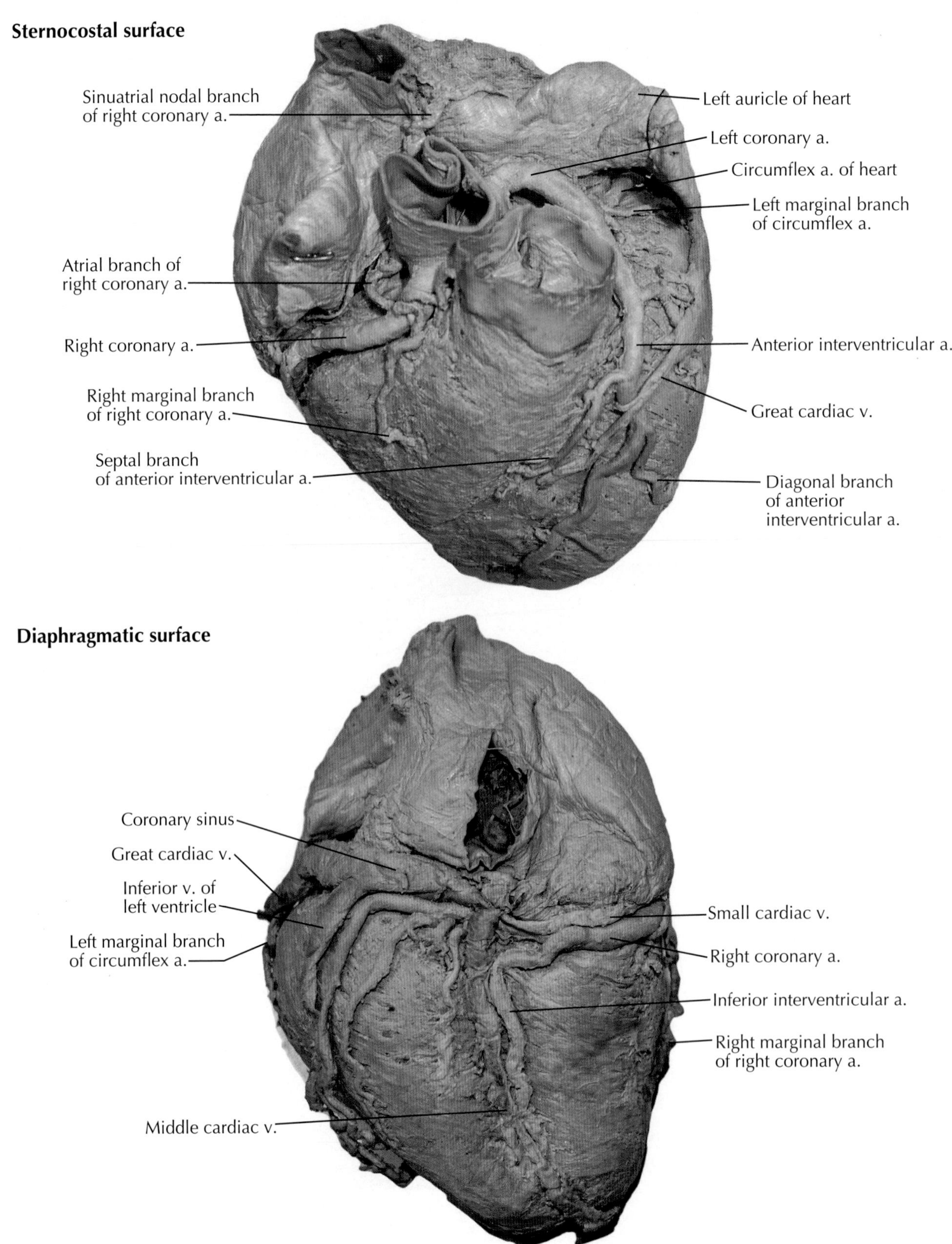
Sternocostal surface
Sinuatrial nodal branch of right coronary a.
Left auricle of heart
Left coronary a.
Circumflex a. of heart
Left marginal branch of circumflex a.
Atrial branch of right coronary a.
Right coronary a.
Anterior interventricular a.
Right marginal branch of right coronary a.
Great cardiac v.
Septal branch of anterior interventricular a.
Diagonal branch of anterior interventricular a.
Diaphragmatic surface
Coronary sinus
Great cardiac v.
Inferior v. of left ventricle
Left marginal branch of circumflex a.
Small cardiac v.
Right coronary a.
Inferior interventricular a.
Right marginal branch of right coronary a.
Middle cardiac v.

Fig. A.7 Coronary Arteries and Cardiac Veins (Photograph) (see Figs. 3.13 and 3.14)

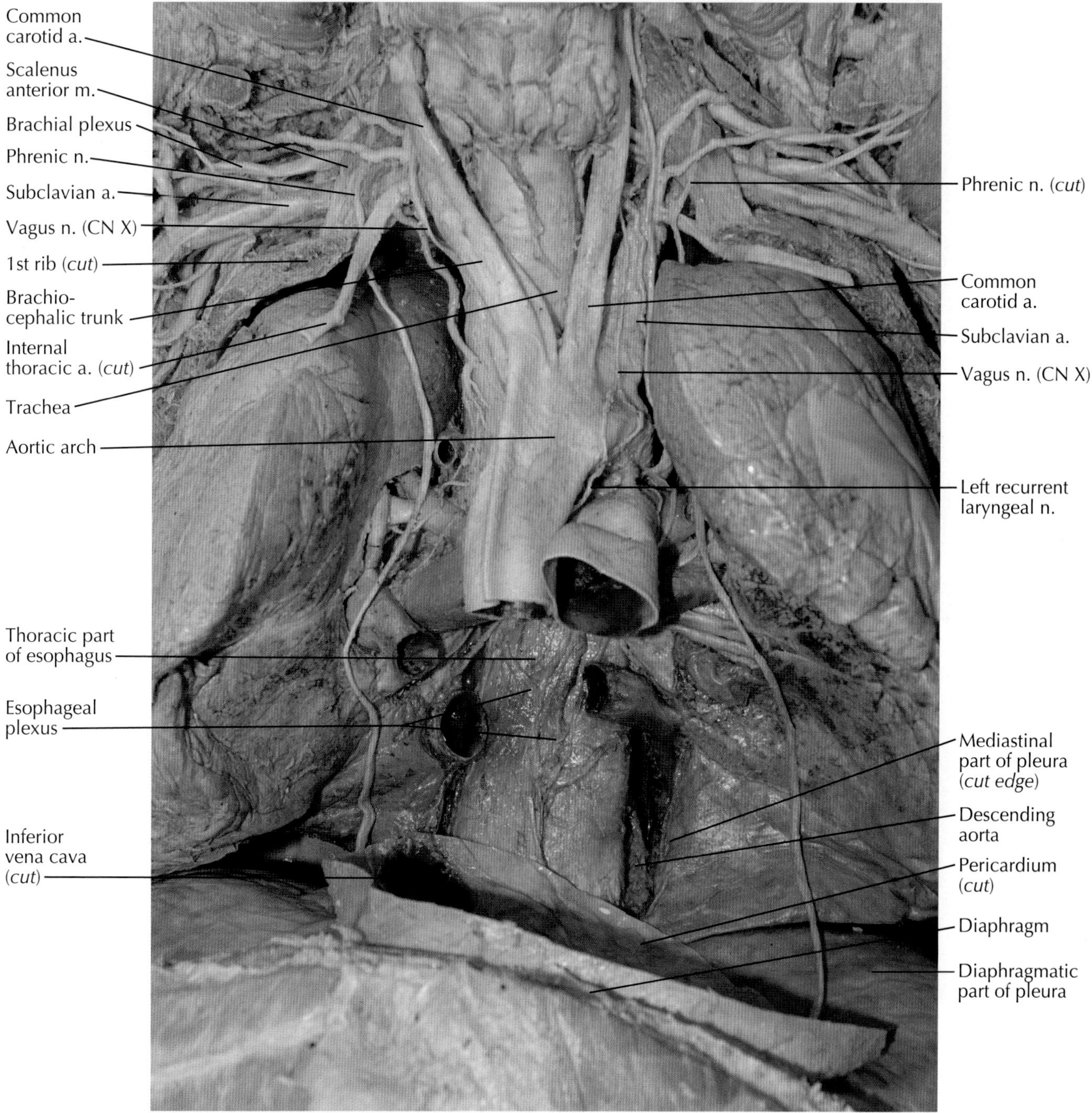
Common carotid a.
Scalenus anterior m.
Brachial plexus
Phrenic n.
Subclavian a.
Vagus n. (CN X)
1st rib (*cut*)
Brachio-cephalic trunk
Internal thoracic a. (*cut*)
Trachea
Aortic arch
Thoracic part of esophagus
Esophageal plexus
Inferior vena cava (*cut*)
Phrenic n. (*cut*)
Common carotid a.
Subclavian a.
Vagus n. (CN X)
Left recurrent laryngeal n.
Mediastinal part of pleura (*cut edge*)
Descending aorta
Pericardium (*cut*)
Diaphragm
Diaphragmatic part of pleura

Fig. A.8 Esophagus In Situ (Photograph) (see Figs. 3.23 and 3.24)

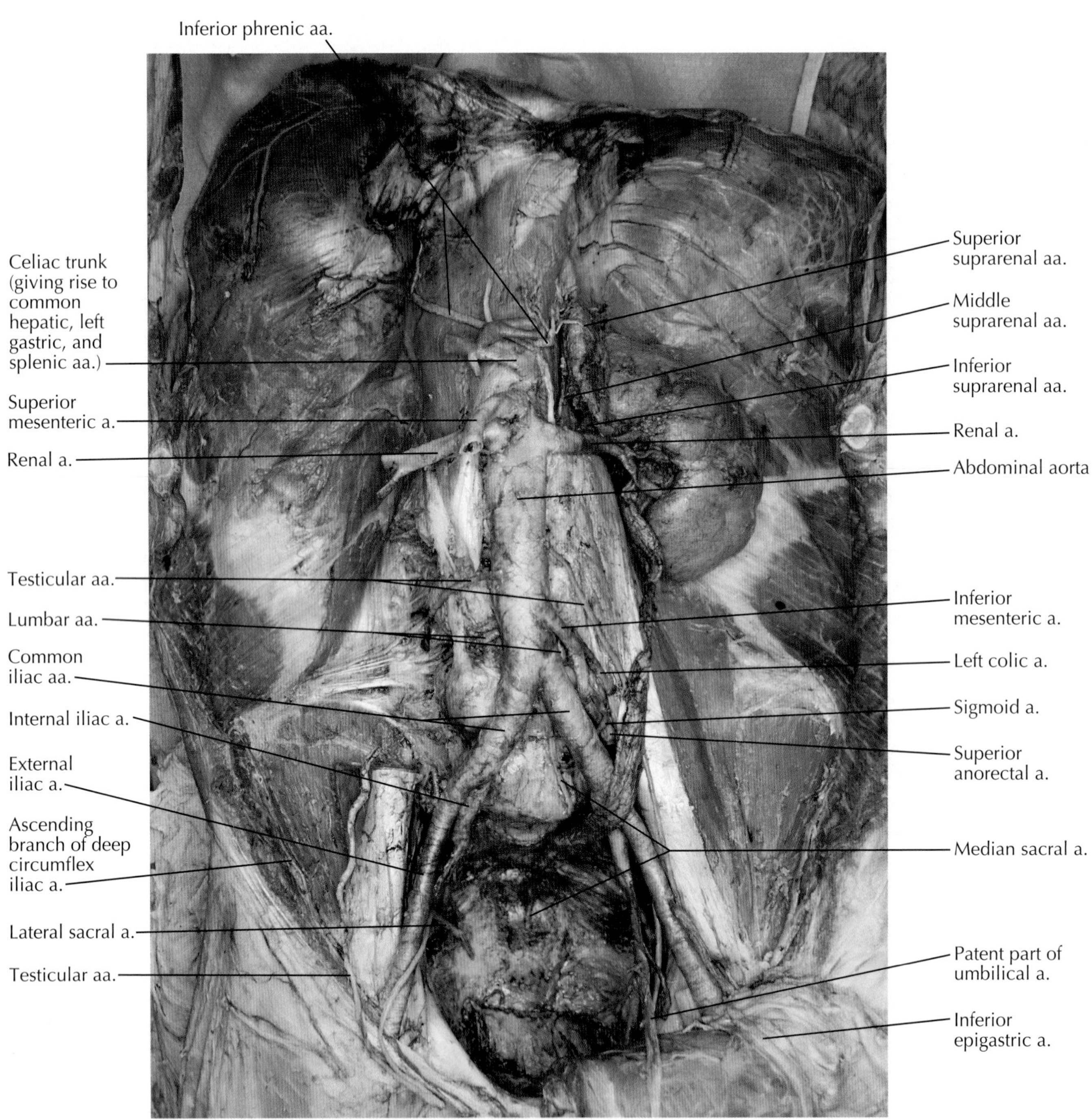
Inferior phrenic aa.
Celiac trunk (giving rise to common hepatic, left gastric, and splenic aa.)
Superior mesenteric a.
Renal a.
Testicular aa.
Lumbar aa.
Common iliac aa.
Internal iliac a.
External iliac a.
Ascending branch of deep circumflex iliac a.
Lateral sacral a.
Testicular aa.
Superior suprarenal aa.
Middle suprarenal aa.
Inferior suprarenal aa.
Renal a.
Abdominal aorta
Inferior mesenteric a.
Left colic a.
Sigmoid a.
Superior anorectal a.
Median sacral a.
Patent part of umbilical a.
Inferior epigastric a.

Fig. A.9 Arteries of Posterior Abdominal Wall (Photograph) (see Figs. 4.3 and 4.4)

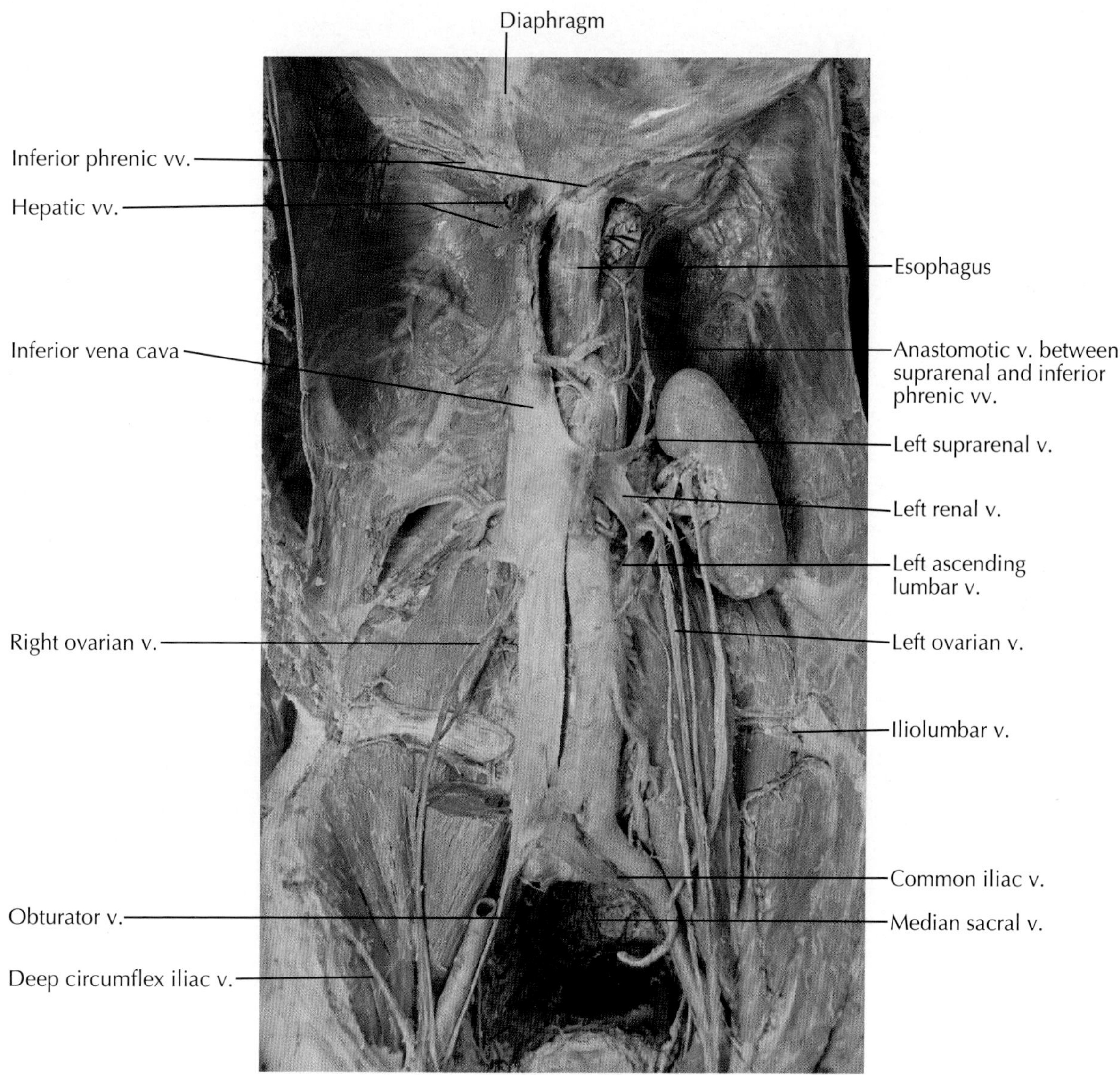
Diaphragm
Inferior phrenic vv.
Hepatic vv.
Inferior vena cava
Right ovarian v.
Obturator v.
Deep circumflex iliac v.
Esophagus
Anastomotic v. between suprarenal and inferior phrenic vv.
Left suprarenal v.
Left renal v.
Left ascending lumbar v.
Left ovarian v.
Iliolumbar v.
Common iliac v.
Median sacral v.

Fig. A.10 Veins of Posterior Abdominal Wall (Photograph) (see Figs. 4.5 and 4.6)

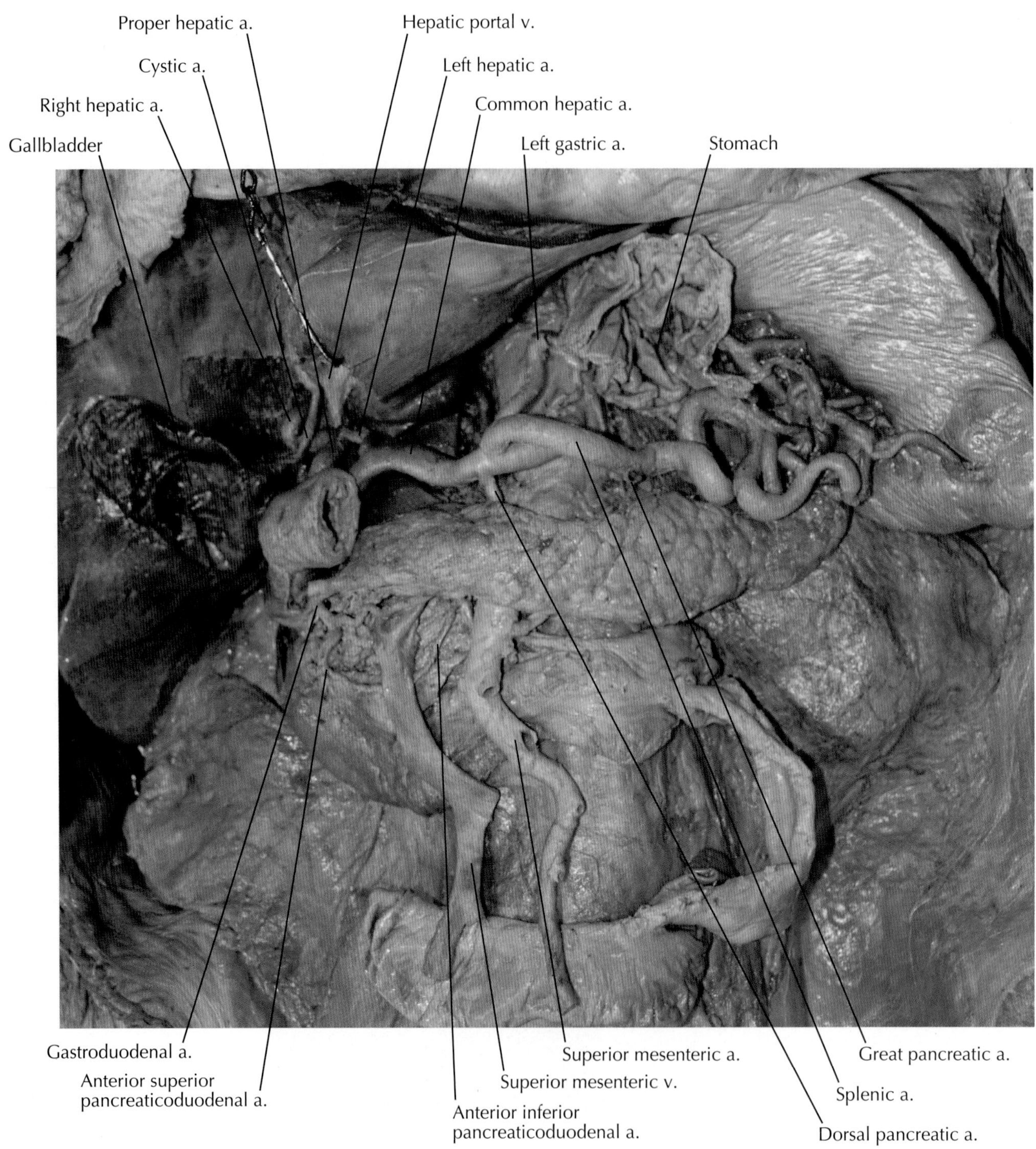
Proper hepatic a.
Hepatic portal v.
Cystic a.
Left hepatic a.
Right hepatic a.
Common hepatic a.
Gallbladder
Left gastric a.
Stomach
Gastroduodenal a.
Anterior superior pancreaticoduodenal a.
Superior mesenteric a.
Superior mesenteric v.
Anterior inferior pancreaticoduodenal a.
Great pancreatic a.
Splenic a.
Dorsal pancreatic a.

Fig. A.11 Arteries of Liver, Pancreas, Duodenum, and Spleen (Photograph) (see Figs. 4.21 and 4.22)

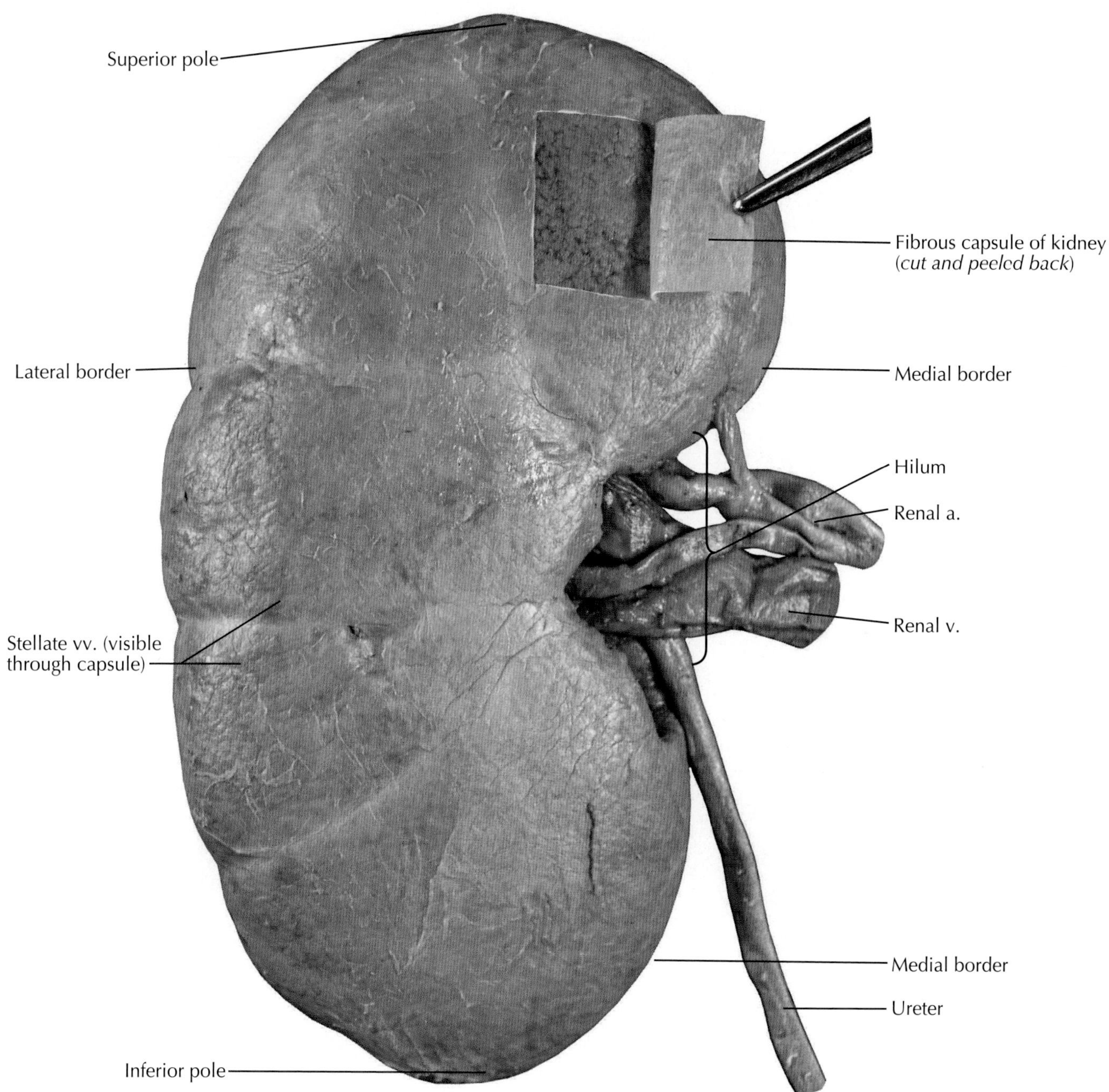
Superior pole
Fibrous capsule of kidney
(cut and peeled back)
Lateral border
Medial border
Hilum
Renal a.
Renal v.
Stellate vv. (visible through capsule)
Medial border
Ureter
Inferior pole

Fig. A.12 Gross Structure of Kidney (Photograph) (see Figs. 4.25 and 4.26)

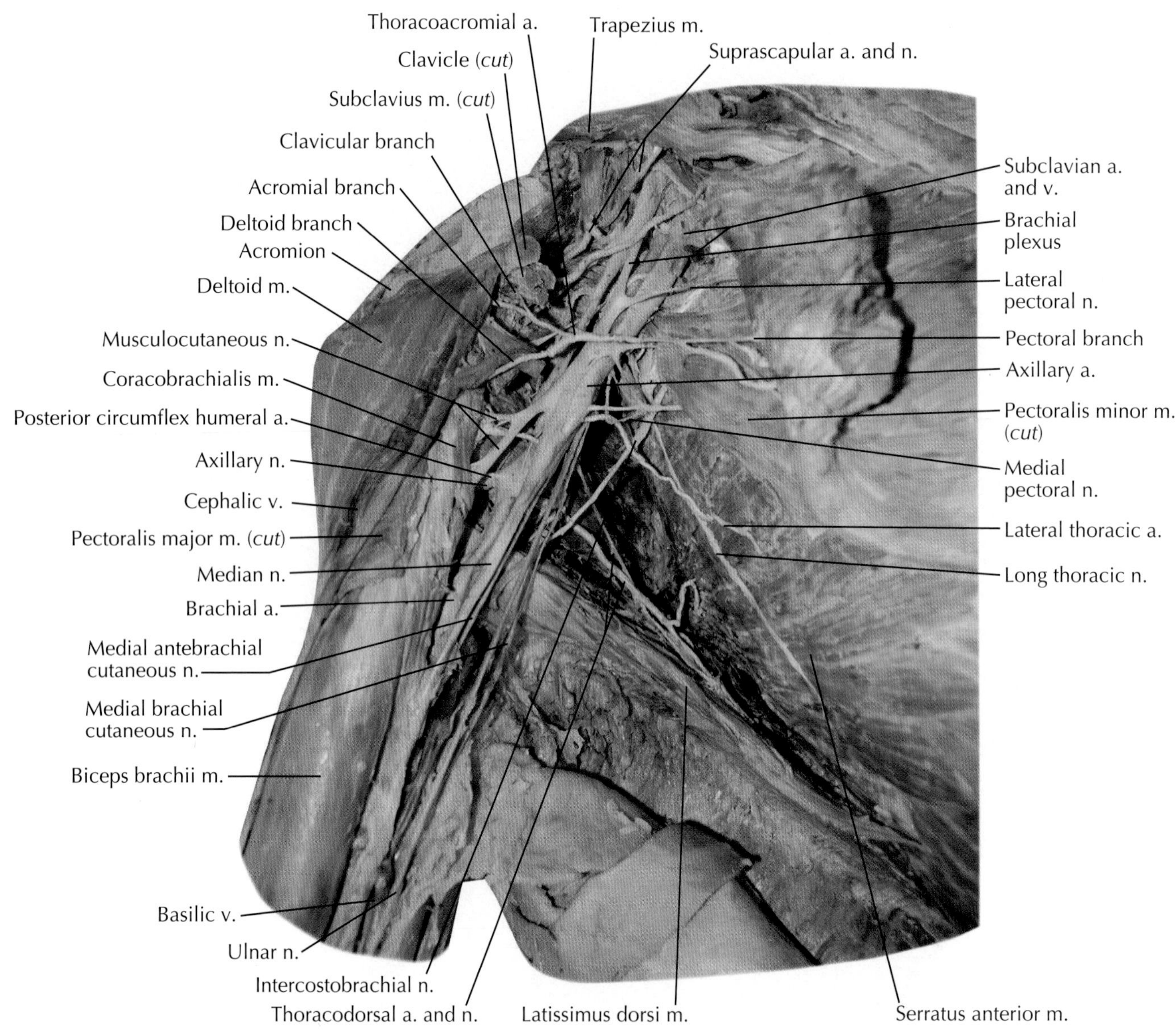
Thoracoacromial a.
Trapezius m.
Suprascapular a. and n.
Clavicle (cut)
Subclavius m. (cut)
Clavicular branch
Acromial branch
Deltoid branch
Acromion
Deltoid m.
Musculocutaneous n.
Coracobrachialis m.
Posterior circumflex humeral a.
Axillary n.
Cephalic v.
Pectoralis major m. (cut)
Median n.
Brachial a.
Medial antebrachial cutaneous n.
Medial brachial cutaneous n.
Biceps brachii m.
Basilic v.
Ulnar n.
Intercostobrachial n.
Thoracodorsal a. and n.
Latissimus dorsi m.
Serratus anterior m.
Subclavian a. and v.
Brachial plexus
Lateral pectoral n.
Pectoral branch
Axillary a.
Pectoralis minor m. (cut)
Medial pectoral n.
Lateral thoracic a.
Long thoracic n.

Fig. A.13 Axilla: Anterior View (Photograph) (see Figs. 6.1 and 6.2)

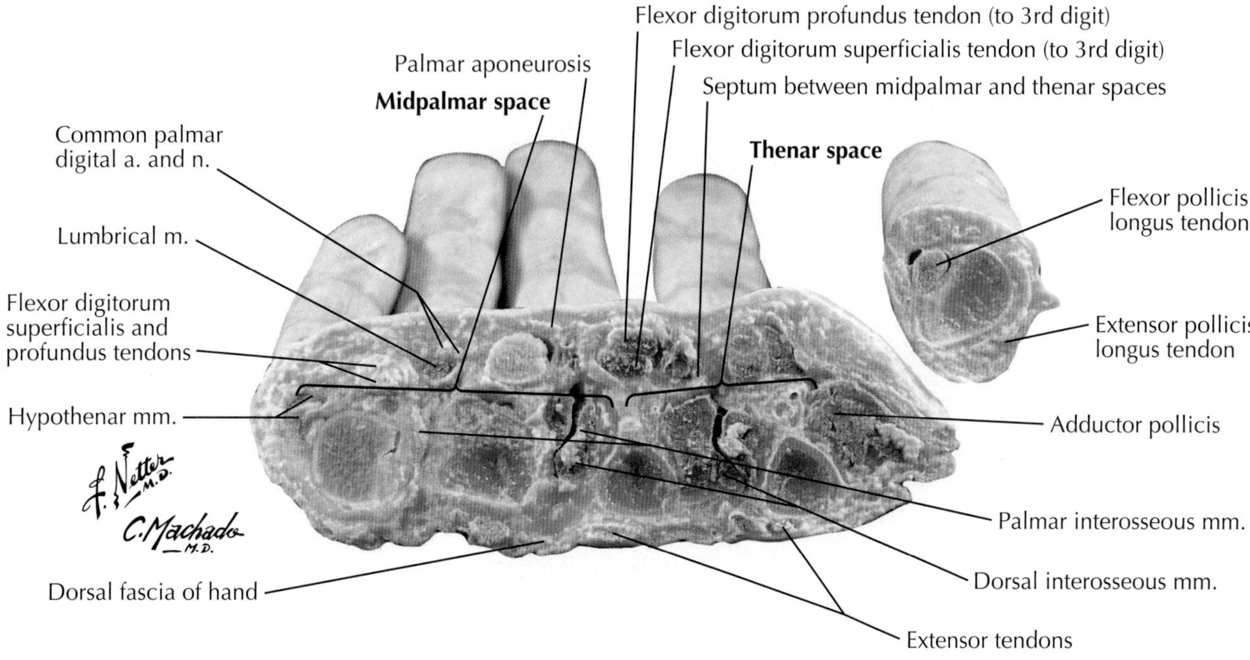
Flexor digitorum profundus tendon (to 3rd digit)
Flexor digitorum superficialis tendon (to 3rd digit)
Palmar aponeurosis
Midpalmar space
Septum between midpalmar and thenar spaces
Common palmar digital a. and n.
Thenar space
Flexor pollicis longus tendon
Lumbrical m.
Flexor digitorum superficialis and profundus tendons
Extensor pollicis longus tendon
Hypothenar mm.
Adductor pollicis
F. Netter M.D.
C. Machado M.D.
Palmar interosseous mm.
Dorsal fascia of hand
Dorsal interosseous mm.
Extensor tendons

Fig. A.14 Spaces and Tendon Sheaths of Hand (Photograph) (see Figs. 6.7 and 6.8)

Superficial dissections

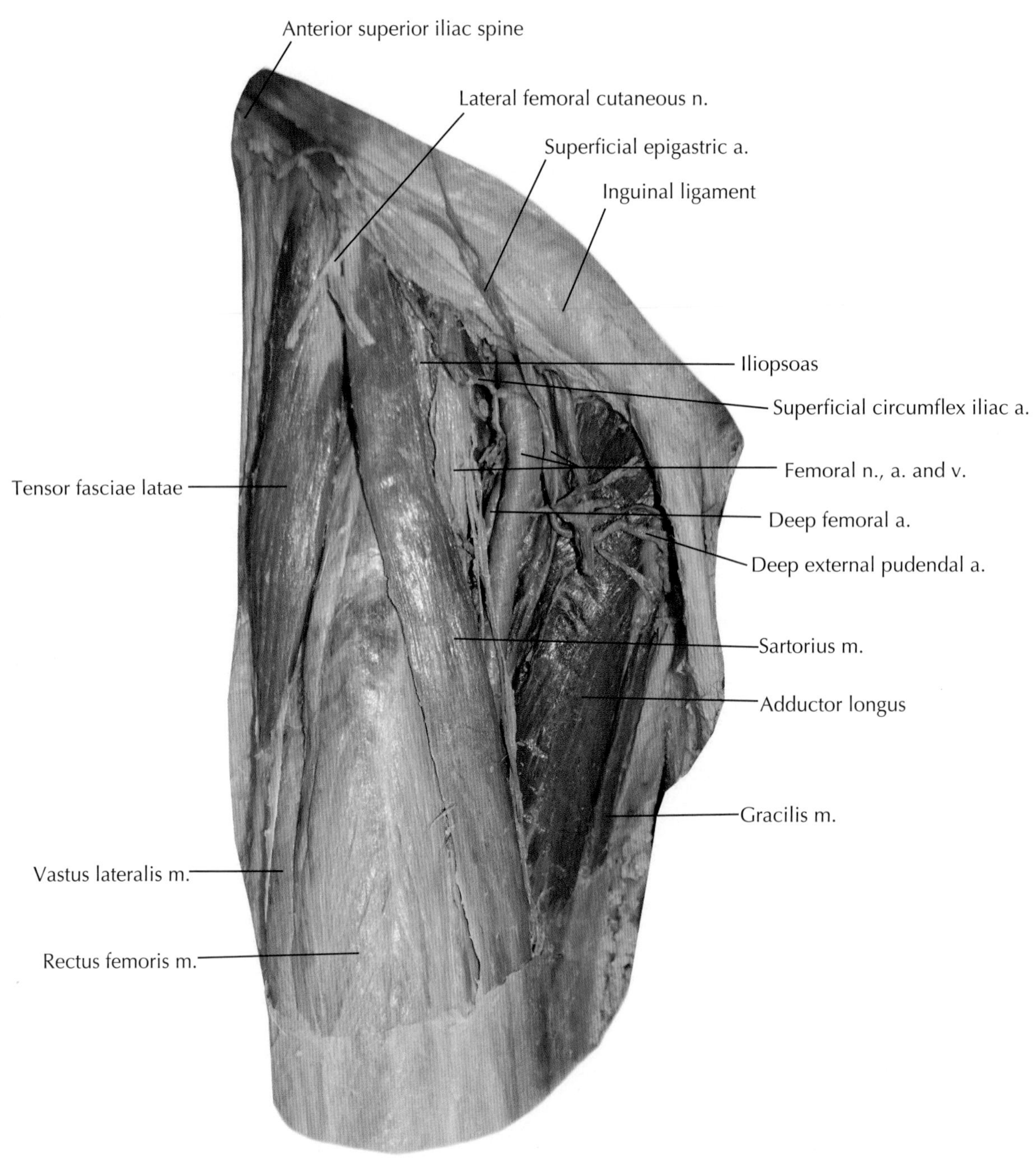
Anterior superior iliac spine
Lateral femoral cutaneous n.
Superficial epigastric a.
Inguinal ligament
Iliopsoas
Superficial circumflex iliac a.
Femoral n., a. and v.
Tensor fasciae latae
Deep femoral a.
Deep external pudendal a.
Sartorius m.
Adductor longus
Gracilis m.
Vastus lateralis m.
Rectus femoris m.

Fig. A.15 Arteries of Thigh: Anterior Views (Photograph) (see Figs. 7.1 and 7.2)

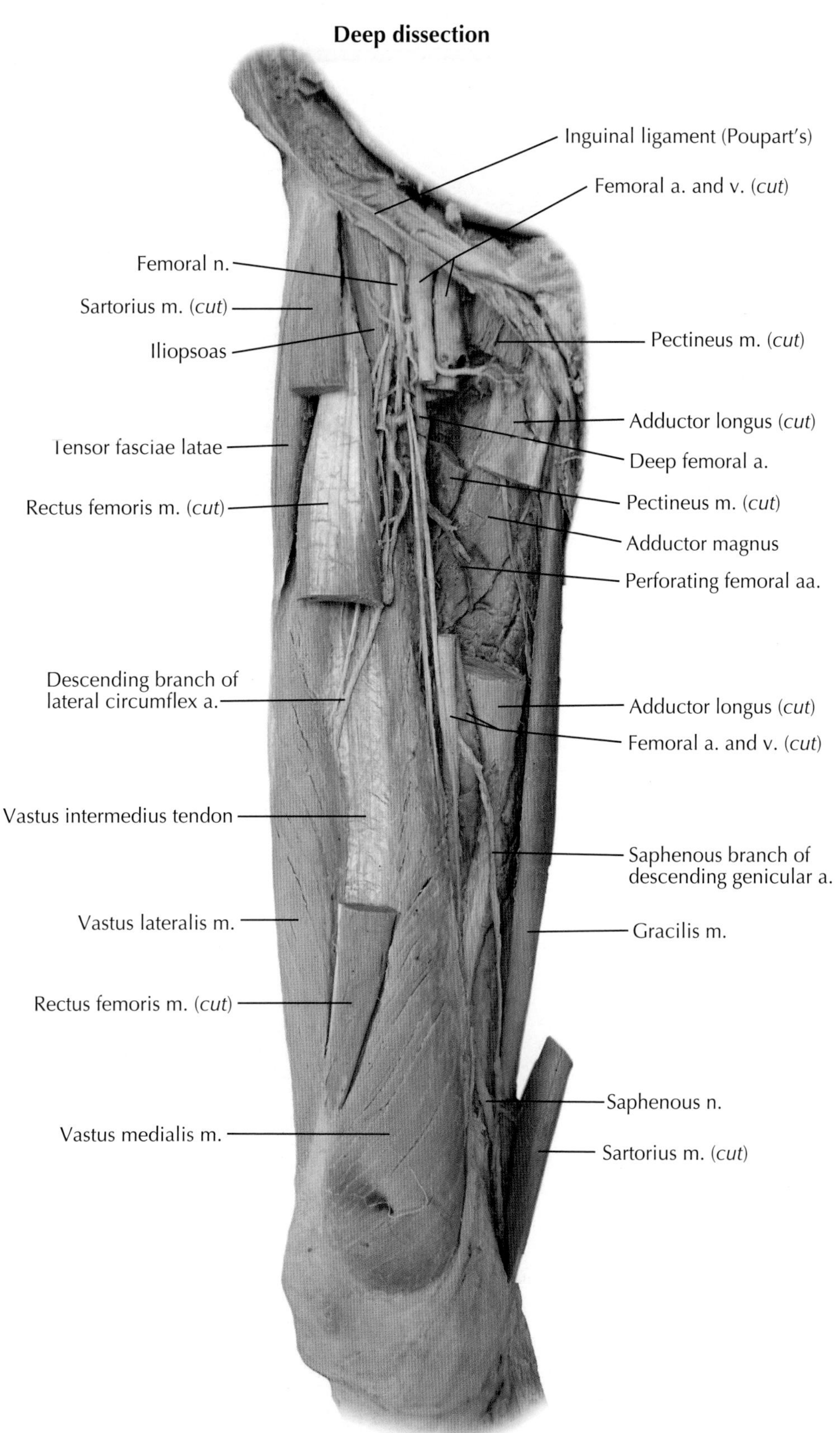
Deep dissection
Inguinal ligament (Poupart's)
Femoral a. and v. (cut)
Femoral n.
Sartorius m. (cut)
Iliopsoas
Pectineus m. (cut)
Adductor longus (cut)
Tensor fasciae latae
Deep femoral a.
Rectus femoris m. (cut)
Pectineus m. (cut)
Adductor magnus
Perforating femoral aa.
Descending branch of lateral circumflex a.
Adductor longus (cut)
Femoral a. and v. (cut)
Vastus intermedius tendon
Saphenous branch of descending genicular a.
Vastus lateralis m.
Gracilis m.
Rectus femoris m. (cut)
Saphenous n.
Vastus medialis m.
Sartorius m. (cut)

Fig. A.16 Arteries of Thigh: Anterior View of Deeper Dissection (Photograph) (see Figs. 7.3 and 7.4)

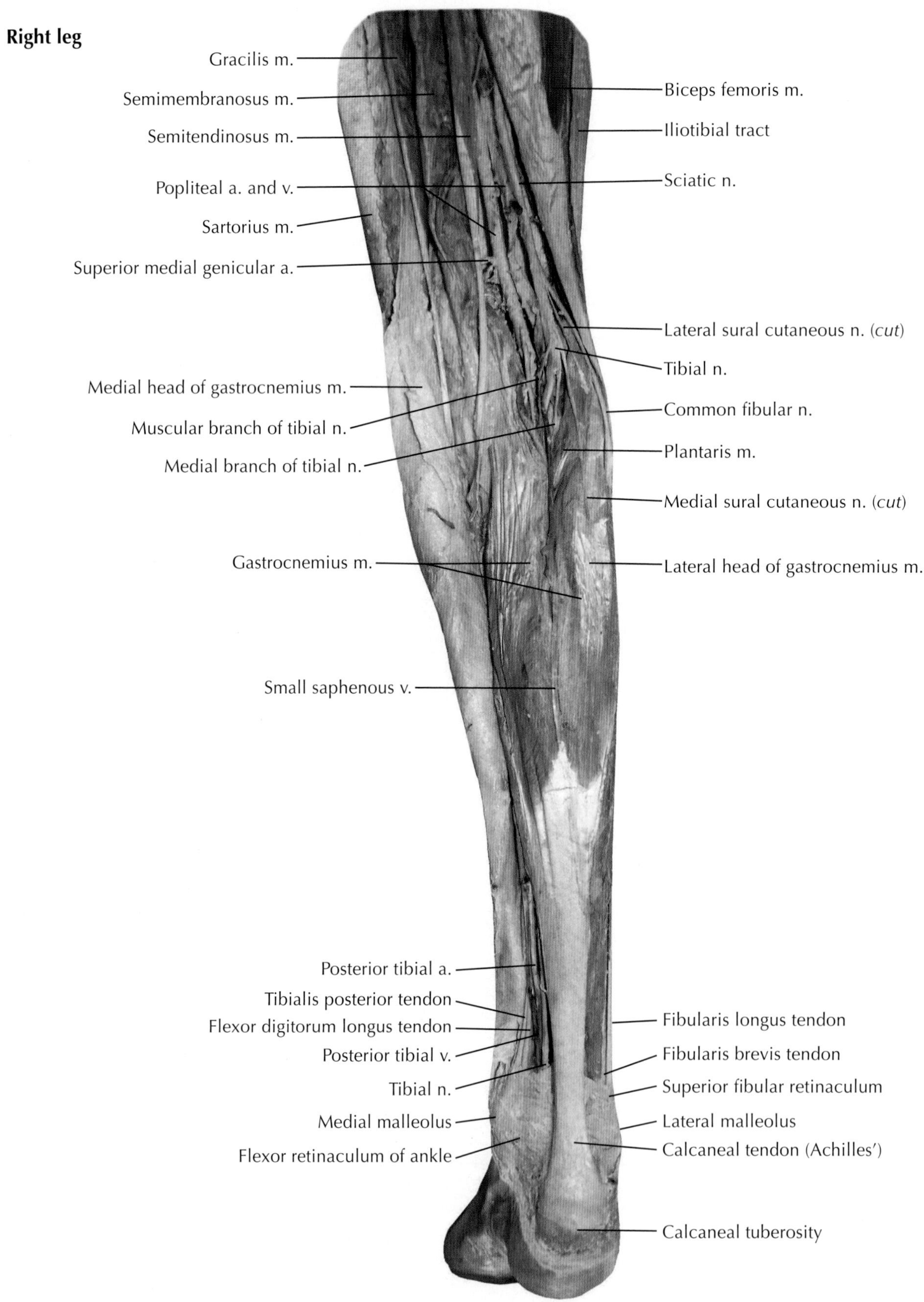
Right leg
Gracilis m.
Semimembranosus m.
Semitendinosus m.
Popliteal a. and v.
Sartorius m.
Superior medial genicular a.
Biceps femoris m.
Iliotibial tract
Sciatic n.
Lateral sural cutaneous n. (*cut*)
Tibial n.
Common fibular n.
Plantaris m.
Medial sural cutaneous n. (*cut*)
Lateral head of gastrocnemius m.
Medial head of gastrocnemius m.
Muscular branch of tibial n.
Medial branch of tibial n.
Gastrocnemius m.
Small saphenous v.
Posterior tibial a.
Tibialis posterior tendon
Flexor digitorum longus tendon
Posterior tibial v.
Tibial n.
Medial malleolus
Flexor retinaculum of ankle
Fibularis longus tendon
Fibularis brevis tendon
Superior fibular retinaculum
Lateral malleolus
Calcaneal tendon (Achilles')
Calcaneal tuberosity

Fig. A.17 Muscles of Leg: Superficial Part of Posterior Compartment (Photograph) (see Figs. 7.11 and 7.12)

INDEX

Note: Page numbers followed by "*f*" indicate figures. *a.* = artery; *m.* = muscle; *n.* = nerve; *v.* = vein

F

G

M

N

O

S

T

U